THERAPEUTICS

THERAPEUTICS

FOURTH EDITION

J. G. LEWIS
M.D., F.R.C.P.
Consultant Physician
Edgware General Hospital

HODDER AND STOUGHTON
LONDON SYDNEY AUCKLAND TORONTO

To my Mother

British Library Cataloguing in Publication Data

Lewis, Jerome Gerald
  Therapeutics. – 4th ed.
  1. Chemotherapy
  I. Title 2. Series
  615'.58   RM262

ISBN 0 340 25166 2 Boards
ISBN 0 340 25167 0 Unibook Pbk

First printed 1968
Second edition 1972
Reprinted (with revisions) 1974
Third edition 1978
Fourth edition 1980

Printed in Great Britain for
Hodder and Stoughton Educational,
a division of Hodder and Stoughton Limited,
Mill Road, Dunton Green, Sevenoaks, Kent
by J. W. Arrowsmith Ltd., Bristol.

FOREWORD

I am glad to welcome another edition of Dr. Lewis's popular book on Therapeutics, for it has become necessary to revise such a practical book in order to keep readers informed of those recent advances in pharmacology and the pharmaceutical industry which are now being applied to the treatment of patients.

As I have said in a previous foreword the subject which we call 'therapeutics' is common ground. Here the patient is at the centre point, and it is to the patient that all our efforts are directed. Only by accurate and painstaking communication between doctor and nurse with the help of the pharmacy can the pharmacological needs of the patient be properly and humanely satisfied.

To do this involves either a ready and full knowledge or the means of quick reference to a text which displays all the aspects of prescription, presentation, usage, abusage and dangers of drugs used in everyday clinical work. Thus a concise text which can easily be carried in the white coat pocket or used in the ward or clinic is invaluable.

Dr. Lewis is an experienced physician and teacher and I am sure that the readers will find helpful, as I do, the specially informative and friendly way in which he sets the clinical scene in each section with words of experience and practical wisdom.

Clinical students in particular will find this a helpful revision companion. This is a subject which they often find to their surprise to be a matter of great moment in the final examinations!

A. J. Harding Rains

PREFACE TO FOURTH EDITION

In the past year I have updated and revised the third edition. My aims have been as before to provide guidance and information for those working in district general hospitals, the backbone of our hospital services. I have tried not to be too parochial; medications likely to be used by travellers have been mentioned and also important drugs in use on both sides of the Atlantic.

Edgware, 1980

J. G. Lewis

CONTENTS

TABLES

FIGURES

1   INTRODUCTION

Medicines in the past were mainly of plant or mineral origin and based on folk-lore or botanical studies. Today, most drugs are synthesized, but some important exceptions are derived from plant, animal or human sources. The pharmaceutical industry has transformed medical practice. Life expectancy has improved; many infections are prevented or conquered, heart disease is better controlled and the mentally ill are more often able to return to or live in the community. Drug therapy has also been extended to the healthy with immunization and the control of fertility.

A **drug** can be defined as any substance which when taken into the body modifies one or more of its functions: or 'a substance used for the diagnosis, treatment or prevention of disease in man or other animal' (W.H.O. definition). It also includes the vehicle, colouring or sweetening agent. This may be clinically important as lactose, gluten, incorporated dyes and added sodium may be harmful at times. The chemical structure of the drug may indicate its likely mode of action, possible side-effects and enable grouping together of related drugs (congeners or analogues) e.g. the tricyclic anti-depressants. Nowadays, often for commercial reasons, many drugs are available with very similar uses and actions and although they will be listed in this book it is impossible for any one person to be familiar with all of them. The original, or prototype, is often as good as the more recently introduced additions (e.g. the beta blockers and the benzodiazepines).

Drug Names
A drug has several names. (1) *Chemical or generic name* based on its structure. This may be too long to remember or pronounce. (2) *Official or approved name* which provides an easier description and indicates the chemical nature e.g. alkaloids end in 'ine' (morphine), antibiotics in 'cillin', 'cycline', or 'mycin' e.g. penicillin, tetracycline and streptomycin. Most official drugs such as those in the British National Formulary become included in the British Pharmacopoeia (B.P.) which contains details of standards of preparation, purity, presentation and a note on doses and uses. B.P. after a drug means it is, or was, in the Pharmacopoeia. Many B.P. drugs are now included in the European Pharmacopoeia (Ph. Eur.) which takes precedence over the B.P. The United States Pharmacopoeia has similar functions, but official names occasionally differ from the B.P. The British Pharmaceutical Codex (B.P.C.) is another source of information about drugs, biological products, investigational agents and some surgical products. Many of its standards are being included in future British Pharmacopoeias and it will no longer be a source of standards. (3) *Proprietary name*: when a drug is made commercially its method of production is patented and it is given a brand name. This protects the company and the merit of the product. Branded prescription medicines account for 95% of the total cost of the N.H.S. pharmaceutical service and 75% of all prescriptions written by general practitioners.

Quality Control
When a drug is discovered, ideally it is marketed therapeutically active, chemi-

cally pure, predictable and constant in performance. Tablets should dissolve in a given period, keep well and have a reproducible performance. Medications are made under strict chemical, physical or biological control. While many official drugs are equally effective and cheaper than the branded product, this is not always so. There is a significant variation in formulation (composition and particle size) and absorption or *bio-availability* between preparations made by different companies. For example with amitriptyline, diazepam, digitoxin, digoxin, ethosuximide, glibenclamide, tolbutamide, metformin, methyldopa and warfarin it is advisable to keep to one make. Oral solutions are better absorbed than tablets. Since branded versions are usually those prescribed outside hospital they are included in this book and given in parenthesis after the official name. In many countries a desk-reference book of ethical products is mailed regularly to doctors and pharmacists.

Identification
It is useful to be able to recognize the commoner drugs and many can be identified by size, shape, colours and markings and matched against charts. Unless instructed otherwise, the pharmacist will write the name, or an identification mark, on the container. When describing a drug in this text *presentation* implies the form in which it is available e.g. tablet, capsule or injection, and the strength. The *mode of administration* is the way and route it is given and the number of times daily (or other interval) it is taken. What happens to the drug in the body is important, namely *absorption,* plasma and tissue *distribution, metabolism* and *excretion.* Other facts to note are for what conditions the medications are given i.e. the *indications,* the *mechanism of action* if known and the *adverse effects.* The expiry date should be noted since certain drugs deteriorate with time. This is important with medications used in emergencies (e.g. cardiac arrest, poisoning). With more recent introductions, it should be evaluated whether the benefit outweighs the extra cost.

Administration
Drugs reach their site of action only after absorption into the blood stream, or by local or topical spread.
Oral: the usual way of giving medicines is by mouth as tablets and less commonly as capsules, powder or fluid. Some drugs when swallowed are unabsorbed and act within the intestine; others are absorbed from the digestive system and distributed by the blood stream. **Buccal** absorption is the method used with trinitrin and isoprenaline. It is speedy and the drug by-passes the liver.
Intragastric absorption occurs with aspirin and alcohol.
Intestine: drugs after absorption go by the portal vein to the liver and then enter the general circulation. Because the liver receives the blood first, drug toxicity commonly involves this organ preferentially. Oral drugs act more slowly than injections. Certain drugs are destroyed by the gastric juices e.g. penicillin G. Others are limited because they produce nausea, vomiting or diarrhoea. Nausea and vomiting may be reduced by *enteric-coated* acid resistant coverings which allow the drug to be liberated in the small gut. Aspirin, sodium chloride and ammonium chloride may be so treated. Another way is to take medicines with food, e.g. iron salts. Better absorption is achieved by taking some drugs such as penicillin V on an empty stomach. *Delayed or prolonged absorption* may be achieved by chemical and physical methods of coating the drug so that it is released slowly, or by altering its surface area. Slow-

release preparations include nitrates, antihistamines, appetite suppressants, antispasmodics, sedatives and potassium salts. Slow-release forms may reduce side-effects from gastro-intestinal irritation, or from a rapid rise in blood concentration, and by reducing the number of tablets be more acceptable to patients.

Injections are indicated in the very ill who cannot swallow or when the oral route is unreliable, or too slow. Injections are necessary when the drug is not absorbed from the gut, and also in children and babies if it is doubtful whether they would take, or be given the medicines. Usual routes are intramuscular i.m., intravenous i.v., or subcutaneous s.c. and less commonly into the dermis, pleura, peritoneum, spinal canal, ventricles, joints or arteries.

Speed of absorption from intradermal, subcutaneous or intramuscular sites depends on the chemical and physical properties of the injected material, the richness of blood supply and the blood pressure. **Intramuscular injections** act faster than subcutaneous or intradermal ones and are given into the lateral aspect of the thigh, the upper and outer part of the buttocks avoiding the sciatic nerves, and into the deltoid and pectoral muscles. Delaying absorption reduces the number of injections needed. This is achieved by suspending or dissolving the drug in oil (e.g. testosterone) or adding gelatin (e.g. corticotrophin gel); adding vasoconstrictors such as adrenaline to local anaesthetics; altering the substance to a less soluble form e.g. with insulin, testosterone and prednisolone and, finally, the implantation of pellets by trocar and cannula e.g. with testosterone which last months by this route.

Intravenous Injections
In peripheral circulatory failure from cardiogenic shock, arrhythmias, diabetic coma or Gram-negative bacteraemia the only reliable injection is intravenous, or possibly deep intramuscular. Intravenous injections are also the quickest way into the blood stream when speed is desirable and achieve a high concentration at once. The rate of administration is important. Fast injections of procainamide, thiopentone and aminophylline are dangerous. Intravenous injections go to organs with high blood flow such as the brain and heart which receive accordingly a relatively large proportion of the drug dose. The only organs to receive all the cardiac output are the lungs and this may explain why they are damaged by a variety of substances (p. 256). Intravenous therapy by continuous infusions, often controlled by infusion pump apparatus, is widely used in coronary care, intensive therapy units and in obstetrics during delivery. Therapy can be slowed, quickened or stopped according to the needs of the patient. It should be remembered that injections contain substances other than the main drugs (e.g. solvents, preservatives) which may cause adverse reactions.

Disadvantages of injections are varied.
(1) *Local pain* from inflammation or direct damage to nerves. With irritants such as paraldehyde, muscles may be damaged and abscesses form. Certain injections given by accident extravenously can harm nerves e.g. thiopentone and colchicine, or destroy tissue e.g. nitrogen mustards or noradrenaline. When i.m. injections are painful (as with tetracycline), a local anaesthetic is added. Iron injections may stain the skin.
(2) *Fear of injections,* and of medical and nursing staff, may occur in children.
(3) *Spread of infection,* especially viral hepatitis. This is prevented by dispos-

able syringes and needles. Special chemical and bacteriological purity is needed for intrathecal injections.

(4) *Drug reactions* may be more severe than with oral therapy.

Distribution of Drugs within the Body

After absorption, drugs enter the plasma and some are attached to and carried by the plasma proteins. The small free or unbound drug is the active form and diffuses between (extracellularly) and within cells (intracellularly). Serum or blood levels are useful as a guide to dosage and effectiveness. They help avoid toxic levels and also ensure that a minimum therapeutic concentration has been obtained. The half-life of a drug 'T½' is the time taken for the maximum concentration to drop to 50%. It is not the same as the biological half-life of the drug in the tissues. The duration of action of a drug depends on the dosage and the half-life. Some drugs enter the C.S.F., others cross into the foetal circulation via the placenta or are secreted in the breast milk. *Inactivation:* after absorption some drugs are excreted unchanged, others are broken down, or inactivated chemically. Hence certain medications must be given frequently to allow for rapid inactivation and excretion. Some drugs combine with chemicals produced in the body and these compounds may be poorly soluble in the urine.

Excretion of drugs is achieved in several ways.

(1) The *kidneys* by glomerular filtration and tubular secretion. With certain drugs an adequate fluid intake is essential to prevent crystalluria. Certain antibiotics are dangerous if renal failure exists (p. 256).

(2) *Bile* is a pathway for the excretion of drugs and this depends on the molecular weight of the drug, its water solubility and its structure. The excreted substance may be re-absorbed (recycled).

(3) Other sites of excretion are the lungs, intestinal wall, sweat and breast milk.

LOCAL OR TOPICAL APPLICATIONS

Examples are: **mouth and pharynx** (gargles, mouth washes, lozenges, paints and surface anaesthetics); **ears** (drops, ointments, powder insufflation); **eyes** (drops, lotions, ointments); **hair** (solutions, lotions); **nose** (douches, drops, inhalations, insufflations, ointments, surface anaesthetics); **rectum** (enemas, suppositories); **skin** (creams, liniments, lotions, ointments, paints, pastes, plasters, poultices, powders, solutions and sprays); **urethra and bladder** (solutions); **vagina** (douches, ointments, pessaries). **Inhalations**: fluid in the form of steam or sprays, aerosols containing antibiotics, antispasmodics and vasoconstrictors may act on the respiratory tract. Gases and volatile substances are used in anaesthesia. Oxygen is given to improve oxygenation of the blood. Drugs such as ergotamine may be absorbed into the systemic circulation.

Precautions

Before giving drugs to a patient by any route it is wise to ask if there has been any previous adverse reaction to any medication. If the patient is allergic to aspirin, penicillin or any other drug, the case notes should be marked accordingly, and whether the diagnosis was made by the patient or a doctor. While the patient is receiving therapy the nursing and medical staff (or relatives) should observe and report any untoward event or symptom. A card stating the dose and name of the medication is useful in patients taking insulin, anticoagulants or corticosteroids. Similarly, the date and type of any vaccination should be noted. Nurses, doctors and pharmacists are concerned with the supervision, administration, stability and storage of drugs, many of which (such as the narcotics) are controlled by legal safeguards (Chapter 32). Ampoules may lose their markings; legibility should be checked and contents. Colourless injections such as potassium chloride may be confused with other solutions; potassium chloride must always be given diluted.

Adverse Effects
There is no such thing as a safe drug, but a drug can be made more dangerous if there is insufficient control of dosage, and insufficient awareness of drug interactions, harmful effects and contra-indications. The therapeutic or beneficial value of a drug should always outweigh its harmful properties. A drug for the treatment of a mild condition should have no appreciable risk. In order to ensure reasonable safety drugs are first tested for toxicity in pregnant and non-pregnant animals before they are given to humans. Reports of the actions and adverse effects are available in the makers' data sheets and medical, pharmaceutical and nursing journals. Dangerous or unsuspected complications are reported to official bodies concerned with the safety of medicines. Overdosage may be difficult to avoid because of variation in absorption, metabolism, excretion and hence plasma levels. Side effects occurring in concentrations below the therapeutic level are unavoidable. The inconvenience has to be balanced against the benefit. Idiosyncratic and anaphylactic reactions are not dose-related, but are related to biological (immunological and genetic) factors.

Drug Abuse
Self-poisoning by soporifics, tranquillizers and analgesics is more common than suicide by violent methods, drowning and carbon monoxide. Deaths from self-poisoning are greater than those from road accidents. Drug abuse by the public with purgatives, analgesics, alkalies, cough medicines, nasal decongestants and iodides is prevalent. The advent of the syringe and needle plus the technology of producing potent mind-altering drugs (chemical 'stoned age') have led to widespread addiction and an easy way of becoming intoxicated.

Prescriptions
Solids are prescribed metrically as grams (g), milligrams (mg) or micrograms (μg). Confusion is possible between mg and μg so microgram should be written in full. When a medication is prescribed in an amount below 1 mg it is written in micrograms to avoid decimal points. The unit of volume is the millilitre (ml). Mixtures in the B.N.F. are usually given in 10 ml amounts (two 5 ml teaspoonfuls) thrice daily (t.d.s.) in water.

Supervision
Medicines prescribed to adults may be fatal if accidentally swallowed by children. Doctors and nurses should point this out especially when drugs acting on the nervous system, heart (e.g. digitalis, quinidine) and quinine, iron, aspirin or paracetamol are prescribed. Elderly or mentally ill persons with paranoia or confusion may fail to take their medicines. Here, administration should be entrusted to a responsible relative or friend. The date on the bottle should be checked since many drugs have an expiry date. Storage conditions should be noted.

Drug Defaulting

Studies outside and inside hospital indicate that patients do not get or take their medicines regularly, or fully for the course. Or if they take them they get the dose, timing or sequence wrong. Others take inappropriate medications intended for other illnesses. Factors contributing to defaulting are:

(1) lengthy treatment (e.g. tuberculosis), poor medical supervision with lack of continuity of medical care;

(2) complex treatment leading to confusion and errors;

(3) an increasing number of concurrent drugs;

(4) lack of clear directions, faulty labelling, poor family supervision. For the elderly the drug regime should be detailed and written instructions given to the patient or supervisor. For the busy mother, school child, worker, and the elderly a once or twice daily regime is a boon;

(5) the formulation, palatability and adverse effects;

(6) the 'clinical setting'—drugs are more likely to be taken in hospital or clinic, but less so at home;

(7) age: children and the elderly may be frightened, unwilling or intolerant;

(8) absence of motivation, such as a desire to get well and return to work, absence of unpleasant symptoms ('feel well today'), failure to relieve symptoms ('drugs don't help'), running out of drugs and not getting a fresh prescription;

(9) illnesses such as psychosis or psychopathy;

(10) inadequate rapport between patient, nurse and doctor so that the patient may not trust the doctor or nurse, or may fear the therapy. Drugs are often 'sold' by the doctor's personality.

(11) lack of money to buy drugs (not in Britain), but prescribers cannot ignore self-audit and economical but effective prescribing.

Drug Combinations

These have the advantage of simplicity for the combination of two or more drugs in one formulation reduces the complexity of the regime, is convenient and at times safer. Combinations are used to treat tuberculosis, infections (co-trimoxazole) and the anaemias of pregnancy (folic acid and iron). Combinations of oestrogens and progestogens are effective and form the basis of the oral contraceptive pill. Their disadvantages are their inflexibility and fixed proportions. However, many people are suited by them and they may cost the patient less to buy.

Harmonization of Information

Regulations have been passed by the European Economic Community to provide a common basis for dealing with the licensing of medical products. Council Directive 75/318 deals with the information needed to license a new medicinal product and covers minimal standards for chemistry, pharmacology, toxicology and clinical trials.

2 ANTIMICROBIALS—PENICILLINS AND ALTERNATIVES

A **chemotherapeutic agent** is a synthetic substance used to overcome, or destroy, invading microbes, ideally without harming the patient. Sulphonamides were the first successful antibacterial agents. Ehrlich (1854-1915) much earlier had used dyes to treat malaria and trypanosomiasis and in 1909 he used by analogy arsenic (because it was similar in the periodic table to nitrogen, a constituent of azo dyes) in the form of arsphenamine to treat spirochaetal infection. 'Prontosil' was also a dye and its introduction by Domagk (1888-1964) led to the discovery of the sulphonamides and thereafter their derivatives such as the thiazides, dapsone and sulphonylureas. **Antibiotics** are substances which act against micro-organisms and originally were derived from fermentation products of living moulds and fungi. Now some antibiotics such as chloramphenicol are manufactured synthetically and others by the action of bacteria. Infections of man are by viruses, rickettsiae, chlamydiae, bacteria, fungi, protozoa, worms and insects; Chapters 2-8 deal with their treatment. Few viruses (but most bacteria, rickettsiae and chlamydiae) respond to antibiotics or chemotherapy.

Use of Antibiotics

The choice rationally is based on isolating the causative organism and determining its sensitivities. In most ill patients it is not possible to wait for a laboratory diagnosis or confirmation, particularly as the best time to treat is early when the microbes are dividing fast. In general practice it may sometimes not be feasible to obtain material for culture.

In other circumstances when fuller information is available it may mean changing the antibiotic (e.g. in Gram-negative bacteraemia, meningitis, pneumonia, osteomyelitis). In ill patients if no material is available for culture and the diagnosis is clinical (as in osteomyelitis) a blood culture must be taken. Antibiotics act in two ways—**bactericidal** directly killing the micro-organisms, and **bacteriostatic** inhibiting or stopping the bacterial growth. The bacteria failing to multiply are then destroyed by the body's natural defences. Antimicrobial drugs are mainly used to cure disease but also at times prophylactically to prevent gas-gangrene after operations, rheumatic fever, malaria, cholera, meningococcal meningitis, recurrent urinary infection, gonorrhoea, syphilis, infection in C.S.F. rhinorrhoea and after Caesarian section and amniotic rupture. They are also given to prevent bacterial endocarditis following dental and surgical operations and to prevent infection in neutropenic patients. Prophylactic antimicrobial therapy is also used after insertion of hip prostheses and recently after colonic and pelvic surgery (metronidazole).

Bacterial resistance arises when microbes (1) produce enzymes capable of inactivating antibiotics e.g. penicillinase produced by staphylococci or (2) develop ways of growing which are no longer blocked by antibiotics. Bacterial resistance is likely when certain antibiotics (e.g. the macrolides) are given alone. (3) Bacterial resistance may be transferred in a *multiple resistance pattern* ('R factor'), an 'infection' passed on to other bacteria in genetic material (usually gut organisms), or as *phage transfer* in staphylococci where the resistance is to one or two antibiotics only.

7

To minimize bacterial resistance, to ensure effective therapy at reasonable cost (avoiding unnecessarily expensive preparations) and to prevent or reduce adverse effects, most hospitals have an antibiotic policy usually jointly formulated by the clinicians, bacteriologist and pharmacist. Antibiotic policies need to be updated regularly to keep in line with pharmaceutical advances and changing patterns of bacterial resistance. Features to note when comparing and choosing an antibiotic are its spectrum of activity, absorption, protein binding, mode of action, resistance, adverse effects and cost. Selection depends on bacteriology (sensitive or resistant organisms) pharmacology and toxicology. Ease of administration, availability and the doctor's experience are also important.

BETA LACTAM ANTIBIOTICS
Penicillins, cephalosporins and the cephamycins all possess a beta-lactam ring or group. Penicillin, the first antibiotic, is still widely used in its various forms. These antibiotics are bactericidal, acting best early in the infection when the bacteria are rapidly dividing, by preventing cell wall synthesis.

NATURAL PENICILLINS
Short-acting **Benzylpenicillin Ph. Eur., B.P.** or **Penicillin G** is available as a highly soluble crystalline sodium or potassium salt. Rapidly absorbed from the tissues when injected i.m., peak blood levels are reached in 1 hour, but because of rapid excretion by the renal tubules frequent injections are needed. Penicillin G may also be given i.v. When injected i.m. or i.v. adequate amounts do not enter the pleural space or joints, so intrapleural or intraarticular injections are given, but in meningitis massive doses i.m. ensure therapeutic concentrations in the C.S.F. Benzylpenicillin is largely destroyed by gastric acid and by bacteria (usually staphylococci) which produce an enzyme *penicillinase* which disrupts the beta-lactam ring. Penicillin G is stable if crystalline, but when made up for injection in aqueous solution lasts only 24h at room temperature and a week in a refrigerator. *Presentation* vials 0.5, 1, 2, 5 and 10 mega units for i.m. or i.v. use. A mega unit or 1 million units is equivalent to 600mg and can be dissolved in 1ml of water. The *dose* varies from 0.5-20 mega units daily; when high levels are needed it can be given i.v. preferably directly via the rubber tubing of an infusion since in some solutions penicillin may lose potency. The dose for intrathecal injection is 10 000-20 000u. Penicillin G 0.5 mega units and streptomycin 500mg are combined for use in 'Crystamycin'. **Oral Penicillin G** is made relatively ineffective by its destruction by gastric acid, though less so in infants. If large amounts are given as sodium or potassium penicillin G as 125 and 250mg tablets, or syrup 125 and 250mg/5ml enough is absorbed if taken before meals to give therapeutic concentrations, but penicillin V is nowadays preferred even though slightly more expensive and slower in action. **Penamecillin** ('Havapen') is resistant to gastric acid and changes to penicillin G in the small intestine. *Presentation* tablets 350mg; *dose* 350mg 8 hourly.

Long-acting forms of penicillin G avoid the need for injections every few hours, but they are more allergenic and contain adjuvants. **Procaine Penicillin Injection B.P** ('Depocillin') is a suspension in Water for Injections when made up containing 300mg or 300 000u/ml and because of its poor solubility is released from the tissues over a period of 12-24h. *Dose* 300-900mg daily i.m. The injection causes little pain, though some patients are intolerant of the procaine. **Procaine Penicillin Injection, Fortified, B.P.** ('Bicillin') combines 60mg of benzylpenicillin with 300mg of the procaine salt for i.m. use and enables a quick action to be followed by a delayed one. **Penicillin Triple Injection B.P.C.** ('Triplopen') contains benethamine penicillin 475mg, procaine penicillin 250mg and benzylpenicillin sodium 300mg. The contents of a single dose vial are dissolved in Water for Injections and given deeply i.m. It finds special use in casualty departments. Repository forms of benzylpenicillin take days (benethamine penicillin) or weeks (benzathine) to be released. They are poorly soluble thick white suspensions which need vigorous shaking before use. **Benzathine Penicillin Ph. Eur., B.P.** ('Penidural L.A.') an aqueous suspension contains 225mg/ml in 10ml vials and the dose is 900mg i.m. every 2-3 weeks. It is used for preventing rheumatic fever, syphilis and streptococcal infections. *Adverse effects* include pain, and allergic reactions in about 1% usually in the second week after injection. Oral benzathine benzylpenicillin although palatable is expensive, poorly absorbed and not long-acting. Penicillin aluminium monostearate (PAM) has been used i.m. in the tropics for the cure of syphilis and yaws. **Phenoxymethylpenicillin** or **Penicillin V Ph. Eur.** as the calcium or potassium salt is an acid resistant natural penicillin and is reasonably, but not predictably, absorbed. Because of this possible unreliability for severe infections such as beta haemolytic streptococcal pharyngitis or bacterial endocarditis penicillin G is injected initially. Penicillin V acts in 30min and lasts about 4h. *Presentation* Capsules B.P. and Tablets B.P. 125 and 250mg, Mixture B.P.C. 125mg/5ml and Elixir B.P.C. 62.5, 125, 150 and 250mg/5ml. *Dose* 250-500mg 4-6 hourly 30min before meals. It is cheaper (particularly in tablet form) and as effective as its semisynthetic derivatives. In general, solid forms of oral penicillin are cheaper than liquid.

SEMISYNTHETIC PENICILLINS
Modification of the penicillin nucleus by adding side-chains has extended the versatility and range of the penicillins, so that some are absorbed taken orally, some are effective against penicillinase-forming staphylococci and others are valuable against Gram-negative bacteria.

(1) Penicillin V Semisynthetic Derivatives
These are likewise acid resistant, orally effective and act like benzylpenicillin. **Phenethicillin** ('Broxil') is quickly absorbed and gives good blood levels. *Presentation* Phenethicillin Potassium B.P. Tablets 250mg, Capsules 250mg and Elixir B.P.C. 125mg/5ml in 100ml bottles. *Dose* 250-500mg 6 hourly. **Propicillin Potassium** after absorption gives high, but ill-sustained blood levels. *Presentation* Tablets B.P. 250mg, Elixir B.P.C. 62.5 and 125mg/5ml. *Dose* 250-500mg 4-6 hourly. The 'oral penicillins' are given 30min before meals. Their main use is when injections of penicillin G (benzylpenicillin) are refused, or are inconvenient as in children and in domiciliary practice. They can cause nausea and bowel disturbance.

(2) Penicillinase Resistant
These are costly and only prescribed when penicillinase-producing staphylococci are present, or are suspected. High levels can be obtained by giving big doses and by blocking tubular excretion with probenecid given orally. **Methicillin Sodium** ('Celbenin', 'Staphcillin') *presentation* vials 1g to be made up with Water for Injections 1.5ml for i.m. and 20ml for i.v. use to make Methicillin Injection B.P. *Dose* 1g 4-6 hourly i.m. or i.v. The drug can only be injected and is excreted quickly.

Isoxazolyl Penicillins include flucloxacillin, cloxacillin, dicloxacillin and oxacillin. Like methicillin they are used against staphylococci, but are several times more potent. Resistance can occur to them and also to the cephalosporins. In such cases gentamicin or rifampicin is useful. **Flucloxacillin Sodium** ('Floxapen') has similar uses to cloxacillin but is absorbed better orally achieving higher blood levels and should supersede it. Both are taken an hour before meals. *Presentation* capsules 250mg, syrup 125mg/5ml, vials containing 250 and 500mg. *Dose* oral, i.m. or i.v. 250-500mg 6 hourly. For i.m. injection 1.5ml of Water for Injections is used to dissolve the powder and for i.v. use 250-500mg is dissolved in 10-20ml of Sodium Chloride Injection. **Cloxacillin Sodium** ('Orbenin') is effective orally and by injection. Blood levels last 4 hours. *Presentation* Capsules B.P. 250 and 500mg, Elixir B.P.C. 125mg/5ml in 100ml bottles, Cloxacillin Injection B.P. vials contents 250 and 500mg dissolved in Water for Injections 1.5ml for i.m. and 10ml for i.v. use. *Dose* adults orally, i.m. or i.v. 250-500mg 4-6 hourly. Children 2-10 years take half and 0-2 years a quarter of the adult dose. Intrathecally 10-40mg daily for adults in 1-2ml of Sodium Chloride Injection B.P., children 3-5mg in 0.5ml of solvent.

(3) **Broad Spectrum**

Carbenicillin Sodium ('Pyopen') must be injected. It is reserved for Pseudomonas species and ampicillin resistant *Esch. coli* and Proteus species. *Presentation* infusion bottles containing 5g, Carbenicillin Injection B.P. vials containing powder 1 and 5g dissolved in Water for Injections. *Dose* 1-2g 6 hourly i.m. for 5-10 days (e.g. for urinary infections), or in severe infections and bacteraemia 5-10g i.v. 4-8 hourly either injected as a bolus, or by infusion over 20-30min. Dose for children is 250-500µg/kg B.W. Intrathecal dose for adults is 40mg. Blood levels of over 25µg/ml are needed to eradicate *Ps. aeruginosa*. Gentamicin may be combined to prevent resistance, but the two must not be given in solution together as they are incompatible. A gram of carbenicillin sodium contains 124mg (5.4mmol) of sodium, a relevant matter for patients with heart failure, or on sodium restriction. An ester of carbenicillin effective orally with similar antibacterial activity and used for urinary infections is **Carfecillin Sodium** ('Uticillin'). *Presentation* tablets 500mg; *dose* 500-1000mg orally 8 hourly. It is changed *in vivo* into carbenicillin and its use should be restricted to avoid increasing bacterial resistance to the parent substance. It is an example of a pro-drug. **Ticarcillin Disodium** ('Ticar') is related to carbenicillin.

Ampicillin ('Amfipen', 'Penbritin', 'Pentrexyl', 'Vidopen') is widely prescribed, but is expected to be superseded for oral use by the better absorbed but dearer amoxycillin. It produces effective tissue and urine levels and adequate amounts reach the C.S.F. in meningitis. It is of no value against staphylococcal infections. *Presentation* **Ampicillin B.P.** anhydrous or **Ampicillin Trihydrate** Capsules B.P. 250 and 500mg, Ampicillin Mixture B.P.C. 125mg/5ml ('Penbritin Syrup'), Strong Ampicillin Mixture B.P.C. ('Penbritin Syrup Forte') 250mg/5ml in 100ml bottles, Ampicillin Tablets B.P.C. ('Penbritin Paediatric Tablets') 125mg, and 'Penbritin Paediatric Suspension' 125mg/1.25ml supplied as a powder to prepare 25ml of the suspension. The sodium salt is used for injections. **Ampicillin Sodium Injection B.P.** is made by dissolving the contents of vials 250 and 500mg in Water for Injections. Ampoules 20mg/ml are available for intrathecal use. *Dose* orally 250-2000mg 6 hourly or i.v. by slow infusion 500-2000mg 6 hourly. Dose for children; 0-2 years 62.5-125mg 6 hourly. Intrathecal dose for adults is 40mg.

'Ampiclox' consists of 250mg ampicillin and 250mg cloxacillin in vials and is made up with 1.5ml of Water for Injections for i.m. use or in 10-20ml for i.v. use. 'Ampiclox Neonatal' contains 50mg of ampicillin and 25mg of cloxacillin in each vial. The dose of 'Ampiclox' is i.m. 1-2 vials 4-6 hourly, i.v. 1-2 vials 8 hourly and of 'Ampiclox Neonatal' is 1 vial 8 hourly. There is also a neonatal suspension for oral use. When made up it contains 60mg of ampicillin and 30mg of cloxacillin in each 0.6ml dose. 'Magnapen' is flucloxacillin with ampicillin in capsules and vials for injection (250mg of each constituent) and a syrup containing 125mg ampicillin and 125mg flucloxacillin per 5ml. These combinations are used for the emergency treatment of severe bacterial infections before bacteriological identification is available. **Amoxycillin** ('Amoxil') is better absorbed than ampicillin with high blood levels irrespective of meals. Adverse effects are similar. *Presentation* Amoxycillin Trihydrate Capsules B.P. 250 and 500mg, syrup 125 and 250mg/5ml, paediatric suspension 125mg/1.25ml and vials 250, 500 and 1000mg (1g) for i.m. and i.v. injection. *Dose* 250-1500mg 8 hourly, children 0-10 years 125-250mg 8 hourly. For typhoid, including the carrier state, doses up to 4-5g daily are given. **Pivampicillin** is an ester of ampicillin and ampicillin is released in the blood by hydrolysis—385mg is equivalent to 250mg ampicillin. **Bacampicillin** is hydrolysed in the gut wall and changed to ampicillin. **Talampicillin** ('Talpen') available as 250mg tablets has similar actions; *dose* 250mg t.d.s.

USES OF THE PENICILLINS
Whenever possible penicillin G (benzylpenicillin) or phenoxymethylpenicillin is used. Both ampicillin and amoxycillin are more expensive and often less effective. A major indication for benzylpenicillin was staphylococcal infection of skin, lungs, heart. kidney, gut, blood and bones. However, bacterial strains both inside and outside hospital have become increasingly resistant to benzylpenicillin. For penicillinase-producing strains of staphylococci methicillin, or one of the isoxazolyl penicillins is used. Other infections for which benzylpenicillin (or phenoxymethylpenicillin at times) may be used are pneumococcal (pneumonia, lung abscess, empyema, pericarditis, meningitis), streptococcal (tonsillitis, scarlet fever, cellulitis, otitis media, mastoiditis, sinusitis, uterine puerperal infection, bacterial endocarditis, impetigo), vulvo-vaginitis in children, *Listeria monocytogenes,* gonorrhoea, syphilis, anthrax, chancroid, gas gangrene, tetanus, Vincent's angina, yaws, relapsing fever, leptospirosis and actinomycosis. The usual dose is 0.5-2 mega units (300-1200mg) 6-8 hourly i.m, or i.v., but more is needed in lung abscess, meningitis, bacterial endocarditis and actinomycosis e.g. up to 20 mega units daily. **Amoxycillin** or **ampicillin** is mainly used for chest infections (bronchitis or pneumonia caused by *H. influenzae* or *Str. pneumoniae),* urinary infections *(Esch. coli, Pr. mirabilis),* meningitis (*H. influenzae* and *Str. pneumoniae)* and infections by *Str. faecalis.* Increasing resistance is occurring with *Esch. coli* and *H. influenzae.* Ampicillin, or amoxycillin is used for chloramphenicol resistant typhoid infections, but is more expensive than the alternative co-trimoxazole. For the severe forms of shigellosis met abroad amoxycillin has not always been as effective as ampicillin. Carbenicillin is used for *Ps. aeruginosa* (aminoglycosides are first choice) and strains of *Esch. coli* and Proteus species resistant to ampicillin. *Prophylaxis* oral phenoxymethylpenicillin or injected depot penicillins (e.g. benzathine) protect against recurrences of rheumatic fever. Penicillin G is given to prevent gas gangrene when amputating ischaemic limbs

and to prevent bacterial endocarditis when performing dental or oral procedures on a patient with valvular or septal heart disease. It may also be used to prevent tetanus in contaminated wounds with other measures.

Adverse Effects of the Penicillins
Although penicillin is virtually non-toxic, anaphylaxis resulting from its use kills more people than any other antibiotic because of its wide use. All patients should be asked about previous reactions to penicillin, since further amounts by any route can be dangerous. Any penicillin can cause a sensitivity reaction since they all contain the same basic chemical nucleus. Rashes are common after topical application, but may follow oral or parenteral administration or if given concurrently with allopurinol. Ampicillin is now a major cause of rashes particularly if given unwisely in infectious mononucleosis, cytomegalovirus infection or in lymphatic leukaemia. Allergic reactions include fever, rash, joint pain, lymphadenopathy, hepatitis and angioneurotic oedema with laryngeal obstruction and respiratory distress and sudden death. (Adrenaline for injection and by aerosol, i.v. antihistamines and hydrocortisone should be at hand.) Anaphylactic shock with circulatory failure is liable with accidental i.v. injections particularly penicillin in oil, wax or procaine. Penicillin G i.v. in massive mega doses (20-40 mega units daily) can cause haemolytic anaemia and convulsions. Renal damage (acute interstitial nephritis with fever, rash, proteinuria, haematuria, eosinophilia) is recorded with methicillin and ampicillin and also occasionally depression of blood formation. Carbenicillin can cause defects in haemostasis by interfering with platelet function and other mechanisms. Nurses preparing injections if they squirt penicillin mist into the air may develop dermatitis. *Drug-interactions* phenylbutazone and salicylates displace penicillin bound to serum proteins so increasing antibiotic activity. Chloramphenicol antagonizes the effect of penicillin.

CEPHALOSPORINS
These were discovered after the penicillins. They are used as an alternative when patients are allergic to, or infected by, organisms resistant to the penicillins. They are semisynthetic derivatives of Cephalosporin C, bactericidal by interfering with bacterial cell wall function. However, because of their shared lactam ring and similar structure a small proportion of patients can be allergic to both the penicillins and cephalosporins. Moreover, the wide choice and range of penicillins restricts the need for, and uses of, the cephalosporins. They have a wide range against bacteria, but the degree of activity varies. The newer cephalosporins (cephamandole and cefuroxime) are more active against Gram negative organisms. Resistance to the penicillinase-producing staphylococci occurs (but not to methicillin type resistance) and the cephalosporins can be inactivated by cephalosporinases which break open the beta-lactam ring (e.g. as produced by *Ps. aeruginosa* which is completely resistant). The cephalosporins are usually excreted by the kidneys unchanged, with the exception of cephalothin which is partly changed to inactive forms in the body and cephaloglycin which is almost all metabolized. In renal failure the dose should be reduced. They are used in undiagnosed severe infection, respiratory and urinary infections and occasionally in the treatment and prophylaxis of bacterial endocarditis. Cephalosporins vary as to the route of administration. Injectable forms are cephaloridine, cephalothin, cephradine, cephazolin, cephacetrile, cefapirin, cefuroxime and cephamandole ('Kefadol').

Cephaloridine is more active than cephalothin. Some forms are painful i.m. particularly cephalothin. They may be injected to combat severe infections by *Staph. aureus, Str. pyogenes, Str. pneumoniae, Esch. coli, Pr. mirabilis. Klebsiella spp, Enterobacter aerogenes* and some strains of *H. influenzae*. When giving an antibiotic i.v. the pharmacist should be consulted about inactivation and incompatibilities with other drugs and infusions. Cephazolin is highly protein bound (60-80%) whereas cephradine (6%) and cephalexin (<30%) have low protein binding. The oral forms are widely used for respiratory infections (cephalexin, cephradine, cefaclor), or for urinary infections in the U.S.A. (cephaloglycin).

Individual Cephalosporins

Cephaloridine Ph. Eur. ('Ceporin') was the first to be introduced in Britain. *Presentation* vials containing 250, 500 and 1000mg dissolved in Water for Injections to make Injection B.P. *Dose* 500-2000mg 8 hourly i.m. or i.v. The maximum daily dose of 6g is only given to those under 50 years (4g if older) and only if the renal function is normal. After operation the dose is restricted to 4g daily. The dose is reduced in renal failure. Children 20-40mg/kg B.W. Intrathecal dose for adults up to 50mg. **Cephalothin Sodium** ('Keflin') is very painful i.m. and gives low blood levels by this route and it is better to give it only i.v. *Presentation* Injection B.P. contents of ampoules 1 and 4g dissolved in Water for Injections; *dose* 500-1000mg i.m. 3-6 hourly and for severe infections 1-2g i.v. 4 hourly. **Cephazolin Sodium** ('Kefzol') *presentation* ampoules 500 and 1000mg; *dose* 250-1000mg 6-8 hourly i.m. or i.v. dissolved in Water for Injections. Children 20-100mg/kg B.W. daily in 2 or 3 divided doses. **Cephacetrile** is not yet available in the U.K. but is less painful i.m. *Dose* 1g 2-4 times daily i.m. or i.v. It is especially suitable for biliary infections. **Cephradine** ('Velosef') can be given both orally and parenterally i.v. or i.m. *Presentation* capsules 250 and 500mg, suspension or syrup 125 and 250mg/5ml; *dose* 250-1000mg 6 hourly orally, For injection there are vials containing 250, 500 and 1000mg which are reconstituted in Water for Injections for i.m., or i.v. administration; *dose* 500-1000mg 6 hourly. Children 25-50mg/kg B.W. daily in divided amounts; in severe infections up to 300mg/kg B.W. but not to exceed adult dose. **Cephalexin** ('Ceporex', 'Keflex') is only available as an oral preparation and is probably more effective than phenoxymethylpenicillin against *Str. pyogenes* infections in children and is more palatable in syrup form. *Presentation* Capsules and Tablets B.P. 250 and 500mg, Mixture B.P.C. (suspension or syrup) 125, 250 and 500mg/5ml in 100ml bottles, paediatric drops 100mg/ml 10ml quantities with graduated dropper. *Dose* 250-1000mg orally 6 hourly and for children 25-60mg/kg B.W. in divided amounts. The oral cephalosporins are much cheaper than the injections but both are more expensive than the corresponding penicillins. *Adverse reactions* hypersensitivity—drug fever, rashes, vulvo-vaginitis, pruritus, eosinophilia; gastrointestinal—nausea, anorexia, diarrhoea, vomiting, oral thrush, abnormal liver function tests. Renal damage can occur with excessive doses e.g. over 6g of cephaloridine, or if there is pre-existing renal disease. The danger of renal failure *is increased by concomitant therapy with potent diuretics such as frusemide and aminoglycosides* such as gentamicin. Features of renal failure include anuria, oliguria, proteinuria and uraemia. Blood changes occasionally seen are neutropenia, thrombocytopenia, and not infrequently a positive Coombs's test. Anaphylactic reactions and fatalities are much less common with the cephalosporins than the penicillins.

CEPHAMYCINS

These may be more resistant to enzyme destruction. **Cefoxitin Sodium** ('Mefoxin') is available in vials containing 1 or 2g to be reconstituted in Water for Injection; *dose* i.m. or i.v. is 1-2g 8 hourly.

AMIDINOPENICILLINS

These are derived from 6-aminopenicillanic acid. **Mecillinam Hydrochloride** is given parenterally and **Pivmecillinam** ('Selexid') orally and by injection. They are used for urinary tract infections and salmonelloses. Synergy is claimed with other penicillins. *Presentation* ('Selexid') tablets 200mg, suspension made from 100mg sachets, vials 400mg to be dissolved in Water for Injections. *Dose* orally 1-2.4g in divided doses 6 or 8 hourly. Parenterally 5-10mg/kg B.W. 6-8 hourly i.v. or i.m.

OCCASIONAL ALTERNATIVES TO THE PENICILLINS AND CEPHALOSPORINS

Fusidic Acid

This is a steroid-like substance absorbed when taken orally and diffuses widely, but not into the C.S.F. Bactericidal, it acts against many organisms, but because of high cost it is reserved for penicillin-resistant staphylococci. *Presentation* Sodium Fusidate ('Fucidin') Capsules B.P. and enteric coated tablets 250mg, Fusidic Acid Mixture B.P.C. ('Fucidin Suspension') 250mg/5ml in 50ml bottles (equivalent to 175mg Sodium Fusidate/5ml). **Diethanolamine Fusidate** is used intravenously; 580mg is equivalent to 500mg of sodium fusidate and it is available as a powder in vials plus 50ml of buffer in a vial. *Dose* orally, adults 500mg 8 hourly; children 20-40mg/kg B.W. daily in 3 divided doses. It is often combined with an oral cephalosporin, penicillin, or erythromycin to enhance its action and prevent the emergence of resistant strains. Intravenously 500mg (as Sodium Fusidate) is infused in Sodium Chloride Injection over 4-6 hours up to 2g daily. The type of infection for which it is given is staphylococcal bacteraemia, pneumonia, or osteomyelitis difficult to eradicate as in diabetics. Topical forms of fusidic acid 2% ('Fucidin Gel') and sodium fusidate 2% ('Fucidin Ointment') are available, but for invasive staphylococcal skin infection the patient should be isolated when in hospital to prevent the spread of fusidic acid resistant strains.

LINCOMYCIN AND DERIVATIVES

Lincomycin Hydrochloride ('Lincocin', 'Mycivin') *presentation* Capsules B.P. 500mg, syrup 250mg/5ml in 100ml bottles, Lincomycin Injection B.P. contained in ampoules 2 and 6.7ml 300mg/ml. *Dose* orally 500mg 8 hourly and, systemically i.m. 600mg 12 hourly, or i.v. 600mg diluted in 500ml Dextrose Injection 5% B.P., or Sodium Chloride Injection B.P. (0.9%) and infused slowly every 8-12 hours. If concentrated forms are given i.v. quickly syncope or cardiac arrest can occur. **Clindamycin Hydrochloride** ('Dalacin C') is a derivative of lincomycin with the advantage that it is better absorbed and several times more active against staphylococci. *Presentation* Capsules B.P. 75 and 150mg, or Clindamycin Mixture Paediatric B.N.F. ('Dalacin C Mixture Paediatric') 75mg/5ml. **Clindamycin Phosphate** injection ampoules 2 and 4ml

('Dalacin C Phosphate Sterile Solution') and in the U.S.A. 'Cleocin' PO₄'.
150mg as clindamycin base/ml for i.m. use, or by slow i.v. infusion. *Dose* orally
150-450mg 6 hourly. *Uses* staphylococcal soft tissue infections and osteomyelitis, as well as streptococcal and pneumococcal infections. Clindamycin
150mg b.d. is an alternative to tetracycline in acne, when the latter is unsuccessful. A special use is against bacteroides (Gram-negative non-sporing
anaerobic bacilli) a cause of wound infection and bacteraemia (Metronidazole
may also be effective). For bacteroides infection of the meninges chloramphenicol is advised. Lincomycin and clindamycin act like the macrolides,
although chemically and structurally different, and they interfere with the protein synthesis of susceptible bacteria. They have good tissue penetration, but
as a group they are expensive. *Adverse reactions* diarrhoea, and a pseudomembranous colitis resembling ulcerative colitis usually following long-term
therapy and if the drug is continued (and not stopped) when diarrhoea first
comes. Occasional fatalities can occur.

Novobiocin ('Albamycin')
This is bacteriostatic and little used in the U.K. When taken orally as the
sodium or calcium salt it diffuses widely, but not into the C.S.F. Excretion is in
the bile and it is safe when there is poor renal function. *Presentation* capsules
250mg; *dose* oral 1-2g daily in divided amounts; children 15mg/kg B.W. daily.
Resistance occurs rapidly so it is often combined with tetracycline (in
'Albamycin T'), or erythromycin. *Adverse reactions* rashes, neutropenia, liver
dysfunction including jaundice.

Vancomycin ('Vancocin')
This is unabsorbed from the gut. It is irritant i.v. and should be used with caution when renal function is poor. The drug does not reach the C.S.F. *Presentation* vials 10ml containing 500mg of Vancomycin Hydrochloride as powder to
be dissolved in 10ml of Water for Injections and then given i.v. in 200-500ml
of Dextrose Injection B.P. 5%, or Sodium Chloride Injection B.P. *Dose* adults
500mg 6-8 hourly, infused i.v. in 200ml of Sodium Chloride Injection 0.9% or
Dextrose Injection 5% over a 30min period; children 20mg/kg B.W. Its use
i.v. is restricted to the treatment of refractory bacterial endocarditis and bacteraemia caused by staphylococci resistant to other antibiotics. Sometimes the
choice is between death untreated, or deafness treated. Vancomycin is occasionally used orally for gut infections including pseudomembranous colitis.
Adverse reactions thrombophlebitis, rashes, renal damage and deafness.

THE MACROLIDES
The macrolide antibiotics are large, cyclical, oxygen-containing lactone rings
with sugars attached and they interfere with bacterial protein synthesis. **Erythromycin** is the most important member and has a wide action against bacteria, rickettsiae, mycoplasmas and large 'viruses', or Chlamydiae. It is a useful
drug, less likely to cause anaphylaxis or rash than penicillin. For instance, it is
suitable for streptococcal, pneumococcal, rickettsial and mycoplasmal infections and for diphtheria carriers. Erythromycin is widely prescribed for cellulitis, soft tissue infections and in contacts of whooping cough (in first year of
life). It is absorbed fairly well providing it reaches the small intestine, but erythromycin base is destroyed by gastric juices and must be enclosed in an acid-
resistant covering and the stearate is inconstant in absorption. Diffusion occurs
widely through the body and excretion is mainly via the bile. Orally it may be
given as tablets, capsules or pleasantly flavoured suspensions. *Oral forms*

Erythromycin Base Ph. Eur., B.P. enteric-coated Tablets 250mg ('Ilotycin', 'Erycen', 'Erythromid', 'Retcin'). Salts and esters of erythromycin improve absorption. **Erythromycin Ethylsuccinate** ('Erythroped') granules when dissolved 5ml contains 250mg erythromycin activity, or for infants 125mg/5ml and for older children 'Erythroped Forte' 500mg/5ml. **Erythromycin Ethylcarbonate** ('Ilotycin Paediatric') suspension 100mg/5ml. The best absorbed is Erythromycin Estolate which can be taken with food; it is available as **Erythromycin Estolate Capsules B.P.** and 'Ilosone' capsules 250mg, tablets 500mg for twice daily use, and suspensions 125 and 250mg/5ml. **Erythromycin Stearate Tablets B.P.** ('Erythrocin Filmtab') 250 and 500mg and Erythromycin Mixture B.P.C. 100mg/5ml. *Dose* orally for adults 2-4g daily in four divided amounts 6 hourly for 7 days or more. Peak levels occur in 1 or 2 hours and last 6 hours. Children take 20-40mg/kg B.W. daily. *Intramuscular Forms* **Erythromycin Ethylsuccinate** ('Erythrocin I.M.') ampoules 2ml, 50mg erythromycin/ml. The dose is limited by pain to 100mg 8-12 hourly. *Intravenous* **Erythromycin Lactobionate** ('Erythrocin Lactobionate') vials 300mg erythromycin *dose* 300mg 4-8 hourly, **Erythromycin Gluceptate U.S.P.** ('Ilotycin Gluceptate') vials 250mg erythromycin. *Dose* 500mg-1g 6 hourly. *Adverse effects* nausea, vomiting and diarrhoea are not infrequent with the oral forms, particularly the base. The frequency of jaundice is 2-4% and occurs after 12 days therapy (quicker if the drug has been taken before) of the estolate derivative and is usually reversible. It is usually cholestatic but can occasionally be hepatocellular. Severe abdominal pain mimicking biliary colic can occur. Unlike the tetracyclines it does not affect the teeth or bones of young children so erythromycin is widely used in paediatric general practice. Injectable forms are suitable for those who cannot swallow (e.g. peritonsillar abscess), those with diarrhoea caused by *Campylobacter* and for very ill patients with pneumonia who may have Legionnaire's disease.

Spiramycin ('Rovamycin') and **Oleandomycin** are rarely prescribed in Britain, but spiramycin is used like erythromycin in France for various infections including gonorrhoea. It achieves good tissue levels and reaches higher concentrations in the prostate than the blood.

New Cephalosporins
Cefuroxime Sodium ('Zinacef') is an injectable cephalosporin introduced for severe infections especially Gram-negative (but not *Pseudomonas aeruginosa, Bacteroides fragilis* or *Streptococcus faecalis*). It achieves high blood levels, with low serum protein binding (40%), slow renal excretion and is not metabolized. *Presentation* vials 250 and 750mg for i.m. or i.v. use, 1.5g for bolus i.v. or i.v. infusion, to be dissolved in Water for Injections. *Dose* 750-1500mg 8h i.v. or i.m. in those with normal renal function. Children 30-100mg/kg B.W.

Cefaclor ('Distaclor') is an oral cephalosporin. *Presentation* capsules 250mg and suspension 125 and 250mg/5ml. *Dose* for adults 250-500mg 8 hourly and children 20-40mg/kg B.W. in divided doses 8 hourly.

3 TETRACYCLINES, AMINOGLYCOSIDES, SULPHONAMIDES AND OTHER ANTIMICROBIALS

TETRACYCLINES AND DERIVATIVES

These were among the earliest orally available antibiotics and their basic structure is made up of four joined rings. They are bacteriostatic for many bacteria, rickettsiae, mycoplasmas and a few large 'viruses'. Whereas they enjoyed great popularity in the past for many common conditions their use has waned as bacteria have become resistant e.g. staphylococci, streptococci and pneumococci, or as serious adverse effects have become apparent. Paradoxically they now find use in many, often rare conditions. They are readily absorbed by mouth and peak levels occur in 2-6 hours. Sustained blood levels required 6 hourly administration with the first generation tetracyclines, but with later forms once or twice daily suffices. They permeate the body, except the C.S.F. and cross the placenta into the foetal circulation. Excretion is via the bile and the kidneys. Oral therapy is best if feasible and is taken 30 minutes before meals. Absorption varies between brands. Tetracyclines combine, complex, or chelate with various metals (divalent or trivalent cations) such as calcium in milk (which should not be taken with it), bismuth, aluminium and magnesium in antacids, and with iron compounds so reducing their absorption.

Chlortetracycline Hydrochloride Ph. Eur. ('Aureomycin') Capsules B.P. 250mg. **Oxytetracycline Dihydrate Ph. Eur.** Tablets B.P. 100 and 250mg ('Berkmycen', 'Galenomycin', 'Imperacin', 'Oxymycin', 'Terramycin'). **Oxytetracycline Hydrochloride Ph. Eur.** Capsules B.P. 250mg ('Unimycin') U.S.P. 125 and 250mg. Oxytetracycline Calcium is available as a syrup 125mg/5ml or a suspension (U.S.N.F.). **Tetracycline Hydrochloride Ph. Eur.** Capsules B.P. 250mg and U.S.P. 250 and 500mg; Tablets 50, 100 and 250mg; syrups 125mg/5ml are available ('Achromycin', 'Economycin', 'Tetracyn', 'Totomycin'). **Tetracycline Phosphate Complex** ('Achromycin V', 'Tetrex') has the same range of capsules, tablets and syrups. There is little to choose in activity between individual tetracyclines but oxytetracycline is one of the cheapest. Twice daily slow-release forms include 'Tetrabid' (250mg b.d.) and 'Sustamycin' 250mg capsules taken 1 or 2 daily. *Dose* for other forms; orally for adults 1-3g daily in 4 equally divided amounts 6 hourly for at least 7 days. There are very few indications for tetracyclines in children (because of teeth and bone problems) but the dose is 20-40mg/kg B.W. daily in divided amounts. Combinations of different tetracyclines exist: 'Deteclo' is tetracycline 115.4mg, chlortetracycline 115.4mg and demeclocycline 69.2mg; tetracycline with novobiocin in 'Albamycin T'; with antifungal agents such as amphotericin B ('Mysteclin Syrup') or nystatin ('Mysteclin' tablets or capsules) and with vitamins ('Terramycin S.F.', 'Tetracyn S.F.').

Derivatives have been introduced with longer action, better absorption or a wider range.

Demeclocyline Hydrochloride Ph. Eur. ('Declomycin' U.S.A., 'Ledermycin') *presentation* Capsules B.P. 150mg and tablets 300mg, aqueous drops 60mg in 10ml bottles, syrup 75mg/5ml 100 and 500ml bottles. *Dose* adults 300mg then 150-300mg b.d.; children 6-12mg/kg B.W. in 2 divided amounts. It is quickly absorbed, effective, gives sustained blood levels and is slowly excreted, but acts as a skin photosensitizer. An occasional use is to treat the inappropriate ADH syndrome and for diuresis in heart failure.

Lymecycline ('Tetralysal') has an added aminoacid which improves absorption and blood levels. *Presentation* Capsules B.P. 204mg equal to 150mg of tetracycline base. *Dose* orally 204mg 6 hourly.

Clomocycline ('Megaclor') is a highly absorbed derivative of chlortetracycline, with a short half life and therefore may be safer in children and suitable for the elderly. Since less remains unabsorbed direct intestinal toxicity should be decreased. *Presentation* capsules 170mg. *Dose* 170mg 6 hourly.

Methacycline Hydrochloride ('Rondomycin') is a slowly excreted compound. *Presentation* Capsules B.P. 150mg, syrup 75mg/5ml. *Dose* 600mg daily divided in 6 hourly amounts.

Doxycycline Hydrochloride ('Vibramycin') taken orally is almost completely absorbed, but is only very slowly excreted and is lipid soluble. It needs to be taken only once daily and good renal tissue levels are obtained. *Presentation* Capsules B.P. 100mg, syrup 50mg/5ml in 30ml bottles. *Dose* 200mg first day then 100mg daily with food. Single dose doxycycline has the advantage of simplicity in tropical situations and has been used effectively in epidemic and scrub typhus. Intravenous Doxycycline Hydrochloride is available in the U.S.A. in vials containing 100 or 200mg powder which is dissolved in 10 or 20ml water for injections and further diluted in Sodium Chloride Injection, dextrose 5% or Ringer's solution. The concentration desired is 0.1-0.5mg/ml and the infusion is up to 12h and should be protected from sunlight. **Minocycline Hydrochloride** ('Minocin') is well absorbed and has a better range of activity than other tetracyclines for it may be effective against *Staph. aureus, Esch. coli, Str. pyogenes* and *N. gonorrhoeae. Presentation* tablets 100mg. *Dose* 200mg then 100mg 12 hourly.

Parenteral Therapy
Intravenous tetracycline and oxytetracycline are used buffered with ascorbic acid. *Presentation* vials 250 and 500mg; 100mg is dissolved in 10ml of Water for Injections and then diluted 10 times in Dextrose Injection B.P. 5% or Sodium Chloride Injection B.P. to make a strength of 1mg/ml. The rate of infusion is up to 5mg/min to a dose of 500mg-1g/24h.

Intramuscular Tetracycline and Procaine Injection B.P.C. is prepared from the contents of a vial containing 100mg tetracycline hydrochloride and 40mg of procaine hydrochloride (a local anaesthetic) because the injection is painful. The contents are dissolved in 2ml of sterile water and used the same day. Injections are made deep into the muscle and no more than 100mg is given at any one site. *Dose* 200-400mg daily. **Rolitetracycline** is available abroad either as the base or rolitetracycline nitrate.

Ointments (and creams) for skin infections include tetracycline ('Achromycin'), chlortetracycline ('Aureomycin') and oxytetracycline ('Terramycin') in 3% strengths. Ointments 1% for eye use and 1% eye drops are available but their stability is restricted in solution to 48 hours.

Uses

Their uses in pneumonia before the organisms have been identified has declined since resistant strains of pneumococci, streptococci and staphylococci are common. They are of value in mycoplasmal pneumonia. Resistance has also occurred with *Clostridium welchii* (gas gangrene) so tetracyclines are not advised prophylactically. A major use in Britain is for chronic bronchitis where they may be used to treat an acute attack, or may be given in small maintenance doses. They are of value in cholera and as supplementary therapy in amoebic dysentery, but in bacillary dysentery in Britain the present trend is not to give antibiotics. Tropical sprue, intestinal blind loops, bacterial overgrowth syndromes and Whipple's disease respond to tetracyclines. Other indications are urinary infections (but beware in renal failure), brucellosis, typhus, psittacosis, Q fever, tularaemia, leptospirosis, actinomycosis, anthrax, lymphogranuloma venereum and gonorrhoea resistant to penicillin. TRIC agents (Chlamydiae) Reiter's syndrome, non-specific urethritis are susceptible and in acne rosacea and acne vulgaris small doses such as 250mg twice daily can be given for months. For systemic infections treatment continues for several days after the fever has settled. *Adverse effects: gastro-intestinal* occur because of incomplete absorption as well as a direct toxic action producing anorexia, nausea, vomiting, epigastric pain and diarrhoea. The intestinal bacteria change in type and alien dangerous organisms (*Proteus spp,* Pseudomonas, staphylococci) or fungi (candida) take over by colonisation or super-infection. Tetracycline-resistant staphylococcal entero-colitis causes a deadly choleralike illness which requires urgent parenteral methicillin or cloxacillin and i.v. fluids. *Muco-cutaneous:* soreness, irritation and inflammatory lesions in the mouth, anus and vagina. The tongue becomes red, sore and beefy. A candida infection is often caused and usually goes when the tetracycline is stopped. Exceptionally, candidosis spreads to the oesophagus or lungs. Light sensitivity or phototoxicity is a particular feature of demeclocycline. *Metabolic:* the tetracyclines are deposited in the dentine, enamel and growing bone and since they inhibit foetal growth they are avoided in pregnancy and in infancy and childhood up to the age of 8 or 9 years. They are not advised in the elderly and those with poor renal function. The smallest dose possible should be given parenterally especially i.v.–doses above 1g may be highly dangerous toxic to the liver and fatal. The danger increases in pregnancy and with renal failure. The expiry date should be noted since time-expired tetracycline has damaged renal tubules. The tetracyclines inhibit bacterial synthesis and possess an antigrowth or catabolic effect in humans. The blood urea rises and there is an increased excretion of nitrogen, aminoacids and riboflavin. In those with poor renal function uraemia, hyperphosphataemia, anorexia, weight loss, vomiting, acidosis and death can occur. If a tetracycline must be given in renal failure doxycycline is the safest. Minocycline causes dizziness and vertigo.

CHLORAMPHENICOL

Chloramphenicol Ph. Eur. ('Chloromycetin', 'Kemicetine') is a synthetic broad-spectrum, bacteriostatic antibiotic, effective against many bacteria, rickettsiae and some larger 'viruses' by inhibiting protein synthesis. It is cheap and widely used in certain countries either because the risks there are slight or unrecognized, or because dearer and safer drugs are not available. It is widely used in Eastern Europe, Italy, Spain and Africa. Tourists may take it unknowingly. In Britain its use is restricted because of its hazards. Bitter tasting, it is absorbed rapidly by mouth, (but absorption varies with brands) diffuses widely and enters the C.S.F. Blood levels with chloramphenicol are higher with oral and i.v. administration than i.m. This is because the enzyme in muscle which splits the ester chloramphenicol succinate to active chloramphenicol acts slowly. The drug is detoxicated by the liver quickly in adults, but very slowly in premature babies. A small percentage of the active chloramphenicol is excreted by the kidneys. *Oral forms: presentation* Capsules B.P. 250mg; *dose* 2-3g daily for 5-7 days. The total should rarely exceed 26g. Children are given flavoured chloramphenicol palmitate suspension either as Chloramphenicol Mixture B.P.C. 125mg/5ml or as 'Chloromycetin Palmitate' which is broken down in the body to chloramphenicol. The dose for premature babies is 25mg/kg B.W. daily; other babies and infants are given twice this amount. Topical preparations are skin and eye ointments 1%, eye drops 0.5% and ear drops 10%. Parenteral injections are given for emergencies (e.g. *H. influenzae* meningitis and epiglottitis or severe typhoid fever). *Presentation* Chloramphenicol Sodium Succinate B.P. ('Chloromycetin Succinate') vials containing 1.2g as powder. For i.m. use 1g is dissolved in 2ml Water for Injections making 2.5ml of a 40% solution which is given deeply. For i.v. or s.c. use a 10% solution is made by adding 11ml of sterile water to a vial of 1g. The dose is up to 1g 6-8 hourly. *Indications* typhoid and paratyphoid fever in an oral daily dose of 500mg 6 hourly continuing for 1-2 weeks after the fever has settled. Occasional resistant strains have been reported abroad. It is probably still the best treatment for *H. influenzae* meningitis and epiglottitis and occasionally severe respiratory infection in the aged and bacteroides infection of the C.N.S. Abroad meningococcal meningitis and some rickettsial infections may be treated with chloramphenicol because of its cheapness, effectiveness and ease of administration by nurses or 'field or foot doctors'. *Adverse effects* nausea, vomiting, diarrhoea, abdominal colic, retrobulbar neuritis, and skin hypersensitivity. Allergy to oral or topical preparations is not uncommon in Eastern Europe. Commonly there is reversible marrow depression. It occasionally causes an aplastic anaemia which is often fatal and not dose related, sideroblastic anaemia and in premature babies given too large a dose a fatal shock-like condition. Although rare, systemic toxic effects have occurred from topical chloramphenicol such as eye medications.

THE POLYMYXINS (Peptide Antibiotics)
This group is produced by bacterial fermentation. They are bactericidal. Of the 5 members only B and E are used and this is mainly against Gram-negative organisms particularly *Ps. aeruginosa* an important cause of infection of the debilitated which can attack the gut, eye, brain, meninges, bloodstream, lungs, kidneys, skin and ears. Polymyxins are also effective against bacillary dysentery. They are well absorbed i.m. but injections are painful. Excretion is by the kidneys. In adults the polymyxins do not enter the C.S.F. so that in meningitis intrathecal injections are needed. They are not absorbed orally.
Polymyxin B Sulphate Ph. Eur., B.P. ('Aerosporin') *presentation* Polymyxin Injection B.P.C. vials of freeze-dried powder containing 500 000u which keep well and are dissolved in water or saline. It is mainly given in topical form as a powder, drops or ointment. For injections the less painful sulphomethyl derivative is best. *Dose* orally 1 mega unit 4 hourly. *Dose* if given systemically is by the i.v. route; 10 000-25 000u/kg B.W. in 24 hours by infusion divided into three 8 hourly doses in Dextrose Injection 5% given each over a period of

1-2 hours. The total daily dose should not exceed 2 million units. **Colistin or Polymyxin E** *presentation* Colistin Sulphate B.P. Tablets 1 500 000u; syrup 250 000u/5ml in 80ml bottles and vials of sterile powder 1 and 5g for oral use. (1mg $\equiv$ 19 500u). The sulphomethyl derivative **Colistin Sulphomethate Sodium Injection B.P.** ('Colomycin Injection') vials 500 000 and 1 million units is a repository form dissolved in 2ml of Sodium Chloride Injection B.P. *Dose* oral 100 000-150 000u/kg B.W. colistin sulphate daily (9-18 mega-units) in 3 or 4 divided amounts. By injection colistin sulphomethate i.m. or i.v. for systemic infections 50 000-100 000u/kg B.W. divided into 6 or 8 hourly injections (adults 1-3 mega-units 8 hourly). Treatment may be for several weeks. The intrathecal dose is 500-1000u/kg B.W. Topical applications and aerosols are available. *Adverse effects* neurotoxic-paraesthesiae (tinglings of the face), ataxia, neuropathy, neuromuscular blockade with respiratory depression (apnoea), kidney damage, rash, fever, nausea, vomiting, diarrhoea, neutropenia, hypokalaemia and ear disturbance. Colistin sulphomethate sodium should not be given concurrently with other medications such as antibiotics with muscle-blockading actions.

AMINOGLYCOSIDES
This class of chemically (hexose containing) and biologically similar broad-spectrum, bactericidal antibiotics are all bases and are used as the water soluble sulphates. They include amikacin, neomycin, paromomycin, framycetin, gentamicin, netilmicin, kanamycin, tobramycin, sissomicin and streptomycin. They are poorly absorbed by mouth and are used topically for skin or ear infections and orally for bowel infections. When injected systemically kanamycin, gentamicin, streptomycin or neomycin can be toxic to the kidneys since they are markedly concentrated in the cortex. They can also cause deafness, vertigo and high frequency hearing loss. They are effective against many bacteria including mycobacteria, but excluding anaerobic bacilli and work best in a slightly alkaline solution e.g. in the urine. Since they have a similar mode of action partial or complete cross-resistance occurs. They may damage normal intestinal mucosa and cause malabsorption. Excretion is by the glomeruli. They may cause neuromuscular blockade and have a curare-like action.
Neomycin Sulphate Ph. Eur. ('Mycifradin', 'Neomin', 'Nivemycin') *presentation* Tablets B.P. 500mg or 350 000u, Neomycin Elixir B.P.C. 100mg/5ml, (70 000u/5ml); *dose* 2-8g daily in divided amounts. *Uses* reduction of bacterial flora before colonic surgery and of the nitrogenous toxic substances formed by them in liver failure. Continued use causes malabsorption and this has been used therapeutically in hyperlipidaemia. Small amounts are absorbed but this is only significant if there is renal failure or with long-term therapy. Neomycin is contained in 'Cremomycin', 'Ivax' and 'Kaomycin'. An important use is topically, either alone, or with gramicidin in 'Graneodin', with chlorhexidine or hydrocortisone in ointments for ear, skin and eye infections and it may be given by inhalation or by injection i.m. in hospital patients. Staphylococcal resistance is increasing as is skin sensitivity to the topical preparations. Topical application in burns may possibly cause deafness.
Paromomycin Sulphate ('Humatin') has been used for anthelmintic, bacterial and amoebic gut infections. It is no longer available in the U.K. but is in the U.S.A. *Presentation* capsules 250mg (250 000 units); syrup 125mg/5ml. *Dose* adults 1-3g daily for 6 days; children 50-100mg/kg B.W. daily.
Framycetin Sulphate ('Framygen', 'Soframycin') *presentation* powder 500mg

in vials, tablets 250mg as solutions for local injection into joints and as an ointment alone, or with gramicidin ('Soframycin'). Eye drops are also available.

Gentamicin Sulphate ('Cidomycin', 'Genticin', 'Garamycin') *presentation* Gentamicin Injection B.P. ampoules or vials 2ml 40mg/ml (as gentamicin base 40 000u = 40mg) paediatric injection vials 2ml 10mg/ml. *Dose* adults 0.8-1.6mg/kg B.W. i.v. or i.m. 8 hourly for up to 7 days which works out at 40-80mg thrice daily for those with normal renal function. In severe infection 120mg 8 hourly has been given for the first 24 hours. In renal failure the drug stays in the serum much longer and 80mg twice daily, once daily or every other day may suffice, since the drug is renally excreted. It must be injected as it is unabsorbed orally and the aim is to avoid sub-therapeutic and also toxic levels. Peak blood levels are measured and they are kept below 10µg/ml. Deafness is more likely if large boluses are given rapidly, or if frusemide or ethacrynic acid is given concurrently. When administered it ought be run in as a rapid infusion in 100ml of Dextrose Injection B.P. 5% since this may be less ototoxic. Vestibular function is tested daily by asking the patient to sit up. *Uses* Gram-negative infections *(Ps. aeruginosa, Proteus spp., Esch. coli)* and it is also effective against staphylococci but not against streptococci or anaerobes. Gentamicin is often part of the regime for bacteraemia before the organism is identified. The *doses for children* initially can be as high as 6mg/kg B.W. daily in neonates and infants and are increased or decreased according to blood levels. Details of administration and drug incompatibilities can be obtained from the hospital pharmacist. Gentamicin is not advised given with a cephalosporin. Topical applications are cream and ointment 0.3% in 15 and 100g tubes, ear and eye drops 0.3% 10ml bottles. Ampoules are available for intrathecal use 5mg in 1ml (Roussel) or 1mg/ml (Nicholas). The *dose* is 1-5mg. Gentamicin is a very widely used drug in hospital practice.

Tobramycin Sulphate ('Nebcin') has a similar range of activity against bacteria as gentamicin although it may be more effective. *Presentation* ready-prepared injections in vials 1 and 2ml 40mg/ml, 10mg/ml as tobramycin base. *Dose* 1-5mg/kg B.W. daily i.m. or i.v. with adjustments in renal disease. *Adverse effects* as for gentamicin. It is not to be given intrathecally.

Kanamycin Sulphate ('Kannasyn', 'Kantrex') is also injected i.m. and effective against some Gram-negative bacteraemias (e.g. *Esch. coli*) and in pyelonephritis, but bacterial resistance is widespread unlike gentamicin. The margin of safety between the therapeutic and toxic levels is said to be wider with kanamycin than gentamicin. *Presentation* Kanamycin Injection B.P. is made from vials 1000mg/3ml and 1000mg/4ml as kanamycin base (1 mega unit = 1g) the contents of which are dissolved in Water for Injections. *Dose* adults 1-2g daily in divided amounts to a total of 10g; children are given 10-15mg/kg B.W. daily in divided amounts 12 hourly up to 6 days. 'Kantrex' is also available in 250mg capsules for gut sterilization; *dose* 250-500mg 6 hourly. **Amikacin Sulphate** ('Amikin') is derived from kanamycin and may prove a valuable alternative. *Presentation* ampoules 2ml 50mg/ml and multidose vials 500mg/ml; *dose* 15mg/kg B.W. i.m. or iv. in two divided doses for up to 10 days. The total dose should not exceed 15g. **Netilmicin** is a new derivative of sissomicin.

THE SULPHONAMIDES
Historically the sulphonamides have been in use since before World War II and from them have been developed diuretics, antileprotics, oral hypo-

glycaemics, anticonvulsants as well as more modern varieties of sulphonamides. They act by stopping bacterial, protozoal and certain fungal (nocardiosis) growth by preventing them utilizing para-aminobenzoic acid an essential food. Because the sulphonamides chemically resemble this nutrient many microbes (e.g. streptococci, meningococci, *Esch. coli*) cannot distinguish between them. When taken orally most are well absorbed from the gut. In the blood they are bound to the serum proteins to a varying extent and they are distributed widely through the body including the C.S.F. The liver inactivates sulphonamides by acetylation. This conjugate is excreted in the urine and is less soluble than the free sulphonamide. *Dosage* high initial blood levels are obtained by giving a loading dose usually twice that of the following doses which are given 4-6 hourly.

There are several types.

(1) Well Absorbed and Rapidly Excreted

Sulphadimidine Ph. Eur., B.P. ('Sulphamezathine') and **Sulphadiazine Ph. Eur., B.P.** are effective and relatively safe. Sulphadimidine is soluble in an acid urine and sulphadiazine readily enters the C.S.F. Suphonamides are **never** given intrathecally. *Presentation* Tablets B.P. 500mg, Sulphadimidine Mixture Paediatric B.P.C. 500mg/5ml, Sulphadimidine Sodium Injection B.P. ampoules 1g/3ml which should be protected from the light. *Dose* orally for severe infections is 3g initially then 1-1.5g 4 hourly and parenterally i.v. or i.m. 1-2g is followed when feasible by oral therapy. Sulphadiazine injection is available in 3ml ampoules containing 1g.

Sulphafurazole (Sulfisoxazole U.S.P., 'Gantrisin') *Presentation* Tablets B.P. 500mg, ampoules of sulphafurazole diethanolamine 2g/5ml for injection but not in the U.K., and syrup 500mg/5ml. It is very soluble and achieves good blood and C.S.F. levels. The *oral dose* is 2g then 1g 4-6 hourly. Injections are by deep i.m. or i.v. routes.

Sulphamethizole ('Urolucosil') *presentation* Tablets 100mg B.P., suspension 100mg/5ml. *Dose* 200mg 4-5 times daily.

Sulphamethoxazole B.P. is available as a constituent of co-trimoxazole, since it can be given 12 hourly.

(2) Long-acting Varieties Well Absorbed But Slowly Excreted

Their advantages are claimed to be prolonged blood levels because of slow excretion, largely because they are reabsorbed renally, a low rate of inactivation and good solubility in acid urine with freedom from crystal deposits. Dosage is usually 2 tablets of 500mg then 1 daily. Severe infections require twice this amount. Preparations include **Sulphamethoxypyridazine B.P.** ('Lederkyn'. **Sulphadimethoxine B.P.** ('Madribon'), and **Sulphaphenazole** ('Orisulf'). **Sulfametopyrazine** ('Kelfizine W') is given in one 2g dose which lasts a week. **Sulfadoxine** ('Fanasil') which is used in malaria also lasts week. Their disadvantages are that if side effects occur they are long-lasting and there is an increased risk of Stevens-Johnson syndrome. On the other hand in some parts of the world single dose regimes are an administrative advantage.

(3) Non-Orally Absorbed Sulphonamides

These have been used pre-operatively to reduce the bacteria in the bowel and in the past for bacillary dysentery. They include succinylsulphathiazole Ph. Eur. ('Sulfasuxidine') and sulphaguanidine *dose* 10-20g daily and phthalylsulphathiazole ('Thalazole') *dose* 5-10g daily. There are few uses for these today.

(4) Sulphasalazine

Sulphasalazine ('Salazopyrin', 'Azulfidine' in the U.S.A.) is used widely and is a combination which is broken down by bacteria in the gut to sulphapyridine and a derivative of salicylic acid. *Presentation* tablets 500mg, and enteric coated tablets 500mg ('Salazopyrin EN-Tablets'); *dose* up to 1-2g 4 times daily then after 2-3 weeks a maintenance dose of 2-4 tablets daily. Suppositories 500mg are available and the dose is 1 or 2 morning and night. It is used for ulcerative colitis and Crohn's disease to prevent recurrence of the disease and is prescribed for at least one year. **Sulphapyridine** is an older sulphonamide and is occasionally used to treat dermatitis herpetiformis 3-4g daily.

(5) Topical Preparations

In general these are rarely prescribed since they cause skin hypersensitivity. However they are applied to the conjunctivae as **Sulphacetamide Sodium Ointment B.P.** 10%, Sulphacetamide Eye Drops B.P.C. 30% and as 'Albucid' 2.5 and 6% ointments, cream 10% and eye drops 10, 20 and 30% in 10ml bottles, or as **Mafenide** ('Sulfamylon') which is applied on burns as a 10% cream to prevent *Ps. aeruginosa* infection.

Uses

Urinary infections, if acute and caused by *Esch. coli,* respond well. *Meningitis* (Chapter 16) has been treated with the sulphonamides (e.g. Sulphadiazine), but resistant forms (e.g. meningococci) occur often enough to restrict their use. The same applies to bacillary dysentery which is often best left to clear naturally. Non-absorbed forms are used for bowel preparations pre-operatively. Trachoma, toxoplasmosis, and malaria may be treated either alone, or in conjunction with other drugs. Some venereal diseases such as gonorrhoea, chancroid, and lymphogranuloma respond, but there are better alternatives. The same applies to streptococcal infections (e.g. tonsillitis) and pneumococcal respiratory infections where in the febrile, dehydrated patient penicillin is superior. A rare use is to treat nocardial infection. To prevent rheumatic fever sulphonamides equal oral penicillin V, but are inferior to long-acting i.m. benzathine penicillin. They are also used in prophylaxis in the contacts of sulphonamide sensitive meningococcal meningitis e.g. a 3 day course of sulphadiazine. For resistant cases minocycline or rifampicin is used.

Adverse effects. The modern varieties have little risk of crystalluria and renal damage, but nevertheless it is wise to ensure an adequate fluid intake and urinary output, and at times to make the urine alkaline with sodium bicarbonate. Allergy is not uncommon and includes rashes (erythematous and morbilliform), plus Stevens-Johnson syndrome (erythema multiforme exudativum) and Lyell's syndrome (toxic epidermolysis). Delayed hypersensitivity and auto-immune reactions may possibly cause peri-arteritis nodosa, vasculitis, erythema nodosum, fixed eruptions and photosensitivity which is a hazard of sunny countries. Depression of the marrow and haemolysis in patients with glucose-6-phosphate dehydrogenase red cell enzyme deficiency are further hazards. While in theory sulphonamides might be hazardous in African negroes in practice they are widely used with little harm, but in Britain screening for red-cell enzyme deficiency should be undertaken. Patients with known glucose-6-phosphate dehydrogenase deficiency are not given sulphonamides. Other complications are anorexia, nausea, vomiting, hepatitis, joint pain and mental depression. *Contra-indications* sulphonamides should be avoided late in pregnancy as they displace bound bilirubin from plasma albumin and excessive levels of bilirubin may damage the brain in the newborn (kernicterus). For the same reason they are not advised in the neonate. The risks of reactions are greater in those who metabolize (acetylate) sulphonamides slowly and if there is renal failure. Sulphasalazine is widely used and gastro-intestinal symptoms are not infrequent. Lung damage, rash, agranulocytosis, Heinz bodies (abnormal red cells) and haemolytic anaemias are possibilities to be considered. Sensitivity reactions are also more liable with the long-acting varieties. Nowadays, sulphonamide rashes are a frequent complication again since a sulphonamide is contained in co-trimoxazole and co-trimazine.

CO-TRIMOXAZOLE ('Bactrim', 'Septrin')

This is composed of **Trimethoprim** (an antifolate) and **Sulphamethoxazole.** The two are bactericidal and kill bacteria by interfering with first folate, then purine synthesis. *Presentation* Co-trimoxazole Tablets B.P. 160mg trimethoprim and 800mg sulphamethoxazole, 80mg trimethoprim and 400mg sulphamethoxazole, and 20mg trimethoprim and 100mg sulphamethoxazole (for paediatric use) and Dispersible Tablets B.P. usually containing 80mg trimethoprim and 400mg sulphamethoxazole. A suspension for adults contains in each 5ml 80mg and 400mg respectively and the paediatric mixture B.P.C. in each 5ml 40mg trimethoprim and 200mg sulphamethoxazole. For i.v. infusions Co-Trimoxazole Injection B.P. a 5ml ampoule contains 80mg trimethoprim and 400mg sulphamethoxazole; *dose* 10-15ml twice daily given in 125ml Dextrose Injection B.P. 5%, or Sodium Chloride Injection B.P.; children are given 6mg trimethoprim and 30mg sulphamethoxazole/kg B.W. daily divided into 2 equal doses. For i.m. use a 3ml ampoule contains 160mg trimethoprim and 800mg sulphamethoxazole. *Dose* adult 1-2 tablets twice daily (up to thrice daily in bacteraemia), or the equivalent in suspension. The course should be restricted to 7 days in the elderly, who for dietary reasons, are often folate-depleted. Children under 6 have 2 Paediatric Tablets twice daily and over this age twice the amount, as syrup, or suspension. *Uses* are wide—streptococcal, staphylococcal, and gonococcal infections, respiratory, renal and blood stream infection by *Proteus spp, Esch. coli* and *H. influenzae.* If sulphonamides alone are effective they are very much cheaper than co-trimoxazole. It has been used in typhoid fever and may be of value in diphtheria, toxoplasmosis, nocardiosis, *Pneumocystis carinii,* and malaria. *Adverse effects* nausea, vomiting, fever, those of the sulphonamides, especially rashes (about 6%), thrombocytopenia (especially in the elderly and in long term therapy) and the precipitation of megaloblastic anaemia. The blood effects are due to hypersensitivity to the sulphonamides plus an antifolate action. *Contra-indications* neonates, pregnancy (though not all authorities would agree), sulphonamide intolerance, glucose-6-phosphate-dehydrogenase deficiency, folate deficiency, megaloblastic anaemia and those taking pyrimethamine or phenytoin.

Co-trimazine ('Coptin') is a similar combination but the sulphonamide is sulphadiazine and it is designed for urinary infections only. *Presentation* Tablets trimethoprim 90mg, sulphadiazine 410mg, suspension 45mg and 205mg/5ml respectively. *Dose* one tablet 12-hourly (or equivalent).

NITROFURANS

Like the sulphonamides they are synthetic, chemotherapeutic drugs, but unlike them they are bactericidal.

Nitrofurantoin ('Berkfurin', 'Ceduran', 'Furadantin', 'Furan', 'Macrodantin', 'Urantoin') is taken orally and because of fast excretion needs to be taken 6 hourly. It is a weak acid and the rate of excretion varies with urinary pH. The main use is for *Esch. coli* urinary infection since high urinary levels are obtained, but lesser concentrations are reached in the renal tissues. *Presentation* Tablets B.P. 50 and 100mg, 'Macrodantin' capsules 50 and 100mg the macro crystal formulation slows the absorption of nitrofurantoin and thus aims to reduce the incidence of nausea; Nitrofurantoin Mixture B.P.C. 'Furadantin suspension' 25mg/5ml. *Dose* 50-100mg q.d.s. taken with food, or for small adults 5-8mg/kg B.W. daily (not exceeding 400mg). Children take up to 1 year 1-2ml 6 hourly; 1-5 years 2.5-5ml 6 hourly and 6-12 years 5ml 6 hourly. *Adverse effects* anorexia, nausea, vomiting, diarrhoea, jaundice, haemolytic anaemia, rashes, eosinophilia, anaphylaxis, neuritis and possibly megaloblastic anaemia. An allergic pulmonary syndrome can cause chills, fever, breathlessness, cyanosis, rales, arthralgia and pleural effusions within an hour or so of taking a tablet. The condition mimics left heart-failure and it is not rare. *Contra-indications* renal failure. To prevent recurrent urinary infection 50 or 100mg nightly is helpful prophylactically, or only after intercourse, when this is relevant.

Trimethoprim alone ('Ipral', 'Trimopan') 100mg at night or twice daily can also be used for prophylaxis and 200mg twice daily for therapy of urinary infection.

Furazolidone B.P. ('Furoxone') is used for bowel infections. *Presentation* Tablets 100mg, suspension 100mg/20ml with kaolin and pectin in 300ml bottles. *Dose* 100mg 6 hourly for 5 days or so.

Nifuratel is used for candida and trichomonas infections as well as bacterial urinary infection, but metronizadole is better for trichomonas infection. It causes less sickness than nitrofurantoin. Nifuratel is especially useful in pregnancy bacteriuria when candidosis may follow conventional antibiotics. *Presentation* tablets 200mg, pessaries 250mg. *Dose* orally 400mg 8 hourly for 5-7 days. *Adverse effects* rashes, drowsiness, occasional nausea, flushing with aicohol, allergic pulmonary syndrome. It is unavailable in the U.K.

Metronidazole ('Flagyl') is a heterocylic nitrogen containing compound introduced in 1960 and unusual in that it contains a NO_2 group. Among its many actions it is active against certain anaerobic bacteria. In the anaerobic cell it is reduced to the active form which binds to DNA so stopping nucleic acid synthesis. The drug enters the body fluids including blood, bile, saliva, breast milk, C.S.F. and pus. It is excreted in the urine largely unchanged. The unique selective activity against anaerobic infection without the serious side effects of clindamycin or chloramphenicol is a distinct advantage. It is also used prophylactically just before and during surgery such as appendicectomy, colon resection and hysterectomy. *Presentation* and *dose* Tablets B.P. 200-400mg 8h, suppositories 0.5 and 1g which are inserted rectally 8-hourly. For i.v. use a 0.5% w/v (500mg) in 100ml 0.9% sodium chloride is infused protected from light over a 20 min period. *Adverse effects* nausea, neutropenia, antabuse effect, interaction with warfarin. If given for long-term use in high dosage peripheral neuropathy can occur which is not always reversible.

4 DRUGS USED MAINLY FOR MYCOBACTERIA

TUBERCULOSIS

Tuberculosis kills several million (about 5) people yearly in the world and 30 million are infected. In Britain more die from it than from any other notifiable disease and more beds are devoted to its cure than all other notifiable diseases. Recently notifications in parts of Britain have increased partly because of immigration.

Streptomycin destroys tubercle bacilli and bacteria causing pneumonia and endocarditis (often given with penicillin), urinary infection, tularaemia, brucellosis (with tetracycline) and plague. However, bacteria quickly become resistant. It is a water-soluble powder which when dissolved keeps for several weeks in a refrigerator. As it is not absorbed from the gut, it is usually given i.m. It diffuses through the body and into the pleural and pericardial cavities, but poorly into the C.S.F. Excretion is by the kidneys. *Presentation* **Streptomycin Sulphate Ph. Eur., B.P.** vials 1g of white sterile powder to be reconstituted in Water for Injections, ampoules 100mg for intrathecal use and containing no stabilizing material or preservative to be freshly prepared dissolved in 10ml of Sodium Chloride Injection. *Dose* for non-tuberculous infections i.m. 500mg-1g b.d. for 5 days if good renal function. In urinary infections the results are better if the urine is made alkaline. *Oral dose* for intestinal infections is 250mg 4 or 6 hourly.

Uses of Antituberculosis Drugs

(1) Treatment of medical forms of tuberculosis e.g. pulmonary and conversion to a sputum negative state.

(2) Surgical tuberculosis can be operated on more safely e.g. lung, kidney, bone, lymph nodes.

(3) Cure of tuberculous meningitis and miliary tubercle, previously fatal.

Mild cases can be treated at home or even at work. Good food is desirable, but even the malnourished can get well if they take their medication regularly. There are problems of treatment in many developing countries and these include patient acceptability of drugs, adverse effects (common among Asians), varying responses of races to treatment, the logistics of mass administration, and daily, or once or twice weekly attendance at clinics, and finally the cost. Streptomycin injections are difficult in rural areas, para-aminosalicylic acid is given in large tablets and causes gastro-intestinal upsets which lead to patient-default, isoniazid is metabolized quickly or slowly in different races, and thiacetazone is cheap but toxic. Many antituberculosis drugs can damage the liver or the brain. Other adverse factors are poor diet, alcoholism, narcotic intake, low intelligence and non-cooperation.

When infants are exposed to open tuberculosis they may be given isoniazid prophylactically. For tuberculosis the *dose* of streptomycin for normal sized adults is 1g daily under *40 years of age,* providing there is no renal or eighth nerve disease; 750mg daily 40-60 years and over 60 years 500mg daily, or 1g thrice weekly. A total course is 80-100g. The control of dosage by blood levels is valuable in the elderly, and essential in renal disease, but it may be better to give a safer alternative such as rifampicin or ethambutol. The dose of streptomycin for children is 30mg/kg B.W. up to 1g daily. For intrathecal therapy the dose is 25mg for infants, 50-70mg for children and up to 100mg in adults. *Adverse effects* are likely in the elderly, in the presence of renal disease, with doses above 1g daily, and if the drug is used for lengthy periods. Toxicity affects the eighth nerve e.g. cochlea and labyrinth causing dizziness, giddiness, deafness, and tinnitus. Other ill-effects are generalized hypersensitivity (see later), nausea, blurred vision, facial tingling, flushing and anaphylactic shock. Nurses, and others, handling streptomycin can become sensitive to it, especially if they do not wear gloves, or if they spray the solution into the air instead of re-injecting bubbles and froth back into the vial. Skin and eye-lid irritation are the usual form of contact hypersensitivity. If a nurse who must handle streptomycin becomes sensitized to it then desensitization with minute doses can be tried.

Types of Antituberculosis Drugs

Para-aminosalicylic Acid (PAS) or **Sodium Aminosalicylate Ph. Eur.** is a weak, but until recently widely used agent, one of the first to be used in the treatment of tuberculosis. Taken orally it diffuses throughout the body, but not into the C.S.F. and is excreted renally most in the acetylated form, Dose and administration; *oral* 10-20g daily in divided doses, an average is 12g; children 300mg/kg. PAS is unpleasant to take and few preparations exist of PAS by itself in the U.K. One is a powder ('Paramisan Powder') available in 100g quantities. Patients often neglect to take PAS and urine tests with ferric chloride will detect defaulters. *Adverse effects* are many and varied. Gastrointestinal effects are anorexia, nausea, vomiting, indigestion, flatulence, abdominal pain and diarrhoea in half the patients. Digestive symptoms may improve by changing the brand or preparation, taking it with meals, or antacids and sometimes, by mere persistence tolerance occurs. Malabsorption of vitamin B_{12} and folates (and isoniazid and rifampicin) can occur and megaloblastic or haemolytic anaemia, as well as thrombocytopenia, leucopenia, lymphadenopathy, splenomegaly, liver damage, jaundice and hepatitis alone or part of a generalized sensitivity reaction. Fluid retention may provoke heart failure with sodium PAS and fever and itching may be a problem as may rashes (erythema, macular, papular, urticarial, exfoliative, erythema multiforme) and mucocutaneous and ocular syndromes. Other features are pulmonary eosinophilia, psychosis, allergic encephalitis, goitre, hypothyroidism, and hypokalaemia.

Isoniazid Ph. Eur. (INAH, 'Nydrazid', 'Rimifon') is chemically a hydrazine (like most monoamine oxidase inhibitors) and gets inside the cells where the tubercle bacilli are difficult to kill with other drugs. It is well absorbed, diffuses widely including into the C.S.F. and is ideal in that it is cheap and comparatively safe. *Presentation* Tablets B.P. 50 and 100mg, Injection B.P.C. ampoules 2ml 25mg/ml. *Dose* orally 200-400mg daily in divided amounts, children 5-10mg/kg B.W.; by injection 100-200mg 6 hourly. In miliary tuberculosis 10-15mg/kg B.W. can be given initially. Isoniazid is used by itself prophylactically when corticosteroids or cytotoxic drugs are given to patients with healed tuberculosis and after adverse reactions to B.C.G. Chemoprophylaxis is also given to Asian immigrants who have strongly positive Mantoux reactions. *Adverse effects* are uncommon. They include allergies, rashes (urticaria, angioneurotic oedema, eczema, erythema purpura), fever, lymphadenopathy, occasionally hepatitis (commoner in fast acetylators), which can be fatal and blood dyscrasias sideroblastic anaemia, eosinophilia, thrombocytopenia; neurotoxicity which occurs either in a dose above 5mg/kg B.W. in slow inactivators, or with large doses, e.g. psychosis, convulsions (pyridoxine deficiency and also by a hydrazine effect), polyneuritis (especially in alcoholics, diabetics and slow inactivators); pellagra-like pigmentation with mental changes, glycosuria, hyperglycaemia, galactorrhoea, lupus erythematosus and rheumatic pain in hands, shoulders and other joints. *Drug inter-reactions* isoniazid given with phenytoin causes toxic levels of the latter by reducing its metabolic breakdown. Cycloserine, PAS and chlorpromazine prolong the action of isoniazid.

It is convenient to combine PAS and INAH for out-patients. Official forms exist as powder or granules. 'Inapasade' is a proprietary form available in the U.K. in two strengths. Each packet contains (for adults) sodium aminosalicylate 6g and isoniazid 150mg and two are taken daily. The paediatric strength is 2g and 50mg respectively.

Rifampicin B.P. ('Rifadin', 'Rimactane') is an expensive semi-synthetic, potent drug which has no cross-resistance. Excretion is mainly in the bile. It has also been used in prophylaxis given to contacts of sulphonamide-resistant meningococcal meningitis, or carriers, and in the treatment of leprosy. Injectable forms have been given for staphylococcal infection. *Presentation* capsules 150 and 300mg, syrup 100mg/5ml; *dose* orally 450-600mg or 8-12mg/kg B.W. once daily 30 minutes before breakfast, children 10-20mg/kg B.W. *Adverse effects* flu syndrome with intermittent therapy, nausea, neutropenia, eosinophilia, abnormal liver function, jaundice, haemolysis, hepatitis, purpura from thrombocytopenia and, rarely, acute renal failure. Jaundice is common in alcoholics and also when high doses of rifampicin with isoniazid are taken intermittently. 'Rimactazid' and 'Rifinah' are a combination in two strengths; 150mg rifampicin with 100mg isoniazid and 300mg rifampicin with 150mg isoniazid. Two tablets of 'Rifinah 300' or 'Rimactazid 300' are taken before breakfast or 3 tablets of 'Rifinah 150' or 'Rimactazid 150' for patients under 50kg. Rifampicin reduces the efficiency of the oral contraceptives. *Contraindications* pregnancy, jaundice. Rifampicin imparts an orange-red colour to the urine (and tears) which can be used as a guide to drug compliance.

Ethambutol Hydrochloride ('Myambutol') also has powerful anti-tuberculous activity without cross-resistance. *Presentation* Tablets B.P. 100 and 400mg; *dose* orally daily 15mg/kg B.W. in one dose. For retreated cases 25mg/kg B.W. is given for 60 days then 15mg/kg B.W. *Adverse effects* paraesthesiae, optic neuritis and sudden visual loss, disturbance of colour vision, or decrease in visual fields. Symptoms improve when the drug is stopped. Ophthalmic checks may be made before and during treatment but in practice it is sufficient if patients are warned to stop therapy if they have eye symptoms. Allergy and liver disease are rare. Ethambutol is combined with isoniazid in varying combinations 200, 250, 300 or 350mg with 100mg of INAH in the 'Mynah' preparations.

Combination Therapy

Initially in all but the mildest cases, triple therapy is recommended. This conventially is streptomycin, isoniazid with a third drug given for 18 months. This used always to be PAS, but because of its defects ethambutol or rifampicin is being used in spite of its cost. In addition ethambutol, isoniazid and rifampicin (an all-oral triple regime) is being increasingly accepted and the treatment course is 9 months. Changes may have to be made when bacteriological guidance is at hand. With sensitive bacilli and the correct regime most patients can be cured clinically. For continuation therapy, isoniazid with either PAS, ethambutol or rifampicin is orthodox. Triple therapy increases the chances of adverse effects. About 10% of patients are hypersensitive to PAS or streptomycin. This sensitization comes on 2-5 weeks after starting treatment and can be fatal, or unpleasant with fever, rashes, hepatitis, brain damage, or anaphylactic shock.

In underdeveloped countries after 3 months triple therapy for pulmonary tuberculosis intermittent supervised chemotherapy can be given in a clinic, hospital, at work, or at home. This consists of twice weekly streptomycin 1g with isoniazid 15mg/kg B.W. and pyridoxine 10mg. Tuberculosis of the spine has been successfully treated by chemotherapy alone, unless complicated by paraplegia, on an ambulant basis. Isoniazid 10mg/kg B.W. daily and PAS 200mg/kg B.W. daily have been given for 18 months. The initial triple therapy has been discarded, unless the patient previously had inadequate chemotherapy or unless initial resistance to the two-drug regime is known to be common in the particular country. When high doses of isoniazid are given weekly results are not so good in those who metabolize the drug quickly.

In Britain (and increasingly abroad) isoniazid and rifampicin together have proved acceptable and easy to take; the period spent in hospital and the time taken to cure the tuberculosis are reduced. The shorter course of treatment and early return to work offset the cost of the combination.

Reserve Drugs (Second or third choice drugs)
These are given when tubercle bacilli are resistant to the more usual therapy, or when toxicity or allergy prevent their use.
Pyrazinamide ('Zinamide') *presentation* Tablets B.P. 500mg; *dose* orally 25-35mg/kg B.W. daily in 3 or 4 equally divided amounts up to 3g. It is used for short term protection, e.g. to cover chest surgery, or for longer periods with isoniazid, rifampicin or ethambutol as primary therapy. Pyrazinamide is a sterilizing anti-tuberculosis agent and is finding increasing use as part of combination therapy. *Adverse effects* 5-10% have evidence of biochemical liver damage; less frequently hepatitis and necrosis, photosensitivity, nausea, vomiting, anorexia, fever, dysuria and gout (because of decreased urate excretion) are observed.
Ethionamide ('Trescatyl') resembles isoniazid in potency. *Presentation* Tablets B.P. 125mg; *dose* 500-1000mg daily. *Adverse effects* drug fever, allergic hepatitis; skin (acne, alopecia, purpura, pigmentation, erythema), gastrointestinal (metallic taste, vomiting, abdominal pain, diarrhoea, jaundice, rise in serum transaminₐses), neuro-psychiatric (headache, drowsiness, insomnia, depression, mania, psychosis, paraesthesiae, peripheral neuropathy, giddiness, increased glare, dreams, optic neuritis, photophobia), hypoglycaemia and electrolyte disturbances. It is better tolerated when taken at night.
Prothionamide ('Trevintix') *presentation* Tablets B.P.C. 125mg; *dose* 500mg-1g daily in one or two doses orally. The preparation is similar to ethionamide, but slightly better tolerated.
Viomycin Sulphate is a weak antituberculous agent now withdrawn.

Cycloserine ('Seromycin' U.S.A.) has a weak action. *Presentation* Tablets B.P. 250mg, Capsules B.P. 125 and 250mg; *dose* 250mg once or twice daily increasing by 250mg every 4-7 days until a maximum of 1g daily. *Adverse effects* neurological ones are common—headache, hyper-reflexia, spastic paralysis, tremors, twitching, dyskinesia, psychomotor stimulation, convulsions, coma, psychosis (depression, drowsiness, confusion, mania, aggression), optic neuritis. *Contra-indications* renal failure, epilepsy, mental instability.

Thiacetazone (thiosemicarbazone) is a useful alternative to PAS. It is no longer available in Britain, but is in other parts of the world e.g. S. America and S. Africa. *Presentation* Tablets B.P.C. 25, 50 and 75mg; *dose* 75mg b.d. Thiacetazone can be combined with isoniazid in a single tablet for adults 150mg thiacetazone and 300mg isoniazid, or as the smaller content of 50mg thiacetazone and 100mg isoniazid ('Thiazina'). This combination is popular in developing countries, since it is cheap, easy to swallow, convenient and keeps well. *Adverse effects* are common and often serious e.g. hypersensitivity, hepatitis, glycosuria, exfoliative dermatitis, Stevens-Johnson syndrome, haemolytic anaemia, agranulocytosis, purpura, nephritis and brain damage.

Capreomycin Sulphate ('Capastat') *presentation* Vials Injection B.P. 1g as a base (equivalent to 1 mega unit) is dissolved in 2ml of Water for Injections. *Dose* 1g i.m. daily. Its antituberculous action is like streptomycin, as are the adverse effects. It is a valuable alternative to it and, similarly, must not be given alone.

Corticosteroids are only used in a few patients, desperately ill with pulmonary or meningeal tuberculosis, when they may be life-saving. They decrease fever and improve the appetite. They must be given with full effective antituberculous therapy. Corticosteroids are also used to suppress hypersensitivity drug reactions and to aid drug desensitization.

In tuberculous meningitis it is helpful to know that pyrazinamide, cycloserine, isoniazid and rifampicin can cross the C.S.F. blood-brain barrier and in coma streptomycin, isoniazid and rifampicin are injectable.

Anonymous Mycobacteria

These organisms may respond to ethambutol, rifampicin, capreomycin or cycloserine but careful testing of drug sensitivity is necessary.

LEPROSY ('HANSEN'S DISEASE')

This disease, which is due to *Mycobacterium leprae,* occurs in millions of people in the tropics and sub-tropics; even in Europe there are sufferers. In Britain expert advice should be sought on treatment. Some protection may be obtained from BCG. Treatment needs judgement, for it may be unwise to give antileprotics in the acute febrile stage. Drugs are always given carefully with gentle increase in dosage.

Sulphones, sulphonamide derivatives, are inexpensive, relatively safe and the mainstay of treatment. They are bacteriostatic and slow to act.

Dapsone ('Avlosulfon') *presentation* Tablets B.P. 50 and 100mg; arachis oil suspension 200mg/ml for i.m. use. *Dose* several schemes are in use. One starts at 5mg daily and slowly increases to 25mg daily. Another consists of 25mg weekly orally, or i.m. for a month, then 50mg weekly for a month with increments of 50mg monthly to a dose of 100-300mg weekly, or divided twice weekly (i.e. 100mg twice weekly), for at least a year. Life-long treatment is given for lepromatous leprosy, often in a smaller dose e.g. 25mg weekly. Children aged 0-6 years have a quarter, and 6-12 years have half adult doses. Problems in its use include dapsone resistance in lepromatous leprosy, and the persistence of drug-sensitive leprosy bacilli in small numbers in spite of years of treatment. 'Avlosulfon Soluble' is water soluble and is equivalent to 200mg/ml of dapsone.

A long-acting form of dapsone called **Acedapsone** in a benzyl-benzoate castor oil suspension 225mg/1.5ml has been given every 77 days to people at high risk of leprosy. It is slowly released from the tissues at a steady rate of 2.4mg daily. No refrigeration is needed and it is cheap. *Adverse effects* exfoliative dermatitis, toxic epidermal necrolysis, erythema, fever; methaemoglobinaemia, Heinz bodies which result from haemolysis and are dose related (people with glucose-6-phosphate dehydrogenase deficient red cells are more sensitive to haemolysis), agranulocytosis, lymphadenopathy, hepatitis, neuropathy, depression and psychosis. (Reactions are more likely in the larger doses used for dermatitis herpetiformis, a non-tropical skin complaint.) A major problem is the emergence of dapsone resistant mycobacteria.

Thiourea compounds or thiosemicarbazones are used when resistance develops to the sulphones or if intolerance occurs.

Thiambutosine ('Ciba 1906')*presentation* Tablets B.P. 500mg; *dose* orally 250 or 500mg daily for 2 weeks increased by 500mg every 2 weeks up to 2-3g or 25-40mg/kg B.W. daily. Although it is quick acting, resistance is likely in 2-3 years. It is less toxic than dapsone. **Thiacetazone** (p. 31) has also been used.

Clofazimine ('Lamprene') is a substituted iminophenazine red dye which suppresses (unlike dapsone) the inflammatory 'lepra reaction' and can be taken alone. *Presentation* capsules 100mg; *dose* 300-600mg weekly, but for lepra reactions up to 600mg daily may be needed. *Adverse effects* gastro-intestinal upsets, pink skin, darkening of leprosy lesions.

Long-acting sulphonamides 500mg twice weekly have been used, but are expensive and the same applies to **Rifampicin** which is rapidly bactericidal in a dose of 600mg daily for several weeks along with dapsone. It can render the patient non-infective within 2-3 weeks.

Reactions such as erythema nodosum, iritis, and neuritis provoked by antileprotics may be controlled if severe by **Corticosteroids**. Thalidomide, if available, can quickly control acute exacerbations of lepromatous leprosy in adult males and females not in the childbearing age at a dose of 400mg daily (Browne, S. G., *Practitioner* **215**, 493, 1975). Clofazimine and apparently i.m. stibophen or i.v. antimony potassium tartrate can also be helpful.

Combined Therapy
In the lepromatous (multibacillary) form rifampicin 600mg daily for 4 weeks, clofazimine 100mg thrice weekly for one year and dapsone 50-100mg daily for life are given. The triple therapy helps to lessen the chances of dapsone resistance. In the paucibacillary form dapsone 25-50mg is given for 3-5 years.

Certain non-mycobacterial infections are of world wide (including tropical) importance namely cholera (p. 178), brucellosis (p. 27), gonorrhoea (p. 35) and the treponematoses (p. 36) and rickettsiae and chlamydiae (Chapter 5).

5 SPECIAL USES FOR CHEMOTHERAPY

ANTIRICKETTSIAL
Rickettsiae are half-way in size between bacteria and viruses and cause epidemic scrub and tick typhus and Q fever. Acute infections respond to tetracycline or chloramphenicol.

ANTIMYCOPLASMA
These organisms have no cell wall and are unaffected by the beta-lactam antibiotics, but are destroyed by tetracyclines or erythromycin.

ANTIVIRAL
The larger viruses now known as chlamydiae such as those causing ornithosis (psittacosis) and lymphogranuloma venereum resemble rickettsiae and respond to the same antibiotics. Other than the prophylactic injection of immuno-globulins (p. 60) there is no effective remedy against the small true viruses causing chicken pox, measles, mumps, poliomyelitis, hepatitis A or B, rubella or influenza, once the disease is apparent.

Methisazone ('Marboran') was used to prevent contacts and suspects from getting smallpox. With the eradication of smallpox it is obsolete. If smallpox is caught from laboratory stored virus, vaccination of primary contacts and potent immunoglobulins are better. Methisazone has no effect on established disease. Other uses have included the treatment of eczema vaccinatum and vaccinia gangrenosum. *Presentation* Methisazone Mixture B.P. is available in sachets containing 15ml suspension or mixture and equal to 3g of methisazone; *dose* in adults is 3g b.d. *Adverse effects* usually nausea and vomiting; as it is a semicarbazone it can cause allergic, marrow and neurological complications. **Idoxuridine B.P.** ('Dendrid', 'Herpid', 'Kerecid') is a halogenated (iodine) nucleoside an analogue of thymidine which inhibits DNA viruses and is poorly soluble. 'Dendrid' and 'Kerecid' are 0.1% solutions used for herpes virus corneal erosions; solutions are also painted on the skin in herpes simplex lesions. For the skin the special solvent used is Dimethyl Sulphoxide B.P. which itself is bacteriostatic and penetrates the skin taking the idoxuridine with it. 'Herpid' is a 5% solution which is brushed on the skin (avoiding the eyes) in herpes zoster for 4 days. Those experienced in this treatment recommend 35 or 40% idoxuridine in dimethyl sulphoxide and that the whole of the dermatome and not just the visible vesicles is treated by frequent (2 hourly) applications (very costly). Ophthalmic ointments 0.5% ('Kerecid', 'Ophthalmadine') are also available and vidarabine ('Vira-A') ointment 3%. For the serious herpes simplex encephalitis systemic idoxuridine has been advocated 100-200mg/kg B.W. given over 2-3 hours i.v. of a 0.5% solution daily for 5 days. It is toxic and difficult to prepare and **cytarabine** or the less toxic **vidarabine** is preferred.

Amantadine Hydrochloride ('Symmetrel') has been used to prevent A2 influenza and modify its course, and also is claimed to help herpes zoster. *Presentation* capsules 100mg, syrup 50mg/5ml in 150ml bottles; *dose* 100mg twice daily up to 7 days for influenza and 14-28 days for herpes zoster. Creuztfeldt-Jakob disease, a possible slow virus infection, may be helped by amantadine.

ANTIFUNGAL

Fungi are of plant origin and physiologically are more complicated than either viruses or bacteria. They may cause topical infection e.g. of the skin, infect the subcutaneous tissues, or produce a serious systemic infection (e.g. candidosis of the heart or brain, or infection by *Cryptococcus neoformans*, histoplasmosis, coccidioidomycosis, blastomycosis, spirotrichosis and *Aspergillus fumigatus*). For topical infections nystatin, candicin, amphotericin, griseofulvin, or tolnaftate ('Tinaderm') are used. Agents used have the ability to selectively destroy fungi since they have a different biochemical system from mammalian cells.

Griseofulvin Ph. Eur. ('Fulcin', 'Grisovin') was originally used for plant diseases and was later shown to be of value when given systemically to humans. When taken orally it is selectively incorporated into newly built keratin of the skin, nails, feet and hair where it kills the fungi. *Uses* tinea capitis, tinea of the hands, nails and feet and some body ringworms. It is not used if simple topical applications such as Whitfield's ointment will suffice. *Presentation* fine-particle Tablets B.P. 125 and 500mg griseofulvin ('Fulcin') suspension 25mg/ml for children; *dose* 1g daily or 10mg/kg B.W. for 3-6 weeks. Absorption is helped by fatty foods. *Adverse effects* gastro-intestinal upsets, headache, urticaria, allergic reactions (particularly in patients allergic to penicillin), gynaecomastia in children.

Polyenes, a subdivision of the macrolides, are a large group of crystalline antibiotics containing a series of conjugated double bonds comprising nystatin (a complex of dienes and tetraenes), natamycin (a tetraene) and amphotericin, candidicin, hamycin and trichomycin (all heptaenes). They bind to the sterols (e.g. ergosterol) and proteins of the fungus wall affecting membrane permeability.

Nystatin ('Mycostatin' U.S.A., 'Nystan',) is used for monilial (thrush or *Candida albicans*) infections. Candidosis follows prolonged use of antibiotics, especially the tetracyclines, altering the body ecosystem (balance of bacteria), cytotoxics (Chapter 9), corticosteroids and the oral contraceptives. Candida also attacks those weakened by tuberculosis, diabetes, leukaemia, cancer, pregnancy or prematurity. Nystatin is used for candida infections of the mouth, skin, vagina and gut but has to be administered in such a way that it will contact the infecting fungus. It is not absorbed from the bowel and is not used systemically. *Presentation* Tablets B.P. 500 000u; *dose* orally 0.5-1 mega units q.d.s. Local preparations; cream, ointment, gel, dusting powder all 100 000u/g usually in 15 or 30g packs, bottles or tubes, and oral suspension 100 000u/ml bottles 30ml; *dose* 1-5ml q.d.s.; vaginal pessaries B.P.C. 1g 100 000u/g and 'Nystavescent' a foaming, quickly-dispersible formulation. There is also a sterile powder 500 000u per vial and a non-sterile powder 3 million units per vial for inhalation.

Candicidin B.P. ('Candeptin') is used as 1g pessaries containing 3mg candidicin B.P.C., or as an ointment 0.6mg/g (0.06%) in 75g tubes for insertion in the vagina twice daily for candida vaginitis.

Amphotericin ('Fungizone') is valuable for many of the systemic yeast and fungus infections (e.g. *Candida tropicalis, Histoplasma capsulatum, Blastomyces dermatitidis, Cryptococcus neoformans*) unless renal failure is present. *Presentation* vials 50mg/20ml (50 000u) for i.v. use. It is crystalline and by itself insoluble in water, but the addition of sodium desoxycholate in the powder converts it into a colloidal solution with Water for Injections. *Dose* i.v. is initially 0.25 mg (250µg)/kg B.W. given in Dextrose Injection B.P. 5%, in a concentration of 100µg/ml over a period of 6 hours daily, increasing if no toxic symptoms up to 1mg/kg B.W. (usually 50-100mg) for several months daily, or every other day. *Adverse reactions* phlebitis, hypokalaemia (so potassium is given concurrently), renal damage, fever. Blood levels can be monitored. Amphotericin can also be given i.m. and intrathecally. *Topical* amphotericin can be used for fungal infections e.g. *Candida granulosa* and has no ill effects by this route. *Presentation* 'Fungilin' ointment 30mg/g in 'Plastibase' and cream 30mg/g(3%) both in tubes of 15g, lotion 30mg/ml in bottles 15ml, 'Fungilin' in 'Orabase' 30mg/g tubes of 10g. Amphotericin ('Fungilin') suspension 100mg/ml 12ml bottles, Amphotericin Lozenges B.P.C. 10mg; tablets 100mg are used for oral and intestinal candidosis and are more palatable than nystatin. *Pessaries* 50mg and a (vaginal) cream 100mg/4g in 60g tubes are used for vaginal thrush.

Natamycin ('Pimaricin', 'Pimafucin') *presentation* vials 20mg, suspension 25mg/ml is used for aerosol inhalation therapy of candida and *Aspergillus spp.* infections; a cream 20mg/g(2%) in 25g tubes is used for candidosis of the skin and orifices and pessaries 25mg for trichomonal and candida vaginal infections. **Sulphonamides** are used against nocardiosis.

Imidazole Derivatives

Clotrimazole ('Canesten') is a broad spectrum antifungal (dermatophytes), anticandida and antitrichomonal agent. *Presentation* vaginal tablets (pessaries) 100mg, cream 1% and spray 1%. The cream is applied once or twice daily for at least a month, the tablets for 6 consecutive days. It has been used in hospital trials orally 60-100mg/kg B.W. for mucocutaneous candidosis. *Adverse effects* of oral therapy are nausea, vomiting, and mental disturbance.
Miconazole Nitrate B.P. ('Daktarin', 'Dermonistat') is an antifungal agent which inhibits cell wall synthesis and is used for skin, nails and vaginal infection as a 2% cream in a water-miscible base. Oral and i.v. forms are available for infections such as *Cryptococcus neoformans*. **Econazole Nitrate** ('Ecostatin', 'Gyno-Pevaryl') is used as a 1% cream or lotion, or 150mg pessaries for antifungal use.

Flucytosine ('Alcobon') acts on the fungal cell membrane and also inhibits protein synthesis. It has been employed when amphotericin cannot be used against *C. neoformans, C. albicans, Torulopsis glabrata* and may be effective for life-threatening systemic infections. *Presentation* tablets 500mg; *dose* 100-200mg/kg B.W. in 4 divided amounts. An infusion for i.v. use is available. *Adverse effects* liver and marrow toxicity.

SEXUALLY TRANSMITTED DISEASES
Gonorrhoea
Single dose regimes are preferred since patients default. However, strains vary in sensitivity to penicillin G. The *dose* is 2.4-4.8 mega units, or even up to 8 mega units of aqueous procaine penicillin i.m. (larger doses are often needed in women) and failure rates are reduced if oral probenecid 500mg is given 6 hourly for 4 doses to ensure high and prolonged blood levels. For women and homosexuals who have rectal gonorrhoea, 3 daily injections of 2.4 mega units are advised. Procaine penicillin may be fortified by adding crystalline penicillin G. An alternative is **Amoxycillin** 2g followed by another 1-2g dose 5-6 hours later. Because of increasing resistance, or allergy to penicillins, alternatives are

needed. They include tetracycline 1.5g stat then 500mg 6 hourly for 16 doses a regime which needs full patient-cooperation, spiramycin 2.5g, kanamycin 2g i.m. as a single dose, or **Spectinomycin Hydrochloride Pentahydrate** ('Trobi- cin') *presentation* 2g freeze-dried powder in a vial with diluent in an ampoule. When made up each vial provides 5ml of solution equivalent to 400mg spec- tinomycin/ml. It acts by inhibiting bacterial protein synthesis and is excreted in the urine in the active form within 24 hours. Chemically it is an aminocyclitol antibiotic related to the aminoglycosides. *Dose* 2-4g i.m. divided into 2 areas for the female buttock (the capacity of which determines the upper limits of individual injections). *Combination therapy* kanamycin with sulphonamides, co-trimoxazole, as well as cephaloridine 2g daily for 2 consecutive days i.m. have been tried.

Syphilis
Primary, or secondary forms, respond to 600 000u i.m. of procaine penicillin daily for 10 days, or if defaulting seems likely 2.4 mega units of benzathine penicillin i.m. can be given at 2 different sites. For those with neurosyphilis, or cardiovascular syphilis, larger doses and longer courses may be needed and this may also be the case in pregnancy. To prevent the Herxheimer reaction in cardiovascular syphilis prednisone should be given 1 day before and concur- rently. In penicillin allergy cephaloridine 500-2000mg daily is suitable (par- ticularly in pregnancy) otherwise, tetracycline 500mg q.d.s. for 2 weeks, or erythromycin in similar amounts for 3 weeks can be given—although for terti- ary syphilis several courses may be needed.

Chancroid or soft sore is treated by sulphonamides e.g. sulphafurazole 4g daily, tetracycline, or streptomycin, or by combinations and **lymphogranuloma venereum** and **granuloma inguinale** by the tetracyclines. **Non-specific urethritis** is treated with fair results by tetracycline 500mg 6h for 10-21 days and genital herpes simplex by 5-40% idoxuridine in dimethyl sulphoxide topically.

Trichomonas infections of the urethra, seminal vesicles, vagina, and cervix are sexually transmitted and are treated by one of the **nitro-imidazoles**.
Metronidazole ('Flagyl') *presentation* Tablets B.P. 200 and 400mg; *dose* 200mg t.d.s. orally for 7 days, or 800mg in the morning and 1200mg at night for 2 days. Both partners are treated. There is a 98% cure rate; the non- responders are either defaulters, or poor absorbers. **Nimorazole** ('Naxogin') is preferred by some. *Presentation* tablets 250 and 500mg; *dose* 250mg after breakfast and after dinner, for 6 consecutive days orally, or 1g stat, 1g later the same day and 1g the next day to reduce defaulting. **Tinidazole** ('Fasigyn') is a more recent member said to be better tolerated and cause less nausea (as in treating *Giardia lamblia*). *Presentation* tablets 150mg; *dose* orally 2g single dose, or 150mg b.d. for 7 days. Similar compounds are moxnidazole and ornidazole. The nitro-imidazoles are also used for amoebiasis, leishmaniasis, ulcerative gingivitis, anaerobic bacteroides infection and giardiasis. *Adverse effects* metallic taste, nausea, vomiting, vertigo, fatigue, hypotension, neuropathy, and antabuse effect. They are not advised in pregnancy (espe- cially the first 3 months, although ill effects have not been reported) nor with neurological disease or alcohol. Vaginitis caused by *Trichomonas vaginalis* can be treated by pessaries e.g. Acetarsol and Di-iodohydroxyquinoline ('Flora- quin') both B.P.C.

EAR, NOSE AND THROAT INFECTIONS

Acute streptococcal tonsillitis, quinsy, otitis media and suppurative sinusitis respond to benzylpenicillin, but the route is important. Viral and *Str. pyogenes* throat infections may be clinically indistinguishable and unless a throat swab is taken a 10 day course of penicillin is advised. While penicillin V 500mg can be taken orally 4-6 hourly, initially, penicillin G injections 600mg b.d. i.m. are better, since oral forms may be unpredictably absorbed. Few children, mothers or doctors will in practice persist in a 10 day course, even though it is the best way to prevent post-streptococcal rheumatic fever. Antibiotics allow greater safety in ear operations, but their indiscriminate use may mask underlying surgical disease such as chronic mastoiditis and enlarged adenoids. Otitis externa is difficult to treat; bacitracin, polymyxin and neomycin help, preferably as a powder and sometimes with local corticosteroids. There is a possibility that certain ear drops when there are large perforations may cause deafness e.g. chloramphenicol, neomycin and gentamicin. Their use is not advised.

EYE INFECTIONS

Methods of applying antibiotics. *Drops* act quickly and penetrate well. Since certain antibiotics decompose in aqueous solution drops should be freshly made and used quickly. Most drops are given hourly except bacitracin, chloramphenicol, framycetin, polymyxin, sulphacetamide and streptomycin which last longer. *Ointments* maintain the stability of the contained antibiotic providing they are water-free. They have a more prolonged action than drops and they do not get into the punctum in the concentrations that drops do. Hence with atropine and adrenaline systemic effects are less, but sensitization can occur to the incorporated bases. Chloramphenicol is one of the best as it is water and lipid soluble. Chloramphenicol Eye Ointment B.P.C. 1%, Chlortetracycline Eye Ointment B.P.C., framycetin 0.5%, and Sulphacetamide Eye Ointment B.P. 2.5, 6, and 10% are examples. *Subconjunctival* injections are useful for highly soluble and diffusible antibiotics. In eyelid infections (blepharitis) relief is obtained from antibiotic-corticosteroid combinations such as neomycin or framycetin with hydrocortisone, prednisolone or dexamethasone. Mild bacterial conjunctivitis responds to sulphacetamide, antiseptic lotions or drops containing zinc, silver, or mercury compounds. Metallic salts find little use and prolonged application leads to scarring and entropion. Severe conjunctivitis needs topical chloramphenicol, tetracycline or penicillin (gonococcal conjunctivitis still occurs). Trachoma, a tropical eye infection (chlamydiae) causing more blindness than any other disease, is treated by oxytetracycline, chloramphenicol or sulphonamides, both locally and systemically.

SKIN INFECTIONS

A major disadvantage of drugs on the skin is that they can irritate, in particular sulphonamides, penicillin, streptomycin and neomycin.**The ideal topical antibiotic** should (1) *not irritate* the skin, (2) *be active* against both Gram-positive and negative organisms (e.g. staphylococcus, streptococcus) and (3) *only be used on the skin* and not systemically. In practice antibiotics used include bacitracin, framycetin, sodium fusidate (even though it is best reserved for serious systemic infections), gramicidin, neomycin and tyrothricin for stapnylococcal and streptococcal infections. Tetracycline 3% and Chlortetracycline Ointment B.P.C. 3% are valuable since topical sensitization is not a problem. Polymyxins and gentamicin are used for *Ps. aeruginosa* infections. *Combinations are popular* e.g. polymyxin and bacitracin ('Polyfax'), neomycin and bacitracin ('Cicatrin', 'Neobacrin'), neomycin, bacitracin and polymyxin B ('Polybactrin Aerosol') and gramicidin 0.025% and neomycin 0.25% ('Graneodin') in 15 and 200g tubes. Sometimes corticosteroids are added. *Impetigo*, if staphylococcal, can be treated topically by neomycin ointment 0.5% (sensitization is not uncommon), or 'Graneodin' or chloramphenicol as ointment or powder, providing there is no fever or malaise. However, with streptococcal impetigo some paediatricians advise systemic penicillin, or erythromycin, for 10 days (as for tonsillitis) because this reduces the risk of subsequent rheumatic fever or of acute nephritis. General practitioners do find this treatment an ideal not often practicable. *Impetigo may also complicate scabies, lice and eczema.* Nasal carriers of staphylococci perpetuate skin infection or act as carriers. Treatment is advised if the strain has caused outbreaks of infection, or is otherwise undesirable, or the person has recurrent sepsis. Topical application of neomycin 0.5%, neomycin and bacitracin ('Neobacrin'), soframycin or neomycin with chlorhexidine ('Naseptin') has been tried.

Systemic antibiotics are prescribed for cellulitis, lymphangitis, lymphadenitis, erysipelas, carbuncles and anthrax. Usually penicillin G, or a cephalosporin suffices or in allergic subjects, erythromycin. In *peri-orbital dermatitis*, often afflicting young women, tetracycline 250mg b.d. is helpful. For *acne rosacea* a 4-6 week course of tetracycline causes a quick improvement as the disease involves the upper dermis and blood vessels. *Acne vulgaris* is an affliction of the pilo-sebaceous follicle, and environmental factors influence sebum production and worsen acne (e.g. androgens, oral contraceptive pill). Therapy involves low dose continuous tetracycline for 6-9 months since the transit time of sebum through the skin takes months. Either tetracycline or oxytetracycline 250mg b.d. is given. Tetracyclines inhibit and alter fatty acid metabolism and suppress secondary infection and kill corynebacteria. Additional measures used include the peeling action of topical sulphur and retinoic acid (avoid eyes). Skin tuberculosis is treated as for other forms, and cutaneous diphtheria by antitoxin and penicillin G.

INSECTICIDES
These have helped by selective toxicity against insects to conquer typhus, relapsing fever, plague, malaria, sand-fly fever, filariasis and enteric infections which are all insect spread, but insects are adapting and becoming resistant.
Dicophane (DDT, called chlorophenothane in the U.S.A.) as a Dusting Powder 10% B.P.C. or Dicophane Application B.P.C. 2% is suitable for lice-ridden children and adults, but resistance occurs and its availability commercially is a problem. It is rubbed into the hair, or the powder is shaken on the skin.
Gamma Benzene Hexachloride Cream B.P. ('Lorexane') 1% strength or 'Lorexane No. 3' 2% gamma benzene hexachloride in detergent base is also used for lice. For resistant lice the organophosphorus compound **Malathion** 0.5% ('Derbac', 'Prioderm') lotion and cream shampoo 1% has proved effective. 'Esoderm' is gamma benzene hexachloride 1% with dicophane 1%. As a shampoo it is used for lice. The hair is washed twice leaving each application on for 2-3 min before rinsing.
Scabies is once again an important infestation and may be atypical. Classic forms exist but also scabies in 'clean people', 'scabies incognito', scabies in

infants and young children, scabies in the bedridden, mentally ill, crusted Norwegian scabies, scabies with syphilis and scabies with acute nephritis from associated streptococcal infection. Expert care is needed and overtreatment dermatitis avoided.

Benzyl Benzoate Application B.P. ('Ascabiol') a 25% emulsion in water is used. The whole family should be treated and the application painted on the skin by a brush after a hot bath. All the body is covered including the soles of the feet, palms and genitalia, but not the head and neck unless involved. Two applications are given, then allowed to dry. The patient dresses, but should not wash for the day. 'Quellada' (1% gamma benzene hexachloride) a lotion in 100 and 500ml bottles or application in 100 and 500ml bottles is a blander alternative and works for pediculosis too. 'Quellada Application P.C.' the detergent containing shampoo can dissolve the keratin around the nits. It is rubbed into the wet scalp and left for 4 min before rinsing. 'Esoderm Lotion' a 1% solution of gamma benzene hexachloride and 1% dicophane like 'Quellada' can be used for scabies as is 'Lorexane' 1% cream. In resistant scabies in patients on immunosuppressives, or corticosteroids, an inunction of 10% sulphur can be used.

Crotamiton ('Eurax') as a 10% lotion or ointment may be valuable for scabies in babies.

Monosulfiram Solution B.P. 25% w/v in methanol ('Tetmosol') in lotion form is used for scabies. If absorbed via the skin, and alcohol (ethanol) is drunk, an 'antabuse-like' reaction with headache can occur.

Diethyltoluamide B.P. applied topically to the skin or clothing in a 50 or 70% solution in ethyl or isopropyl alcohol is an insect repellent.

6 DRUGS FOR PROTOZOAL INFECTIONS

'Tropical' diseases are increasingly seen in temperate areas. Their management requires skill and expertise and if there is time help should be sought from Tropical Medicine Hospitals. Because of varying resistance to drugs in different areas those going abroad should seek local information (e.g. on suitable antimalarials). The treatment of tropical illness abroad on a mass scale is involving problems of logistics, administration and cost. Moreover, drugs should be long-acting with high acceptability, low cost and little toxicity. This ideal is rarely achieved and mortality from prophylaxis is a deterrent to eradicative measures. Other forms of control involve dealing with parasitic life cycles in water supplies, humans and animals and in modifying agricultural methods and irrigation.

PROTOZOAL INFECTIONS

Unicellular organisms, spores and cysts are difficult to eradicate and are not killed by antibiotics or chemotherapy in the minute concentrations which destroy or inhibit bacteria. Sensitivity tests are not possible. Living animals, or volunteers, have to be used to test efficacy. Moreover, immunization, either active or passive, is ineffective. Protozoa may live in harmony or symbiosis with their hosts who act as carriers, or they can cause chronic, or even acute fatal disease.

Important protozoal infections are malaria, amoebiasis, trypanosomiasis, leishmaniasis, giardiasis, trichomoniasis and toxoplasmosis. Protozoa invade the blood and tissues e.g. malaria (blood, tissues, including liver), *Entamoeba histolytica* (bowel, liver, occasionally brain), *Giardia lamblia* (bowel), *Trichomonas vaginalis* (genital tract), leishmaniasis (blood and tissues, including liver, spleen, marrow or skin), trypanosomiasis (blood, lymphatics and brain) and *Toxoplasma gondii* (blood and tissues).

MALARIA

In about 1200 million people malaria has been partially eradicated. In 500 million people no attempt has been made at eradication and malaria kills about 1 million yearly. It is the commonest blood infection. With air travel it appears everywhere. It harms non-immunes, but this term also includes Asians and Africans born in temperate countries, or expatriated for a long time who 'go home to visit their relatives'. Malaria also kills native infants and children before they become immune. The unicellular spore-like organisms of the *Plasmodium* genus occur in 4 pathogenic varieties: *P. vivax* (benign tertian malaria; *vivax* malaria), *P. falciparum* (malignant sub-tertian malaria; *falciparum* malaria), *P. ovale* (tertian malaria; *ovale* malaria), *P. malariae* (quartan malaria; *malariae* malaria). Drugs act at various points of the life cycle (Figure 1). Man is bitten by the female mosquito Anopheles whose salivary glands contain *sporozoites*. These immediately leave the blood stream, enter the liver cells and multiply for several days (liver or pre-erythrocytic stage). This clinically silent phase ends by the liberation of the parasites now called *merozoites* into the blood stream from disrupted liver cells and which now enter red blood corpuscles. Here they will multiply, until they burst the cell and this disruption is accompanied by the clinical features of fever, rigors and in some forms anaemia.

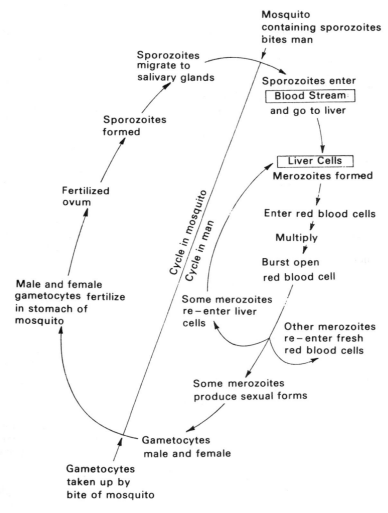

Fig. 1
Life cycle of the malaria parasite

Suppression of Acute Attacks
Schizontocidal drugs kill the dividing merozoites or schizonts within red cells, so preventing further red cell invasion and multiplication, and so symptomatically cure. The main ones chemically are **4-Aminoquinolines.**
Chloroquine is available as Chloroquine Phosphate ('Aralen', 'Avloclor',

'Resochin') Tablets B.P. 250mg equivalent to 155mg of chloroquine base, or Chloroquine Sulphate ('Nivaquine') Tablets B.P. 200mg equal to 146mg base. Both salts are available as Chloroquine Injection B.P. equivalent to 40mg/ml in 5ml ampoules. *Dose* oral 600mg as base (4 tablets) then 300mg after 6 hours; thereafter, 300mg daily for 2 days. 'Nivaquaine' syrup 15ml is equivalent to one tablet. Patients who are severely ill with shock, coma or vomiting as in *P. falciparum* cerebral malaria require injections; 400mg is given i.v. dissolved in 20ml of Water for Injections very slowly because of the risk of hypotension, or is infused in 500ml of Dextrose Injection B.P. 5%, or Sodium Chloride Injection B.P. over a period of 1 hour. Alternatively, half is given i.m. and half (200mg) i.v. If all is injected i.m. there is a risk of abscess formation. Children are given 5mg/kg B.W. Treatment is also given for shock, hyponatraemia and hypotension (i.v. fluids, protein albumin fraction), renal failure (dialysis), coagulation defects (heparin use is debatable), anaemia (packed red cells), cerebral oedema (dexamethasone 10mg then 4mg every 6-12 hours, or hydrocortisone sodium succinate 100mg 8 hourly). Too much i.v. fluid can cause pulmonary oedema. Administration should be metered carefully.

Amodiaquine Hydrochloride ('Camoquin') is less popular since it occasionally causes agranulocytosis. *Presentation* Tablets B.P. 200mg as the base; *dose* 600mg on the first day then 400 or 600mg daily for 3 days. It is no longer available in the U.K.

The problem of varying resistance to chloroquine e.g. with *P. falciparum* has led to the re-use of older drugs and the adoption of combinations. **Quinine Ph. Eur.**, an alkaloid used for centuries (1633), is a rapidly acting preparation useful for chloroquine resistant strains. Evidence from Africa also suggests that even with chloroquine sensitive *P. falciparum* it may be more effective. Different antimalarial regimens have to be compared on the basis of efficacy, toxicity and cost which includes cost of actual drugs, i.v. infusions that may be required and the time needed in hospital for cure. Quinine at least in the Far East has scored on all counts. *Presentation* Quinine Bisulphate Tablets B.P. 300mg (approx. equals 200mg quinine base), Quinine Hydrochloride Tablets B.P. 300mg (equal to 290mg base). *Dose* orally to suppress acute malaria 4-8 tablets (1200-2400mg) in divided doses. Quinine serum levels should be 4-8mg/dl. In iller patients Quinine Dihydrochloride Injection B.P., available in ampoules 2ml 300mg/ml, is given in a dose of 500-600mg in 20ml of Water for Injections injected slowly i.v. (e.g. 10min), or preferably in 500ml of Sodium Chloride Injection B.P., or Sodium Chloride and Dextrose Injection B.P. and infused over 4 hours. The next infusion is in 12-16 hours. Paradoxically, the sicker the patient the less quinine may be required. *Adverse effects* nausea, tinnitus, deafness, blackwater fever, hypotension if given rapidly i.v., abscesses if injected i.m. Children may find the bitter taste of the above tablets unacceptable; quinine ethylcarbonate available abroad is less bitter although quinine sulphate is sugar coated.

Mefloquine, a quinoline derivative, has been on trial since 1975.

Combined therapy attacks the resistant malarial parasite at different sites and may provide a radical cure. Quinine (e.g. 2 tablets 8 hourly for 3-10 days) with pyrimethamine and sulfadoxine at the onset, or preferably sequentially, have been tried successfully. Pyrimethamine 25mg is combined with 500mg of sulfadoxine in 'Fansidar' and 3 tablets are given. Ampoules containing 500mg sulfadoxine and 25mg pyrimethamine for deep i.m. use are available. Their prolonged action (the half life of sulfadoxine is 200h and pyrimethamine nearly 100h) provides for better eradication than the alternatives pyrimethamine with dapsone, or diformyldapsone, or multidose therapy with tetracycline or clindamycin (see *Brit. med. J.* **2**, 15 (1975)) for a 3 drug 3 day regimen. For quinine and chloroquine resistant strains **Sulfadoxine B.P.** ('Fanasil') 1g can be given with 50mg of pyrimethamine.

Eradicative Therapy

In falciparum malaria chloroquine, amodiaquine or the quinine-pyrimethamine-sulfadoxine regimen above will cure completely since this form has no exo-erythrocytic tissue reservoir of liver parasites. In other forms eradication of liver tissue parasites is obligatory after the acute attack has subsided. This eradication is achieved by the **8-Aminoquinolines** which also kill gametocytes. **Primaquine Phosphate** is the best. *Presentation* Tablets B.P. 13.2mg equivalent to 7.5mg primaquine base (obtained from I.C.I., or stocked in district hospital pharmacies). *Dose* 7.5mg base (1 tablet) 2 or 3 times daily for 2-3 weeks. Some strains of *P. vivax* need a longer period. *Adverse effects* preferably it is given in hospital since vomiting, abdominal pain, cyanosis, and haemolysis occur especially in Negroes and Mediterranean people with glucose-6-phosphate-dehydrogenase deficient red cells. Africans are not usually given this drug. **Pamaquine** is more toxic; *dose* 10mg t.d.s. for 10-14 days.

Prophylaxis

Suppression or prevention of acute attacks is employed for persons not native to a malarial district (non-immunes) when they are at risk. They prevent clinical malaria by killing merozoites and some destroy *P. vivax* and *P. falciparum* in the pre-erythrocytic phase. Prophylaxis is advised 2 weeks before going to malarial areas (but not absolutely essential) and continues for 4-8 weeks after leaving. This applies to all, including the pregnant.
Daily regimes are **Proguanil Hydrochloride** ('Paludrine') *presentation* Tablets B.P. 100mg; *dose* 100 or 200mg daily and for children 0-5 years 25mg, 6-12 years 50mg. *Adverse effects* nausea, vomiting, diarrhoea. **Quinine** 300-600mg daily has also been used. It is highly poisonous to children in accidental overdose. **Weekly regimes** should be taken on the same day each week, otherwise they may be forgotten. Preparations used are **Chloroquine** 300 or 450mg as the base weekly (or 150-300mg twice weekly in very malarious areas), **Amodiaquine** 400mg base once weekly (or 200mg twice weekly), or **Pyrimethamine** ('Daraprim') *presentation* Tablets B.P. 25mg; *dose* 25-50mg weekly and for children 0-5 years 6.25mg, 6-12 years 12.5mg. The synergistic combination of pyrimethamine and sulfadoxine 'Fansidar' 2 tablets once weekly, fortnightly or monthly is effective especially in chloroquine resistant areas. Pyrimethamine is also used to treat toxoplasmosis together with sulphonamides. Pyrimethamine crosses the placenta and also into the breast milk. *Adverse effects* such as nausea, vomiting or diarrhoea are reduced by taking the prophylactics after meals and with fluids.

In some parts of the world strains resistant to proguanil, pyrimethamine or chloroquine are met. Local opinion should be sought. Combinations are prescribed such as chloroquine base 300mg, pyrimethamine 50mg and dapsone 25mg weekly. 'Daraclor' is chloroquine sulphate equal to 150mg as base, and pyrimethamine 15mg. 'Maloprim' is pyrimethamine 12.5mg with dapsone 100mg. Chloroquine and primaquine can be given together weekly without the risk of haemolysis (from primaquine) plus dapsone as an alternative prophylactic regime. There is a risk of retinopathy when over 100g of chloroquine has been taken.

AMOEBIC INFECTIONS

Treatment depends on site (gut, liver, brain), severity (acute, chronic or asymptomatic), the patient's condition and the local experience. *Entamoeba histolytica* causes dysentery by involving the large bowel. In the active stage motile amoebae are seen and with chronicity and slow transit non-motile cysts. Infection may spread from the colon to the liver and beyond. Treatment has been simplified by the introduction of **Metronidazole** and the other nitro-imidazoles (see p. 36) at an oral *dose* of 400-800mg t.d.s. for up to 10 days for amoebic dysentery and liver abscess with a high cure rate (90% or more). An injectable form will be available. The lower dose causes less giddiness and 'antabuse' reaction. A high dose 2g repeated for 2 nights has been tried in India. For *liver abscess* 2g can be given as a single dose, but it is safer to assume associated gut infection and give a 10 day course as above. Metronidazole interferes with nucleic acid synthesis and reaches the amoebae via the blood stream, when they are in the intestinal or liver cells, or by being excreted in the gut after absorption. The role of metronidazole for the treatment of chronic cyst passers is not clear. Nor, it seems, do all forms of amoebic dysentery in different areas respond equally well.

In acute dysentery non-responders usually do well with **Emetine Hydrochloride**, an alkaloid of ipecacuanha. *Presentation* Emetine Injection B.P. ampoules 1ml containing 30 or 60mg in Water for Injections; *dose* 30-60mg daily s.c., or i.m. (never i.v.). Injections are painful and liable to cause abscesses and are best administered in hospital, and in bed. In acute dysentery the diarrhoea may settle with 2 or 3 injections, but for severe disease up to 12 daily injections are needed. Relief of diarrhoea is quick, but although mobile amoebae disappear the cysts do not. Some, otherwise well subjects will excrete cysts and become carriers. *Adverse effects* tachycardia, hypotension, ECG T wave changes, nausea, vomiting, abdominal distension.

The role of **supplementary drugs** is to eradicate the bowel or liver disease, or the carrier state. **Diloxanide Furoate** ('Furamide') can be used with few side effects for both the acute and chronic forms of amoebic dysentery including mass therapy for the carrier state. *Presentation* Tablets B.P. 500mg; *dose* 500mg t.d.s. It is suitable for out-patients. **Di-iodohydroxyquinoline** has decreasing use. It is given for asymptomatic cyst passers (and also acrodermatitis enteropathica, a rare childhood disease). *Presentation* Tablets 650mg; *dose* 650mg thrice daily for 20 days. Taken orally little is absorbed. *Adverse effects* nausea, vomiting, optic atrophy, severe furunculosis (iodide toxicoderma), thyroid enlargement, dermatitis, fever, headache, and irritation. **Phanquone** ('Entobex') and the arsenicals **Carbasone, Acetarsol B.P.** and **Bismuth Glycollylarsanilate** ('Milibis') are largely superseded. Amoebicides may be more effective when the bacterial content of the gut has been modified by **antibiotics** such as oxytetracycline, tetracycline, erythromycin or paromomycin. For chronic bowel infection there are various schemes and combinations depending on the skill, experience and preference of the physician and they employ metronidazole with the supplementary drugs and antibiotics.

In *amoebic hepatitis or abscess*, if metronidazole is ineffective and surgery is not the correct measure, then chloroquine, or emetine hydrochloride, may still be required. Cases of amoebic abscess have developed after orthodox courses of metronidazole have been used to treat bowel infection. Chloroquine is safe and markedly concentrated by the liver and the dose is 600mg base, followed by 300mg 6 hours later and then 300mg daily for 2-3 weeks. It should be remembered that amoebic dysentery mimics ulcerative colitis and may appear years after leaving an endemic country and that **Corticosteroids** by enema, or mouth, *may seriously exacerbate the disease.*

TRYPANOSOMIASIS
African sleeping sickness or trypanosomiasis is caused by *Trypanosoma gambiense (T. gambiense)* or *T. rhodesiense* and is spread from infected animals, or man, by the tsetse fly. At least 100 million Africans and S. Americans are at risk from it. The disease has three stages: (1) blood stream infection, (2) lymphatic infection, (3) brain infection with mental deterioration, fits, tremor and coma. Medications used are called **Trypanocides.**
(1) **Early disease without C.N.S. involvement**
Suramin is most effective against *T. rhodesiense* and is a urea derivative introduced over 50 years ago which does not enter the nervous system. *Presentation* powder 5 and 25g in bottles and ampoules 1g. The powder is poorly soluble and the Water for Injections needs to be warmed. *Administration* is slowly i.v. as a freshly made-up 10% solution. *A test dose* of 200mg is given and if all goes well. 800mg the next day. Thereafter, 1g is given weekly for 5-10 weeks. For children the dose is 20mg/kg B.W. *Adverse effects* circulatory failure, renal damage, peripheral neuritis, blood disorders, vomiting, rash, diarrhoea. It is advisable to test for proteinuria before each injection.
Pentamidine Isethionate and **Pentamidine Mesylate** have similar uses and can be used if suramin causes harm, or is ineffective. *Presentation* ampoules containing 200mg of powder. The B.P. Injection is made up in Water for Injections 2-3ml for i.m. and 10ml for i.v. use. *Dose* 2-4mg/kg B.W. daily, or alternate daily injections, for 5-15 injections. An average dose is 250mg daily. Repeated courses can be given. For prophylaxis the dose is 300–400mg every 3-6 months, but is only effective against the Gambian form of the disease. Other uses are for Kala Azar, cutaneous leishmaniasis and *Pneumocystis carinii. Adverse effects* vertigo, sweating, salivation, epigastric pain, nausea, vomiting, diarrhoea, tachycardia, hypoglycaemia, hyperglycaemia, megaloblastic anaemia, rash, itching and abortion; i.v. pentamidine can cause hypotension, dyspnoea and chest pain (Adrenaline should be available).
(2) **Central Nervous System Involvement**
Tryparsamide, an organic arsenical, enters the brain. *Presentation* 1, 2 and 3g ampoules; the contents are dissolved in 10ml Water for Injections just before use. *Administration* i.v. is preferred to i.m.; *dose* 20-40mg/kg B.W. A test amount of 1g is followed by 2-3g every 5 days up to a total of 10-12 injections. *Adverse effects* circulatory failure, pain and watering of eyes, photophobia, blurred and restricted vision, blindness, vomiting, hepatitis and rashes. Arsenic toxicity can be treated by dimercaprol. **Melarsoprol** (Mel B, Melarsen Oxide-BAL) is an arsenical chelated with dimercaprol. Since it acts against *T. gambiense* and *T. rhodesiense* in all stages it is replacing tryparsamide. *Presentation* 3.6% solution in propylene glycol. *Dose* 1-3.6mg/kg B.W. i.v. with care with a maximum of 200mg daily for 3 days which can be repeated after 10 days. *Adverse effects* vomiting, abdominal pain, diarrhoea, brain damage (in part a reaction to killing the parasites in the brain), confusion, excitement, mania,

tremor, ataxia, stupor, convulsions, hepatitis and rashes.
Melarsonyl Potassium (Mel W) has similar uses, but has the advantage of being water soluble and so can be given i.m. or s.c. *Presentation* powder in vials which is dissolved in Water for Injections and given in a dose of up to 4mg/kg B.W. and for children 2mg/kg B.W. *Adverse effects* fatal brain damage may occur.

LEISHMANIASIS
Leishmaniasis is a disease of the tropics, the Far East and Mediterranean area and is spread by sandflies. Some 7 million people are said to suffer from it. The systemic form (Kala Azar) affects the blood, lymphatics, liver, spleen and marrow, and is caused by *Leishmania donovani*. Cutaneous forms are caused by *L. tropica* (oriental sore) and *L. braziliensis* (espundia). **Antimony compounds** are used such as **Sodium Stibogluconate Injection B.P.** ('Pentostam') which is widely used for Kala Azar and the cutaneous forms. *Administration* is of a 33% solution equivalent to 100mg/ml of pentavalent antimony in Water for Injections, given i.m. or i.v. *Dose* 2-6ml daily for 10-30 days, a course which may be repeated after 7-14 days. Indian and Brazilian strains respond better than Mediterranean. Other substances sometimes used include **Antimony Sodium Tartrate Injection B.P.**, **Pentamidine Isethionate Injection B.P.**, and **Hydroxystilbamidine Isethionate Injection B.N.F.** an aromatic diamidine available in vials 250mg dissolved in Water for Injections and given slowly i.v. 250mg (or 5mg/kg B.W. adults; 3mg/kg B.W. children) daily in 10 day courses, which may be repeated 3 times, with a week's interval between.

GIARDIASIS
The drug of choice for diarrhoea due to *G. lamblia* is metronidazole 2g stat, then 2g daily for the next 2 days. Also useful is mepacrine 100mg t.d.s. for 5 days, or furazolidone 100mg q.d.s. for a week.

7 ANTHELMINTICS (DRUGS AGAINST WORMS)

Worm infestation is world wide and the number of people exposed to, or infected by, intestinal helminths such as hookworm is thought to include 1000 million people. It is common among recent immigrants to Britain. The important intestinal infestations are by roundworms, flatworms and flukes, but spread to the circulation, lymphatics and lungs can occur. The skin can also be involved. Worms are multicellular with a cuticle or protective coat which drugs must be able to penetrate to paralyse the neuro-muscular system. As with protozoal or mycobacterial infections, there are great problems in mass treatment, or even deciding in asymptomatic and symptomatic disease whether, because of cost or adverse effects, treatment should be given at all. Associated anaemia and malnutrition may handicap the patient further. Not all the drugs mentioned are available in Britain though they may be made here. The conquest of worm infestation is more likely to be achieved by sanitary engineering, good nutrition and health education than chemotherapy because of the inevitability of re-exposure in tropical countries.

ROUNDWORMS (Nematodes)
In some countries roundworm or ascaris infection affects nearly everybody, and when heavy, can cause intestinal obstruction so treatment is desirable.

Threadworms *(Enterobius vermicularis)*
Threadworms are the commonest worm infestation in Britain and usually involve the whole family, who should be treated. Hygiene is important, the nails are clipped and hands are kept clean since the eggs are deposited around the anus by the female living in the large bowel and so auto-infection is possible.

Viprynium Embonate is a dye and some paediatricians prefer it to the piperazines for threadworms. It is given in a single dose, which can be repeated after 2 weeks. *Presentation* as the base Tablets B.P. 50mg, Mixture B.P.C. 10mg/ml; *dose* (as base) 5mg/kg B.W. which as the suspension is 25-30ml for an adult, 5ml for a child 0-2 years, 7.5ml 2-4 years and 20ml at 12 years. *Adverse effects* red stools, nausea, vomiting, diarrhoea.

Piperazine compounds are used mainly for *Ascaris lumbricoides* (roundworms), *E. vermicularis,* and *Trichuris trichiura* (whipworm). They paralyse worms which are then expelled by intestinal peristalsis or purgation. Preparations are **Piperazine Adipate Ph. Eur., B.P.** Tablets 300mg equal to 250mg of piperazine hydrate, **Piperazine Phosphate Ph. Eur., B.P.** ('Antepar') Tablets 520mg equal to 500mg piperazine hydrate, **Piperazine Citrate Ph. Eur., B.P.** ('Antepar', 'Helmezine') Elixir B.P.C. 5ml contains the equivalent of 750mg piperazine hydrate. 'Pripsen' granules contain in each 10g 4g of piperazine phosphate, plus standardised senna, *Dose* (as piperazine hydrate) as tablets, syrup or elixir: *roundworms* 4g single dose for adults, children 2-3g according to age; *threadworms* 2g daily, in divided amounts, for adults for 7 days, children 2-6 years have half, and under 2 years, quarter doses. 'Pripsen' can be taken as a single dose regime for either roundworm or threadworm infections; the granules are mixed with water or milk at bed-time. *Adverse* *effects* gastrointestinal disturbances, allergy, neurotoxic effects in children— hypotonia, ataxia, myotonic contractions, incoordination, nystagmus, muscle weakness and choreiform movements. These 'worm wobbles' are rare but are more likely if the normal excretion of piperazine is reduced by renal failure.

Imidazole Derivatives

Thiabendazole ('Mintezol') *presentation* Tablets B.P. 500mg; *dose* 50mg/kg B.W. in 2 divided amounts, morning and evening, after meals up to a maximum of 3g for 2-3 days. *Uses Strongyloides stercoralis, Ascaris lumbricoides, Trichuris,* threadworms, hookworm and toxocara infestation. *Adverse effects* nausea, vomiting, diarrhoea, fever, vertigo, flushing, abdominal discomfort, angioneurotic oedema. *Contra-indications* pregnancy and lactation.

Mebendazole ('Vermox') is a broad spectrum anthelmintic with a standard dose, irrespective of age and weight. A single 100mg tablet or suspension 100mg/5ml repeated after a week radically cures *E. vermicularis* and *A. lumbricoides* infestation. Two tablets daily for 3 consecutive days are said to be effective against *Necator americanus, Ancylostoma duodenale* and *T. trichiura* and may be useful against tapeworms and *Strongyloides stercoralis.*

Levamisole Hydrochloride B.P. ('Ascaridil', 'Descaris', 'Ketrax') is effective, cheap and available abroad. *Presentation* Tablets 20mg; *dose* in adults 2.5mg/kg B.W. in a single amount, after food; children 0-3 years receive 40mg, 3-9 years 60mg and over 9 years 80mg. It is used for *Ascaris lumbricoides.* **Tetramisole Hydrochloride,** is a racemic mixture of levamisole and the dextrorotatory form; *dose* 2.5-5mg/kg B.W. for *Ascaris lumbricoides.*

Other anthelmintics. Pyrantel Embonate ('Combantrin') as a 5% suspension has also been tried for ascaris, threadworm and hookworm in a dose of 10mg/kg B.W. and for heavy infestations 20mg/kg B.W. for 1-3 days. Whipworms respond poorly; thiabendazole cures about a third, mebendazole may prove better. For strongyloidosis thiabendazole is best, with mebendazole as an alternative. **Difetarsone** has been introduced for *T. trichiura*, and so too has **Dichlorvos**, an organophosphorus compound (an insecticide which alters cholinesterase activity) as a single-dose regime.

Hookworms

Drugs for hookworm (*Ancyclostoma duodenale, A. braziliensis* and *Necator americanus)* are as follows.

Bephenium Hydroxynaphthoate B.P. ('Alcopar') although used principally for hookworm especially *A. duodenale* also kills *Ascaris* and *Strongyloides.* It is well tolerated and has been used in pregnancy. *Dose* 5g of Granules B.P.C. of bephenium hydroxynaphthoate equivalent to 2.5g of bephenium base in single sachets taken first thing in the morning on up to 3 successive days in 60ml of water. It is a bitter insoluble powder which may cause vomiting, so it is best given after fasting overnight, and sweetened for children. No purgation is required. Children under 2 years take half adult doses. **Pyrantel Embonate** is said to be superior for *N. americanus.*

Tetrachloroethylene is inexpensive, effective and suitable for mass therapy but is a toxic colourless liquid. *Dose* 3-5ml (U.S.P.) on an empty stomach in the morning in an emulsion in Capsules B.P. 1ml, *dose* 1-3ml or as a draught 2.5ml/50ml. Purgation is no longer considered desirable. Children take 0.1ml/kg B.W. or 0.2ml/year of age. *Adverse effects* nausea, vomiting, diarrhoea, abdominal pain, vertigo, liver and renal damage.

Hexylresorcinol B.P. acts against hookworm, *Ascaris*, *Enterobius* and intestinal flukes. *Dose* for adults 1g, children 100mg/year of age. It is given for hookworm in cachets so that it is liberated in the small gut and is followed by a saline purge. Enteric-coated capsules have been used for threadworms and roundworms. It irritates the mouth should children bite open the contents.
Bitoscanate ('Jonit') one capsule 100mg given 12 hourly after meals for 3 doses has had success in treating hookworm. *Adverse effects* abdominal pain, dizziness, anorexia, nausea, vomiting. As mentioned above, thiabendazole, mebendazole, levamisole and pyrantel embonate have also been used. A major problem in treating hookworm is *iron deficiency anaemia* from chronic blood loss. Iron salts by mouth are needed as well as parasite eradication.

Filariasis
Filaria is an invasive worm infestation; about 250 million people live in contact with it. The adult worm lives in the lymphatics *(Brugia malayi* and *Wuchereria bancrofti*), or under the skin (*Loa loa* and *Onchocerca volvulus*). The larvae or microfilariae invade the blood stream and lungs causing pneumonia, asthma, blood eosinophilia and elephantiasis of the legs. **Diethylcarbamazine Citrate** ('Banocide', 'Hetrazan') is used primarily to kill microfilariae of *W. bancrofti* or *Loa loa* on reaching the liver or skin. Taken orally it is rapidly absorbed with maximum blood levels in 2 hours. It is excreted renally. *Presentation* Tablets B.P. 50mg; *dose* 3-12mg/kg B.W. daily in 3 divided amounts after meals for 2-4 weeks. The daily total is usually 150-600mg. For tropical eosinophilia with lung infiltration seen in S. E. Asia a large dose of 300mg t.d.s. is given for a week. Small doses are given when allergic reactions are likely.

    Onchocerciasis is a major cause of blindness, with about 20 million people at risk and 300 000 blinded yearly by it. Without eye lesions the dose of diethylcarbamazine is 3mg/kg B.W. increasing over a week to 12mg/kg B.W. If there are eye lesions the starting dose is 0.5-1mg/kg B.W. daily and allergic reactions are suppressed by antihistamines and topical and systemic steroids. The drug has little effect on the adult worm, but it has on the microfilariae, and itching and sleepiness occur after its use. It may need to be given for life. The adult worm is treated with **Suramin** 1g i.v. weekly for 6 weeks after a test dose of 100mg, but it may have to be stopped if renal complications occur. While **Melarsonyl Potassium** (p. 46) kills the adult worm with one injection, fatalities with its use have occurred. *Adverse effects* of diethylcarbamazine are from allergic reactions to dead larvae, namely fever, nausea, pruritus, rashes, eosinophilia, dizziness, headache, body pain *(Brugia)*, encephalitis, a tissue reaction to heavy infestation (*Loa*) and in ocular forms (onchocerciasis) blindness and alopecia.

    Guinea worms (*Dracunculus medinensis*) have been treated with niridazole (p. 51) for 7-10 days.

FLATWORMS (Cestodes, Trematodes)
Cestodes (tapeworms)
Taenia saginata the beef tapeworm, is of importance in Britain, *T. solium* (pig), *Hymenolepis spp* (dwarf) and *Diphyllobothrium latum* (fish) are problems abroad. Only the adult forms can be treated. The larval forms of *T. solium* (cysticercosis) and of *Echinococcus granulosa* (hydatid) have no specific therapy.
Taeniacides are preparations to eradicate tapeworms.
Dichlorophen ('Anthiphen') is suitable for out-patients, because no fasting or

purgation is necessary, since the tablets are laxative. *Presentation* Tablets B.P. 500mg; *dose* adults 6g, children 500mg-4g before breakfast with fluid. The dose can be repeated the next day. The worm is destroyed and is unrecognizable in the stools. Hence proof of cure requires no evidence of tapeworm segments within 4 months. A high success rate is claimed. Neither it, nor niclosamide, kill the escaping eggs though they rupture the segments of the worm so if there is poor hygiene in *T. solium* infestation auto-infection can lead to cysticercosis which is a systemic invasion of the larvae to body tissues e.g. brain. Hence, dichlorophen is better for *T. saginata* (as is niclosamide) and *D. filix mas* is still used for *T. solium*. *Adverse effects* diarrhoea, nausea, vomiting, urticaria.

Niclosamide ('Yomesan')*presentation* vanilla flavoured chewable Tablets B.P. 500mg. *Dose* after fasting overnight for 12 hours adults are given 1g in the morning and 1g an hour later which is thoroughly chewed with water. Purgation is advised 2 hours after. Children under 8 years have half adult doses.

Mepacrine Hydrochloride Ph. Eur. ('Atabrine', Quinacrine Hydrochloride U.S.P.)*presentation* Tablets B.P. 100mg; *dose* 1g in 2-3 divided amounts followed by a purge, or because of the risk of vomiting (caused by the bitter taste) which may induce cysticercosis the tablets are best dissolved in 100ml of water and injected via a duodenal tube and an anti-emetic is prescribed. The tube is removed after 30-60g of magnesium sulphate is given. The worm can be recognised by the yellow colour it has absorbed. For 24 hours beforehand the patient should only take fluids. *Adverse effects* diarrhoea, vomiting. It can also be used for giardiasis.

Male Fern Extract is obtained from *Dryopteris filix mas* and is an ether extract of the root, a thick, smelly, green oil of unpleasant taste given as an emulsion with water, or as a draught. It paralyses the worm which is then expelled (with eggs in situ) by purgation. Good results demand a strict regimen. The patient is starved for 48 hours taking clear fluids only and purged once or twice daily. On the morning of the third day he is kept in bed and given 4g or approximately 4ml of the extract in 3 divided doses every 30 minutes. The B.P.C. Draught contains 4g of the extract in 50ml suitably flavoured. Strong coffee also helps to prevent nausea. Two hours later 15-30g of magnesium sulphate is taken, plus if needed, an enema. The stools are saved and the head of the tapeworm identified. Oily purgatives e.g. castor oil must not be used as they increase the absorption of the toxic constituents of *D. filix mas*. *Adverse effects* nausea, vomiting, colic, diarrhoea, yellow vision. The treatment is lengthy, unpleasant, and is unpopular but may have advantages in *T. solium* infestation.

Paromomycin (p. 21) has been found effective against *Diphyllobothrium latum*, *T. solium* and *Hymenolepis nana* 4g over 1 hour before breakfast. It can cause abdominal pain and diarrhoea.

Trematodes (flukes)
Schistosomiasis or bilharzia is one of the most important fluke infestations and there are over 200 million people exposed to it (with it or at risk) in the world and with irrigation and dams this figures is increasing. *S. haematobium* involves the bladder from the blood stream and *S. mansoni* and *S. japonicum* the liver and large bowel. *S. haematobium* is easiest to treat. Drugs used to kill the egg-laying flukes are antimonials, thioxanthones and niridazole.

Antimonials
Antimony Sodium Tartrate B.P. (A.S.T.) *presentation* ampoules 60mg/ml;

dose 30mg diluted in 20ml Water for Injections, Dextrose Injection 5%, or Sodium Chloride Injection and given very slowly i.v. preferably with the patient in bed. The dose rises by 30mg every other day to 120mg daily. A total course is 1.5-2g or 25mg/kg B.W. given over a period of 20 days. The cure rate approaches 100%. *Adverse effects* for safety daily E.C.G.'s are advocated as they precede other toxic effects—(pain in the vein and shoulder during injection, cough and vomiting are minimized by slow injection), fever, muscle and joint pain, headache, liver damage with raised enzymes S.G.O.T., S.G.P.T., and jaundice, nervous symptoms; cardiac pain, arrhythmias, circulatory failure, hypotension and cardiac arrest. It is the most effective but it is also the most toxic of available remedies.

Stibocaptate ('Astiban') or antimony dimercaptosuccinate *presentation* ampoules containing powder 500mg to be dissolved in Water for Injections. *Dose* 500mg i.m. weekly, twice weekly or even monthly up to a total of 2.5g or 30-40mg/kg B.W. It is available abroad only. It has the advantage of i.m. administration and a shorter treatment time. *Adverse effects* are due to allergy, or toxicity, vertigo, headache, vomiting, abdominal pain, nausea, fever, bad taste, anorexia, cough, arthralgia, backache, myalgia, insomnia, constipation, cloudy vision, E.C.G. changes.

Stibophen ('Fuadin') *presentation* vials 25, 50 and 100ml, 64mg/ml; *dose* i.v. or i.m. 1.5-5ml daily or every other day to a total of 70ml. Others include **Sodium Antimonylgluconate B.P.** and **Antimony Lithium Thiomalate** ('Anthiomaline').

Thioxanthones

Lucanthone Hydrochloride ('Miracel D') is a synthetic oral, non-antimony compound effective mainly against *S. haematobium*. *Presentation* Tablets B.P. 500mg; 'Miracel D' 200mg. *Dose* 1g b.d. for 3 days repeated monthly, or 500mg daily for 20 days. *Adverse effects* nausea, vomiting, abdominal pain, mental upsets, giddiness, vertigo, tremor and insomnia. **Hycanthone Mesylate** ('Etrenol') is a derivative. This has the advantage that for mass administration only a single i.m. injection is given. *Presentation* vial containing powder equal to 200mg hycanthone; *dose* 3mg/kg B.W. *Adverse effects* vomiting, anorexia, nausea, abdominal pain, ECG T wave changes, liver function disturbance. Some deaths have occurred from acute liver toxicity, when the drug has been given on a mass basis. It is effective against *S. mansoni* and *S. haematobium*.

Niridazole ('Ambilhar') is an imidazole derivative. *Presentation* Tablets 100 and 500mg; *dose* 25mg/kg B.W. daily for 4-10 days in divided amounts 12 hourly, or 750mg b.d. is used for schistosomiasis especially *S. haematobium* in children, amoebiasis and guinea worms. The total daily dose should not exceed 1.5g; half taken in the morning and half in the evening with, or after, meals. *Contra-indications* epilepsy, mental disorders, liver disease e.g. portal hypertension, severe cardiac disease, concurrent isoniazid administration. *Adverse effects* some are common—brown urine, headache, abdominal distress and pain, diarrhoea, nausea, vomiting, anorexia, drowsiness, insomnia and ECG T wave changes (like antimony). Others are EEG changes, mania, convulsions, confusion, apprehension, hallucinations, excessive salivation, ocular pain, jaundice, allergy, rashes, blood eosinophilia and haemolytic anaemia (glucose-6-phosphate-dehydrogenase deficiency). Niridazole is taken up by the germinal cells ova (schistosomes as well) and testes in man with a temporary anti-fertility action. The drug is available in the U.K. by special request only (Ciba). It is available abroad.

Metriphonate ('Bilarcil'), an organophosphate, has been given as a single dose 7.5mg/kg B.W. or 2.5mg/kg B.W. at fortnightly intervals for 3 doses for *S. haematobium* with few side effects. It is suitable for the large scale treatment of schistosomiasis and is highly effective, cheap, well tolerated and suitable for oral therapy. While taking metriphonate it is best to avoid suxamethonium as metriphonate like other organophosphorus compounds depresses cholinesterase activity.

Paragonimiasis is a fluke infestation seen in S.E. Asia and **Bithionol** and **Bithionol Sulphoxide** are used, 30-50mg/kg B.W. on alternate days for 10-15 days. The same treatment is used for *Fasciola hepatica. Clonorchis sinensis* has recently been treated with niclofolan 1mg/kg for 3 days, and in China hexachloroparaxylol 30mg/kg daily for 10 days or alternate days for 10 doses (*Brit. med. J.* **3**, 767 (1975)).

8 IMMUNIZATION

Protection against infection can be conferred artificially by injecting, inhaling or swallowing vaccines of antigenic substances made of *killed whole organisms* (typhoid, pertussis, cholera, plague, typhus, anthrax, poliomyelitis or influenza), *toxoids* which are chemically treated toxins made harmless (diphtheria, tetanus) or *living viruses* (poliomyelitis, yellow fever, rubella, mumps, smallpox, measles) or bacterial strains (B.C.G.). These make the body form protective antibodies hence 'immunization'.

Active immunization has largely been responsible for eradicating many diseases. Vaccines may be given by mass administration and ideally for this they should be cheap, efficient, long-lasting and safe. With jet injection large numbers of people can be dealt with, but they must individually be asked about their health beforehand. The occasional fatalities get publicity and as some diseases become rare, or mild, vaccination policies must be reviewed. Schemes for administration, types of vaccine and dose-spacing vary between countries and with migration and tourism unvaccinated people may meet new infections (e.g. poliomyelitis in Africa).

Protection starts early in most countries: pertussis, tetanus, diphtheria and poliomyelitis vaccines are given at 4-6 months in Britain and at about 3 months of age in the U.S.A. In under-privileged groups exposure to disease may make earlier vaccination advisable. Further vaccinations are made in infancy, during school, on leaving school and in adult life. The baby at birth has protection gained from maternal antibodies (passive protection) which may prevent successful active vaccination against some diseases. The injection of live viruses should not be given to the pregnant, or those with poor resistance because of malignancy, reticulosis, leukaemia, active tuberculosis, corticosteroid therapy, immunosuppressives, radiation, or allergy to hen's eggs (e.g. smallpox, measles, mumps, rubella).

The unwanted effects of vaccination can be grouped as follows: (1) severe local and constitutional reactions e.g. to typhoid, tetanus, plague or measles vaccines and which may be from constituents in the medium, chicken proteins, or adjuvants; (2) extraneous bacterial or viral contamination; (3) allergy and serum sickness; (4) neurological — neuritis, convulsions, encephalomyelitis; (5) abnormal sensitivity of patient to B.C.G. or smallpox, and a rare death with pertussis, yellow fever, typhoid, smallpox and rabies vaccines. These rare reactions must be balanced against the enormous benefits of vaccination.

BACTERIAL AND RICKETTSIAL VACCINES
Killed or Toxoids. These are stored at 2-10°C unless otherwise stated.

Diphtheria
Diphtheria has been virtually eradicated from Britain and vaccinations are recommended in all infants from 4-6 months of age as well as pre-school and school children.

Diphtheria Vaccine B.P. (Dip/Vac/FT or Dip/Vac/Ads Ph. Eur.). Formol toxoid (FT) is a formalin treated toxin unsuitable for primary vaccination, but the use of mineral carriers improves the antibody response e.g. aluminium salts making purified toxoid aluminium phosphate (PTAP), or purified toxoid aluminium hydroxide (PTAH). The aluminium salts as gels make a large surface on which the toxoid is adsorbed, retaining and slowly releasing the toxoid. *Dose* 0.2-0.5ml deep s.c. or i.m. for children, 0.2ml for adults and given in 2 doses at 1 month's interval in the second 6 months of life, with re-inforcing or booster doses at school entry and later at school or university. Preparations are expected to keep 2 years stored under the conditions specified by the makers. *Adverse effects* local pain, fever, headache and malaise are infrequent.

Toxoid-Antitoxin Floccules (TAF) a mixture of toxoid and antitoxin has a mild action with few reactions and is useful in adults, but since it contains horse serum, sensitization can occur. *Dose* 0.5ml s.c., or i.m. 3 injections 4-6 weeks apart.

Tetanus

This is not a communicable disease (i.e. not infectious to others), but infections result from contaminated wounds and it kills more people than diphtheria in many countries. Unlike diphtheria, people infected with tetanus are not a risk to the unvaccinated. All infants, children, soldiers and farmers should be actively immunized. A booster dose should be given at 15-19 years to prepare for adult life. In countries where tetanus neonatorum is a problem tetanus vaccination of mothers provides passive immunity to the baby, or Human Tetanus Immunoglobulin could be given if availability and cost permit.

Tetanus Vaccine B.P. (Tet/Vac/FT or Tet/Vac/Ads Ph. Eur.). Like diphtheria vaccine it is available as the formol toxoid, as purified toxoid aluminium phosphate (PTAP), or purified toxoid aluminium hydroxide (PTAH). Tetanus vaccine can be given alone, but is usually part of a combined injection. An advantage of the adsorbed preparations is that they are not neutralized by antitoxins (immunoglobulins) so that they can be given concurrently unlike the plain tetanus toxoid where a 6 weeks wait is necessary to allow the antitoxin levels to fall. *Dose* 0.5 or 1ml, 2 injections at 6 week intervals given i.m. or deep s.c. Further doses are advised 6-12 months later and then every 5 years.

Whooping Cough (Pertussis)

Pertussis vaccine is a suspension of whole killed bacteria of selected strains of *Bordetella pertussis.* Whooping cough can kill in the first few months of life and causes much morbidity. At present it is hotly debated whether more lives are saved by the vaccine than die from it, but it does reduce the severity, incidence and the duration of attacks. Proof either way is difficult to obtain, but many parents now refuse it although it is still officially recommended.

Pertussis Vaccine Ph. Eur., B.P. (Per/Vac) is made plain, or adsorbed (Per/Vac/Ads). *Dose* 0.5ml or 1ml i.m. 3 injections 1 month apart. Immunization starts at 4-6 months. The response improves with maturity (vaccination is started earlier in U.S.A.). Stored as directed it lasts 2-3 years. *Adverse effects* minor reactions occur in 20-40% e.g. fever, local erythema, and settle in 48 hours; rarer complications are persistent screaming, pallor, flaccidity, convulsions and brain damage which may be persistent. Immunization should be avoided if the child is unwell, has had previous convulsions or has a family history of epilepsy or reactions to the vaccine.

COMBINED VACCINES

Diphtheria and Tetanus Vaccine B.P. (DT/Vac/FT) and (DT/Vac/Ads) is available as the plain or the adsorbed preparation. *Dose* 0.5ml deep s.c., or i.m. of the formol toxoid. For primary vaccination 3 injections of the adsorbed product are given a month apart starting from 4-6 months. Both forms are given later in booster doses at school entry.

Diphtheria, Tetanus, Pertussis Vaccine B.P. (DTPer/Vac) or (DTPer/Vac/Ads) is the popular triple vaccine. *Dose* 0.5ml deep s.c., or i.m. in 3 injections 4-6 weeks apart in the second 6 months of life. Reactions are due to the pertussis vaccine. Booster doses are advised at 18 months.

Tetanus and Pertussis Vaccine B.P. (TPer/Vac) is a mixture of formol toxoid and pertussis vaccine. *Dose* 0.5 or 1ml; the first interval is 6-8 weeks between the first and second dose and 4-6 months between the second and third.

Typhoid

This is a common infection abroad including Continental Europe and the vaccination is advised for tourists and others at risk such as hospital staff. Protection is by no means complete. It reduces the attack rate only by about a fifth.

Typhoid-Paratyphoid A and B Vaccine Ph. Eur. (TAB/Vac). For military use tetanus or cholera vaccines may be added. The *dose* of phenol and heat-treated vaccines is 0.5ml then 1ml a month later, followed after 6-12 months by booster doses and yearly if at risk. Acetone treated vaccines are 0.5ml per dose. Route s.c., i.m. or intradermally (military use) 0.1ml. *Adverse effects* local swelling, pain and fever as a rule and, occasionally, nervous system involvement. Injections are best avoided in pregnancy. Alcohol should be forbidden for 24 hours. The doses of typhoid-paratyphoid A and B and tetanus vaccines are 0.5ml then 1ml. **Typhoid Vaccine Ph. Eur., B.P.** (Typhoid/Vac), a monovalent vaccine of heat-killed *Salm. typhi*, should have less adverse effects as it does not contain paratyphoid and the protection afforded against the latter by vaccines is unproven. *Dose* 0.5ml s.c. or i.m. twice at intervals of 4-6 weeks.

Cholera

Cholera is a world-wide problem and is now invading Europe. In epidemics the immunity gained from mass vaccination is small and the expense great. Public health measures and perhaps prophylaxis with co-trimoxazole or tetracycline are better.

Eltor Vaccine B.P. (Eltor/Vac) is prescribed if the endemic strain is known to be an Eltor biotype, otherwise **Cholera Vaccine Ph. Eur., B.P.** (Cho/Vac) is given which always contains classical strains, but may also contain the Eltor biotype. It is given to those at risk or travelling to endemic areas. The heat-killed phenol vaccine is given s.c., or i.m., 2 doses 0.5 and 1ml 1-4 weeks apart and a booster dose of 1 ml after 6 months. Under fives get half these doses. Immunity lasts 5-6 months.

Typhus and Plague

These are both vaccines like cholera given selectively to those at risk, or travelling to endemic areas.

Typhus Vaccine B.P. (Typhus/Vac) is given as three 0.2-1ml injections 10-28 days apart. It protects mainly against louse-borne typhus. **Plague Vaccine B.P.** (Plague/Vac) is formalin-killed and phenolized; *dose* 0.5ml and 1ml with 10-28 days between.

Anthrax
This is rare in Britain, but some workers handling infected material (wool, bones, hides) are liable to it. The dose of the specially prepared vaccine (Porton) is 0.5ml i.m., a second is given 3 weeks later, a third 3 weeks after the second and there is an interval of 6 months between the third and fourth doses. Thereafter, boosters are given yearly.

LIVING BACTERIA
Protection against Tuberculosis
Bacillus Calmette Guérin Vaccine Ph. Eur., B.P. (Dried Tub/Vac/BCG) is a freeze-dried vaccine of attenuated bovine tubercle bacilli. It is used specially for Mantoux- negative hospital staff, dentists, children and contacts of tuberculous families and in special risk groups e.g. certain immigrant children. In Sweden all babies are vaccinated in the maternity units and it protects them against miliary and meningeal tuberculosis. Depending on the prevalence of tuberculosis BCG may, or may not, be worth the trouble. In Britain it is offered to tuberculin negative school children aged 10-13 years. (10 000 vaccinations have to be given to prevent 1 case).The contribution of BCG to eradicating tuberculosis is diminishing and in the future will be given to special risk cases. The preparation can be kept for a year below 10°C in the dark. To make a suspension 1 or 5ml of Water for Injections is added respectively to the 1 or 5ml multi-dose bottles. It should be used immediately. *Dose* 0.1ml intradermally. A stronger percutaneous BCG is used abroad with a jet injector. *Adverse effects* local ulceration, rarely granulomata of internal organs.

LIVING VIRUSES
Smallpox
World eradication has been achieved, but some countries still require visitors to be vaccinated. Laboratory workers handling smallpox virus and those who may visit such laboratories are vaccinated. Immunity is not permanent so that those at risk should be regularly and effectively immunized. Mass vaccination is possible and the use of the jet injector and bifurcated needle has helped to increase the take rate.
Smallpox Vaccine Ph. Eur., B.P. (Var/Vac). To produce lymph, vaccine or cowpox (vaccinia) is inoculated into the skin of calves, sheep, buffalo or goats. A blister results from which the fluid or lymph is obtained, filtered and purified. This protects humans against smallpox. Stored at −10 to −20°C it remains potent for 1 year, below 10°C 14 days, and at 10-20°C a week. It can also be freeze-dried. Alternatively, a freeze-dried suspension of vaccinia grown in hen's eggs or rabbit kidney cell cultures may be used, which when kept below 4°C in the dark lasts 5 years. The stable freeze-dried vaccine is suitable for the tropics and lasts unrefrigerated for 9 months. Glycerolated lymph is no longer kept in the U.K. and has been replaced by freeze-dried vaccine. When made up it should be used at once. *Vaccination* lymph is expelled from the tube by a rubber teat, usually over the deltoid which is cleaned with soap and water. One tube suffices for several subjects. With a flame-sterilized needle, either multiple pricks, or several scratches are made into the lymph-covered skin. *Adverse reactions* should be of historic interest only when all countries no longer require smallpox vaccination. Vaccination should be

avoided if the subject has eczema, dermatitis, impetigo, herpes zoster, or is pregnant. Smallpox vaccination is highly dangerous and sometimes fatal in patients taking corticosteroids, cytotoxics, having radiation, or who have altered immunity as in agammaglobulinaemia, leukaemia and Hodgkin's disease. The vaccinated site is not usually covered, except in children, who by scratching can spread the living virus to the cornea and damage the eye. Here, a light non-waterproof dressing is safe. Some lymph node enlargement and skin redness are normal; infection with lymphadenitis is common. Serious complications infrequently occur: vaccinia may generalize and patients with eczema may die from chickenpox-like, eczematous or gangrenous skin eruptions. Death may occur also from encephalitis. An attenuated strain grown specially has been tried for use in atopic (eczematous) children. If vaccination must be done in atopics it should be under the cover of human antivaccinial immunoglobulin. Most countries require that certain vaccinations (cholera, smallpox, yellow fever) should have the procedure, date and batch number recorded and an official stamp on a valid document to prove this.

Other vaccines are grown in tissue cultures from specially protected domesticated animals (dogs, monkeys, guinea-pigs, rabbits, ducks) or human diploid cells.

Poliomyelitis
Poliomyelitis has been preventable since 1954 when a killed vaccine was introduced. It is a rare disease in Western countries, but can be contracted in the Mediterranean area and Africa, and recurrences have occurred in the U.K. in 1977. The first preparation of poliomyelitis types 1, 2 and 3, was grown in monkey kidney tissue, and killed by formalin (Salk vaccine). Later, a safe living oral vaccine was introduced by Sabin and is preferred in Britain.
Poliomyelitis Vaccine (Inactivated) Ph. Eur., B.P. (Pol/Vac/Inact) is imported from abroad and is given in a dose of 1ml i.m. twice at monthly intervals and a booster dose 6-9 months later. Its use is restricted to special cases, such as pregnant women, or anyone on immunosuppressives. **Poliomyelitis Vaccine (Oral) Ph. Eur., B.P.** (Pol/Vac (Oral)) contains all 3 types of strains. Three doses each of 2 or 3 drops on a lump of sugar are given monthly. Oral vaccine keeps 6 months at 0-4°C and a week at 18-22°C. Very rarely the virus can become wild and infect contacts. Consideration should be given to vaccinate non-immunized parents if their children are immunized.

Rabies
Rabies-carrying animals (wolves and many other animals) have spread westward through the continent of Europe and now Britain is at risk. Protection is indicated for kennel workers in quarantine camps, and probably all animal attendants, and also those bitten by known or suspected rabid dogs. Active vaccination is possible because of the long period of incubation of rabies.
Rabies Vaccine B.P. (Rab/Vac) is prepared from suckling rabbit brains—before the myelin has developed—infected with a strain of attenuated rabies virus. A series of injections is given into the abdominal wall (because of the volume), plus anti-rabies serum up to 4000u (20ml) prepared from goats. A special organic solvent has reduced the neuronal protein and side effects: the chance of encephalitis resulting is now only 1:1000. Rabies virus can now be grown in human diploid cells and the vaccine made from this has far less risk to those needing protection. It is made in France, Germany and U.S.A.

Yellow Fever
This is indicated in all those who visit endemic areas.
Yellow Fever Vaccine B.P. (Yel/Vac) is a specially modified strain (17D) of yellow fever virus and protects for 6 years. Obtained from special centres it is given s.c., or i.m. not less than 1000 LD_{50} virus particles. *Adverse effects* occasional encephalitis. It is not given to babies under nine months or to the pregnant. It is advised that smallpox and yellow fever vaccination be separated by 21 days. If this cannot be done, both have been given together, and this has become common practice with safety in France and Africa.

NEWER LIVE ATTENUATED VIRUSES
Rubella
Rubella Vaccine (Live Attenuated) B.P. (Rub/Vac(Live)) 'Almevax', 'Cendevax' is given in Britain to young adolescent girls between the 11th and 14th birthdays and in the U.S.A. from 1-5 years. Women who wish to be vaccinated should be tested serologically first. If sero-negative they should be offered vaccination, but only on the understanding that they will not become pregnant within 3 months of receiving the vaccine. If sero-negative in pregnancy women should be offered vaccination in the post-partum period providing that pregnancy is avoided for 3 months. Women at risk of rubella are teachers, nurses, nursery staff and female doctors. The vaccine is 95% effective. If given to girls the object is to prevent rubella embryopathy. *Presentation* vials with separate 0.5ml diluent for reconstitution; *dose* 0.5ml s.c. *Contra-indications* pregnancy and those listed earlier in the chapter. It is not to be given within 4 weeks of other vaccinations, or 6 weeks of immunoglobulin therapy. *Adverse effects* radiculo-neuritis, fever commonly 6-7 days after vaccination, adenopathy 9-13 days, arthralgia 21-28 days later.

Measles
Deaths from measles could be reduced still more and vaccines are needed in countries like India, Africa or S. America where the disease can be serious or fatal. In Britain and the U.S.A. it is relatively mild, but it is still the most frequent and severe of childhood infections with ear and lung complications.
Measles Vaccine (Live Attenuated) Ph. Eur., B.P. (Meas/Vac(Live)) is safe and potent and recommended in the second year of life. A freeze-dried attenuated vaccine is injected 0.5ml s.c., or i.m. after it is reconstituted with the diluent. *Adverse effects* such as fever and rashes are rare.

Mumps
The Jeryl Lynn live attenuated mumps vaccine is well tolerated, immunogenic, but the antibody response is less than with the natural infection. It is available as 'Mumpsvax', a freeze-dried powder with a diluent in a dose of 0.5ml s.c.
    Live Measles, Mumps and Rubella Vaccine U.S.P. combines all three.

KILLED VIRUSES
Influenza
Vaccines are moderately effective, the antigens of influenza vary, immunity is short and it is difficult to prepare a suitable vaccine quickly in severe epidemics. Protection is indicated in patients at risk with chronic heart and lung disease, the young and the elderly as well as doctors, nurses and those

working in vital industries. Trivalent influenza vaccines available in Britain are a saline suspension containing virus strains A and B killed by formalin or β-propiolactone. The virus is grown on the allantoic fluid of the fertilized egg. Prophylactically it is given in the autumn. Immunity takes 1-2 weeks to achieve and lasts several months. Public health policy is to review influenza vaccine formulations and to allow for major antigenic changes and antigenic drift. In the U.S.A. a trivalent inactivated preparation was used in 1978-79.

Influenza Vaccine Ph. Eur., B.P. (Flu/Vac) and **Adsorbed Influenza Vaccine, Ph. Eur., B.P.** ('Admune', 'Fluvirin', 'Influvac') *presentation* ampoules and disposable syringes 1ml, multidose vials 10 and 100ml; *dose* adults 1ml, children 0.1-0.5ml. The vaccine is shaken then given s.c. deeply, or i.m.

Russia is using live attenuated influenza vaccines by the nasal route and in 1975 a live attenuated 'Alice' strain was introduced in the U.K. **Influenza Vaccine, Live (Intranasal) B.P.** is an aqueous suspension of a suitable live attenuated strain either type A or B. The reconstituted vaccine is dropped into each nostril.

FUTURE VACCINES
In the U.S.A. combinations of viruses have been given so reducing the cost of administration. Future research promises to provide vaccines against hepatitis, syphilis and gonorrhoea. Immunization is also being tried against leukaemia and cancer.

DENSENSITIZATION
Desensitization against allergy is possible for many ingested or inhaled allergens such as pollens, house dust, house mite, moulds and animal fur. Vaccines are made in graduated strengths and some in delayed acting forms.

MALIGNANCY
Non-specific enhancement of immunity has been tried in cancer and acute leukaemia using BCG, whooping cough vaccines and *Corynebacterium parvum* and with levamisole which may restore delayed hypersensitivity.

PASSIVE IMMUNITY
This is conferred by protective immunoglobulins obtained from serum, either by natural, or artificial means. They are prepared from horses injected with vaccines or from humans. Their advantage is immediate protection, their disadvantage is short lived immunity. As foreign proteins when made in animals, they cause frequent hypersensitivity reactions. Early serum reactions are urticaria, asthma, and anaphylactic shock within minutes or hours of the injection. When giving horse sera adrenaline, antihistamines, hydrocortisone and an airway should be handy. Delayed reactions occur 4-12 days later namely, urticaria, arthralgia, joint swelling, fever, proteinuria, lymphadenopathy, nerve and brain damage. Local redness and swelling are common at the injection site 7-10 days later.

Precautions Patients must be asked about previous horse serum injection, reactions to injections, a past or family history of allergy, asthma, urticaria, hay fever or eczema. With a positive history, a test dose of 0.1ml of a 1 in 10 dilution is given intradermally or by the same route as the intended main injection. A local skin redness indicates slight sensitivity. If no general reaction occurs after 30 minutes the full dose is given. The risk of the injection is balanced against the possibility of the disease occurring.

IMMUNOGLOBULINS

Human Normal Immunoglobulin Injection Ph. Eur., B.P. contains the natural antibodies and is derived from pooled adult plasma or convalescent sera. The concentration is 250mg/1.7ml. It gives some protection against Type A viral hepatitis, measles and the risks of smallpox vaccination. Another use is in patients who fail to make their own globulins and become abnormally liable to infection. Given i.m. there is little risk of serum hepatitis (Type B). *Dose* 500-1500mg i.m. for adults.

Human Specific Immunoglobulins are hyperimmune globulins produced artificially by actively immunizing donors or by natural means. They have been produced against rhesus D factor, tetanus, mumps, varicella, zoster, vaccinia and HB$_s$ Ag (Type B) hepatitis.

Human Antitetanus Immunoglobulin Injection Ph. Eur., B.P. ('Humotet') is derived from the sera of healthy human donors who have high levels of tetanus antitoxin after being immunized with tetanus vaccine. It has replaced horse tetanus antitoxin because of the risks of anaphylaxis. *Presentation* vials 1ml containing 250u. *Dose* for prophylaxis 250u i.m., or 500u if the wound is liable to be contaminated. Protection lasts 4 weeks. It is given to those with inadequate immunization or who have never been immunized. Active immunization with adsorbed toxoid should be started at once injecting with a separate syringe at a different site. If an injured person has already been efficiently immunized only a booster dose of toxoid is needed. For the treatment of tetanus the dose is 30-300u/kg B.W. i.m. For many countries the cost is such that for the treatment of tetanus animal derived sera would still be used. The preparation is stored at 2-10°C. *Contra-indications* history of anaphylaxis to human gamma globulin. Other measures see p. 127.

Human Antivaccinia Immunoglobulin Injection Ph. Eur., B.P. is given in the presence of contra-indications to vaccination such as eczema when smallpox protection has to be given, as in the rare event of exposure to laboratory stored smallpox virus. *Dose* 500mg for children under 1 year, 1g 1-6 years, 1.5g 7-14 years, adults 2g (1g = 7000u).

Anti-D (Rh₀) Immunoglobulin Injection B.P. is used to prevent rhesus sensitization. Passive immunization of Rhesus-negative women liable to have Rhesus-positive babies may prevent erythroblastosis foetalis. They are given anti-D globulin 200µg i.m. shortly (within 60 hours) after delivery of their first pregnancy, or after abortion when 50-100µg is given. The antibody coats the antigenic sites on the baby's Rhesus-positive red cells that may possibly have entered the maternal circulation before they have had a chance to sensitize the mother. It may also be given if Rhesus-positive blood has been given to a Rhesus-negative person and the transfusion is incompatible. The dose is 10µg for each ml of blood infused.

Human Anti HB$_s$Ag Immunoglobulin is a preparation containing a high titre of antibodies to hepatitis B$_s$ surface associated antigen (HB$_s$Ag). It is used for those inoculated, or injected accidentally with infected material. Before giving it the blood of the person should be examined for the antigen and the antibody. If neither is present then 500mg is given. The material contaminating the person should be examined also. The present dose is an arbitrary one.

Herpes Zoster Antivaricella Immunoglobulin Injection is used to prevent herpes zoster in a dose of 500mg i.m.

Transfer factor is a product obtained from freezing peripheral white blood cells, which are thawed, disrupted and the juice dialysed. The material it contains is suitable for immune deficiency of the type where lymphocytes are present. The preparation is safe, but its nature is unknown. It is not an antigen. The factor is contained in fresh blood. *Uses* are Wiscott-Aldridge syndrome, cutaneous or mucocutaneous candidosis and vaccinia.

Antilymphocyte Immunoglobulin (Horse) ('Pressimmune') *presentation* ampoules 5 and 10ml 50mg of equine immunoglobulin/ml has been used in organ transplantation under specialist care in hospital.

Human Antirabies Immunoglobulin (HRIG)
HRIG has been produced commercially from vaccinated donors and has been available for supply from the U.S.A. since 1974. Although it is a powerful suppressor of antibody formation it is replacing antirabies serum. *Dose* 20u/kg B.W.; 1500u are contained in 10ml. Human antirabies immunoglobulin is now being produced in the U.K. by the Blood Products Division at the Lister Institute, Elstree and 450u/1.1ml are contained in each vial.

Pre-Exposure Treatment. In the U.K. HRIG has been used with the more potent Human Diploid Cell (HDC) vaccine rather than the duck embryo rabies vaccine (DEV). This is available commercially from l'Institut Merieux, Lyons. It is a whole virion vaccine inactivated by β-propiolactone. *Dose* an initial course of 4 doses 1ml i.m. is given at spaced intervals during the first 14 days (0, 3, 7, 14) followed by 2 boosters on days 30 and 90. For those nursing cases of rabies where aerosol spread is a possibility, 0.1 intradermally in each limb (4 injections) on the first day is given.

Post-Exposure Treatment. Combined serum-vaccine treatment is offered to the non-immune patient. The wound is washed with soap and water and iodine or 40-70% alcohol applied. The dose of rabies antiserum is 40u/kg B.W. and up to half is given locally into the wound and the rest i.m.. In the U.S.A. a combination of HRIG and DEV is advised; because of immunosuppression produced by HRIG the number of doses of DEV given is increased to 23 or 24. The human diploid cell vaccine is now available in the U.S.A. on a limited experimental basis, (C.D.C. Atlanta).

IMMUNOSERA

These are obtained from native (unpurified) sera and then refined.

Diphtheria Antitoxin Ph. Eur., B.P. (Dip/Ser) is given to those possibly incubating diphtheria or who actually have the illness. It should be given early before bacteriological confirmation. Protection lasts 3 weeks. It cannot neutralize toxins attached to organs. *Dose* 10 000-100 000u according to site, duration and severity of the infection. Doses up to 30 000u are given i.m., larger amounts half i.m. then 30 min later the rest i.v. Prophylactic dose 500-2000u s.c. or i.m.

Mixed Gas-Gangrene Antitoxin Ph. Eur. at a dose of 25 000u in the proportions stated is given prophylactically i.m. and therapeutically not less than 75 000u i.v. 4-6 hourly. No antiserum should be given without adrenaline being handy.

Special antitoxins and antisera are available against *Clostridium botulinum* toxins, anthrax, leptospirae and the venom of snakes and scorpions. Zagreb antiserum is advised for adder bites. The contents of 2 ampoules 10.8ml are given in 100ml of isotonic saline for severe cases with hypotension.

Scorpion Venom Antiserum B.P. is usually made in horses and the species of scorpion venom against which the serum is effective varies according to the area in which it is given.

The Centre for Disease Control (C.D.C.), Atlanta, U.S.A. contains medicinal products not commercially available, or those which are under strict control as well as sera against rare diseases, arbovirus, viral haemorrhagic fever and snakes.

Newer Vaccines
Polysaccharide
With the resurgence of bacterial resistance to certain important infections interest has shifted back to pre-war ideas namely immunological control. The pneumococcus, meningococcus and *H. influenzae* contain antigenic polysaccharide substances, vaccines can be made if the polysaccharides can be identified in the various strains.

Polyvalent Pneumococcal Vaccines
Recently infections of multiply resistant pneumococci have occurred in different parts of the world especially S. Africa. The repertoire of antibiotics which can be used has been reduced to rifampicin, vancomycin, bacitracin, fusidic acid and novobiocin. To protect adults and children over 2 years a 14(poly) valent pneumococcal polysaccharide vaccine has been prepared which contains types 6A and 19F. 'Pneumovax' is stated to give protection to 80% of pneumococcal disease isolates in the U.S.A. and Europe. A single dose is contained in a pre-filled syringe and there is 50µg of each polysaccharide type derived from the capsules of the 14 most prevalent pneumococci. The indications are for those at risk from pneumococcal infection and this includes the splenectomised patient, and those with reticulosis, sickle cell anaemia and nephrotic syndrome. It is given i.m. Pregnant women should not be given the injection. The usual precautions against anaphylaxis should be observed and 1:1000 adrenaline should be kept handy. Patients with a recent history of pneumococcal infection should not be given the vaccine. Some selectivity is essential since the injection is about £5 per shot.

Meningococcal A and C Vaccines
Monovalent A and C vaccines have been made (A in France, C in U.S.A.) and also bivalent containing both. The vaccines are made from purified cell wall polysaccharide. Their use has curtailed epidemics in U.S.A., Brazil and Finland where an extensive vaccination scheme has been achieved. Close communities such as military establishments are given vaccination.

Other Vaccines
Protection is possible against tularaemia with a live attenuated *Francisella tularensis*. One drop is placed on the skin and multiple local pressure applied (as with smallpox vaccination). Rocky Mountain Fever is prevented by formalin killed *Rickettsia rickettsii* 0.2-1.0ml every week for 3 doses s.c., or i.m. For typhus prophylaxis formalin killed *Rickettsia prowazekii* is grown on chick embryos. The dose is 0.2-1.0ml every week for 3 doses s.c., or i.m.

9 CYTOTOXIC THERAPY

Cytotoxics are used to treat malignancy and as immunosuppressives. The aim is to kill the cancer cells by selective toxicity without unacceptable harm to the patient. Cytotoxic therapy rarely cures and it is mainly used for palliation to prolong worthwhile life and in terminal disease. Its use has to be considered in relation to surgery or radiotherapy. If a cancer is removable this is the treatment of choice. When radiotherapy is unsuitable or unavailable, as in the poorer countries, cytotoxic therapy is valuable. In developed countries the trend is to specialize in cancer therapy (oncology) and the best results are obtained in special centres e.g. in Hodgkin's disease and in leukaemia.

These agents act at different phases of the cell cycle and interfere with the ability of cancer cells to synthesize nucleic acids or undergo mitosis and hence prevent their growth and division. Normal fast growing and dividing cells are also suppressed. The marrow (red cells, neutrophils and platelets), intestinal cells, gonads, hair and skin are suppressed, but adverse effects extend to the liver, lungs, coagulation processes, metabolism of uric acid, chromosomes (mutagenesis), the foetus (teratogenesis) and the induction of cancer (carcinogenesis). They act like X-rays and likewise cause nausea, sickness, vomiting and diarrhoea, and increase the liability to infection by immunosuppression. Limitations of cytotoxic therapy are therefore general toxicity, suppression of immunity, teratogenicity and possibly genetic damage. The trend is to give cyclical pulse therapy with large doses which allow the non-tumour tissue such as the marrow to recover and, hopefully, not the tumour. The drugs are powerful with severe side effects so the maker's literature as regards dosage and precautions should be studied.

Illnesses treated include reticuloses (generalized Hodgkin's disease, Burkitt's lymphoma, lymphosarcomata, reticulum cell sarcoma, mycosis fungoides), myeloproliferative disorders (acute and chronic leukaemia, myelofibrosis, polycythaemia rubra vera, thrombocythaemia), plasma cell disorders (multiple myeloma, Waldenstrom's macroglobulinaemia), and choriocarcinoma. Treated with less success are embryonal carcinoma of the testis or ovary, rhabdomyoma, Wilms' and Ewing's tumours, retinoblastoma and cancer of the breast, colon and ovary. Solid tumour therapy uses methotrexate, fluorouracil, vincristine, cyclophosphamide, doxorubicin and prednisone singly or in various combinations. Many common cancers are unresponsive, or poorly so, e.g. stomach and lungs. Deposits in brain or liver are also resistant. *Administration* is by mouth, i.m., or i.v., into body cavities (pleura, peritoneum, joints) or intrathecally. By direct infusion into an artery supplying the head, a limb, pelvis or an organ such as the liver a more precise effect can be obtained. Dosage is controlled by frequent blood counts. Individual agents lose their effect so that it may be preferable to combine drugs which act by synergism at different sites in the cell, or at different phases, as in leukaemia and in Hodgkin's disease where alkylating agents, antimetabolites, prednisone and vinca alkaloids are given. DNA synthesis is impaired by purine, pyrimidine and folate antagonists, mitotic spindles by vinca alkaloids, alkylating agents cross-link strands of DNA, antibiotics bind with DNA and interfere with replication and RNA. The nitrosoureas and procarbazine work by unknown means.

ALKYLATING AGENTS
Nitrogen Mustard and Derivatives
Alkylating agents attach groups of carbon and hydrogen atoms (alkyl radicals) to the organic molecules of the nucleus thereby destroying them and inhibiting cell division. (They stick chromosomes together.)

Nitrogen Mustard (Mustine Hydrochloride, Mechlorethamine Hydrochloride) is rapid in action, unstable in solution and supplied as a powder which when dissolved is used at once. It is highly irritant when given accidentally outside a vein. *Presentation* vials 10mg. Mustine Injection B.P. is a sterile solution in Water for Injections. *Administration* as a bolus i.v. dissolved in 20-50ml of sterile water, or the solution may be injected into the tubing of a fast-running i.v. saline infusion. It is best given at night with an anti-emetic and hypnotic before. The patient should not have eaten. *Dose* i.v. 400-600μg/kg B.W. as a single injection, or more customarily 100μg/kg B.W. up to a maximum of 8mg daily for 4 days in one course which may be repeated after a month. It is used when rapid action is needed, as in mediastinal obstruction from reticulosis, or cancer, or as part of the quadruple therapy for Hodgkin's disease. Mustine 20-50mg may be directly injected into malignant pleural and peritoneal effusions.

For safety and convenience derivatives which can be taken orally or i.m. have been introduced. Orally the drugs take several weeks to work.

Oral Nitrogen Mustards
Chlorambucil ('Leukeran') is used against chronic lymphatic leukaemia, macroglobulinaemia, ovarian cancer, follicular lymphoma and lymphosarcoma e.g. chronic lymphocytic type. *Presentation* Tablets B.P. 2 and 5mg; *dose* 5-15mg orally daily (200μg/kg B.W.) as a single dose, usually 10mg for a course 4-8 weeks which can be repeated later, or a maintenance dose of 2-4mg daily (30-100μg/kg B.W.) is given. *Adverse effects* marrow depression, anaemia, thrombocytopenia, nausea, vomiting, abdominal pain.

Cyclophosphamide ('Cytoxan', 'Endoxana') is a phosphoric acid derivative of nitrogen mustard which is changed into the active substance by hydroxylation in the liver. *Uses* Hodgkin's disease, as part of a quadruple therapy, along with vinblastine (or vincristine), prednisone and procarbazine; leukaemia, lymphosarcoma, and in bronchial cancer where it may be the sole therapy. *Presentation* Tablets 10 and 50mg, vials 100, 200, 500 and 1000mg; the Injection B.P. is made by dissolving the contents in 5-10ml of Water for Injections. It is sparingly soluble in water and needs to be shaken vigorously. If given extravenously, by accident, it causes no pain. *Dose* 15mg/kg B.W. i.v. weekly, or 1-1.5g/m² (see note, p. 267) i.v. every 3 weeks or 1.5-3mg/kg B.W. daily. A usual daily dose is 100mg rising to 200mg for 2-3 weeks, then an oral maintenance dose of 50-100mg daily. A similar dose is used for immunosuppressive therapy. *Adverse effects* baldness, haematuria and fibrosis from chemical cystitis which may be helped by drinking plenty of water and frequent emptying of the bladder. It is usually reversible, but fatal bleeding has occurred. Testicular germinal damage with decreased sperm count and sterility can occur with long-term use. Intermittent (e.g every third week) therapy may reduce the risk of marrow suppression. Diffuse lung fibrosis, water retention can occur.

Uramustine ('Uracil Mustard') is relatively non-toxic and is used in chronic leukaemia and the reticuloses. *Presentation* capsules 1mg; *dose* 3-5mg daily for 1-2 weeks then 1mg daily.
Melphalan ('Alkeran') *presentation* Tablets B.P. 2 and 5 mg, Injection B.P. made from vials containing 100mg with ampoules of solvent and diluent. *Uses* multiple myeloma and by local perfusion for malignant melanoma. *Dose* adults 2-10mg daily orally for 1-2 weeks, or i.v. as a single dose 1mg/kg B.W. and for maintenance 2-4mg orally daily. Dangerous accumulation readily occurs. *Adverse effects* nausea, vomiting, marrow depression (especially thrombocytopenia), mouth ulcers, gastro-intestinal bleeding. Either alkylating agent melphalan or cyclophosphamide is used in myelomatosis, in intermittent dosage, with corticosteroids. Pain, infection, hypercalcaemia, hyperuricaemia and plasma hyperviscosity also require therapy.

Nitrosourea Derivatives
Carmustine ('BCNU') and **Lomustine** ('CCNU') which is better have been used in Hodgkin's disease resistant to usual therapy. Carmustine is lipid soluble and poorly ionized so therefore crosses readily into the CSF and brain. The dose is i.v. up to 300mg/m^2 body surface. Lomustine is taken as capsules 40mg; *dose* orally up to 2mg/kg B.W. or 120-130mg/m^2 once every 6-8 weeks. **Semustine** ('Methyl CCNU') and streptozotocin are nitrosoureas.

Ethyleneimines
Thiotepa is a useful alternative to nitrogen mustard and causes less nausea and vomiting but marrow suppression can occur. *Uses* Hodgkin's disease, leukaemia, breast and ovarian cancer and malignant effusions. *Presentation* vials 15mg; to make Thiotepa Injection B.P. the contents are dissolved in Water for Injections; the solution also contains sodium chloride and sodium bicarbonate. *Dose* i.m., or i.v. 200μg/kg B.W. daily for a 5 day course and then a maintenance dose of 5-20mg weekly. For local injections into the pleural and peritoneal cavities 10-50mg in 20-60ml volume of solution is given. It is less vesicant then mustine; before local injections the effusion is almost completely aspirated.

Methane Sulphonates (Alkyl-Sulphonates)
The main example is **Busulphan** ('Myleran') used for long-term therapy against chronic myeloid leukaemia, myelofibrosis and polycythaemia rubra vera. *Presentation* Tablets B.P. 500μg and 2mg: *dose* 2-6mg orally daily (65μg/kg B.W.) until the white blood count reaches 20 000/mm^3 then a maintenance dose of 500-3000μg (3mg) is given daily. *Adverse effects* pigmentation, amenorrhoea, thrombocytopenia, and hyperuricaemia are common; cataracts and lung fibrosis are rare. Piposulfan and Treosulfan have similar uses.
Mitobronitol ('Myelobromol') chemically is a bromine derivative of mannitol, a polyhydric compound. It is used for chronic myeloid leukaemia when busulphan fails, or by some, as first therapy from the start. It is absorbed, excreted by the liver and re-absorbed. This recycling leads to high and prolonged blood levels. Excretion is also renal. *Presentation* tablets 125mg; *dose* 500mg initially then 125mg daily, or every other day so that the white cell count does not fall below 20 000/mm^3. *Adverse effects* as for busulphan; it should not be given if thrombocytopenia is present or occurs.
Pipobroman U.S.P. ('Vercyte') has also been used for myeloproliferative dis-

orders. *Presentation* tablets 10 and 25mg; *dose* initially 1-3mg/kg B.W. and later reduced to 100-200µg/kg B.W. **Hydroxyurea** ('Hydrea') is not an alkylating agent, but has been used as an alternative to busulphan. It may work by inhibiting DNA synthesis. *Presentation* capsules 500mg; *dose* 20-30mg/kg B.W. as a single dose daily or 80mg/kg B.W. every third day. **Dacarbazine** ('DTIC', imidazole carboxamide) may work as an alkylating agent or a purine antagonist. It has been used for cutaneous malignant melanoma in a daily dose of 250mg/m² i.v. for 5 days. *Presentation* vials containing powder 100 and 200mg.

ANTIMETABOLITES OR METABOLIC ANALOGUES
These disturb the formation of essential purines, and pyrimidines needed for the synthesis of DNA and RNA as well as coenzymes such as tetrahydrofolic acid needed for nucleotide synthesis. They closely resemble natural substances.

Antipurines
Mercaptopurine ('Puri-Nethol') introduced in 1952 a hypoxanthine analogue is used for acute leukaemia and for immunosuppression. *Presentation* Tablets B.P. 50mg; *dose* orally 2.5mg/kg B.W. in divided doses averaging about 100-200mg daily. *Adverse effects* marrow suppression, mouth ulcers and gastrointestinal symptoms. Mercaptopurine is metabolized by xanthine oxidase and allopurinol a xanthine oxidase blocker potentiates its action. **Azathioprine** ('Imuran') is slowly converted by the body to mercaptopurine and then metabolized into thio-inosinic acid. It is used in leukaemia and because of its sustained action to suppress auto-immune and hypersensitivity reactions and renal transplant rejection. *Presentation* Tablets B.P. 50mg; *dose* 2-5mg/kg B.W. orally. Vials containing 50mg of the freeze-dried sodium salt are available for injection. The toxicity may be increased if allopurinol is taken concurrently (as with mercaptopurine). **Thioguanine** ('Lanvis') a guanine analogue is occasionally used for acute leukaemia. *Presentation* tablets 40mg; *dose* initially 2mg/kg B.W. orally daily which may be increased to 3mg/kg B.W. after 4 weeks. *Adverse effects* marrow depression, jaundice, nausea, vomiting, anorexia, stomatitis.

Antifolates
Methotrexate Ph. Eur. (Amethopterin) is used in acute childhood leukaemia, testicular cancer and choriocarcinoma. It is bound to plasma albumin and can be displaced by salicylates and sulphonamides. *Presentation* Tablets 2.5mg., Methothrexate for B.P. injection preservative free and suitable for i.v., i.m., intrathecal and intra-arterial administration ampoules 1 and 2ml 2.5mg/ml and ampoules 1, 2 and 10ml 25mg/ml; vials containing 50mg lyophilized powder to be dissolved in 2ml Water for Injections. This contains preservative and is for i.v. use suitably diluted. Another vial is available containing 500mg for high dose without preservative. *Dose* orally 120µg/kg B.W. for 5 days then 60µg/kg B.W. An average adult dose is 2.5-7.5mg daily. The injected dose is 5-100mg i.v. or i.m. daily and 5-10mg intrathecally. In choriocarcinoma treatment is only in specialized units; 20-25mg can be given daily for short courses, or pulses or 750µg/kg B.W. is given i.m. with 300-600mg daily of mercaptopurine. Methotrexate is also prescribed for severe psoriasis, steroid resistant myopathy and dermatomyositis. For the serious, potentially fatal conditions it is at first given daily for 7-10 days, then

weekly. In osteogenic sarcoma 6 hourly i.v. infusions of doses as high as 2-7g/m² have been given, preceded by vincristine 1.5mg/m² body area and followed by calcium folinate. Methotrexate is excreted renally and large amounts may precipitate in the kidney if the urine is acid. *Adverse effects* mouth ulcers, hair loss, marrow depression, megaloblastosis, hepatic fibrosis and jaundice; intrathecal-paraplegia. Methotrexate combines with the enzyme dihydrofolate reductase so preventing synthesis of tetrahydrofolic acid which is essential for DNA synthesis. **Calcium Folinate** ('Calcium Leucovorin') is an antidote which prevents or minimizes the systemic and unwanted effects of methotrexate on normal cells without preventing the anti-tumour action ('rescue programme'). It may therefore be given concurrently. *Presentation* ampoules 1 and 10ml containing 3mg/ml; *dose* 3-21mg i.m. 6 hourly, or up to 120mg by i.v. infusion up to 12 hours when large doses of methotrexate have been given. Also available are 15mg tablets as an alternative to the injection to counteract folic acid antagonists.

Pyrimethamine is another folate antagonist (see p. 43) which has a prolonged action and so can lead to cumulation. It can be used for CNS leukaemia and is given once weekly. The adverse effects on the marrow can also be prevented by calcium folinate. An occasional use is primary·thrombocythaemia.

Antipyrimidines
Cytarabine Hydrochloride U.S.P. ('Cytosar') gives an encouraging chance of remission in acute myeloblastic leukaemia. *Presentation* vials containing 100mg and an ampoule with 5ml of solvent. *Dose* 500μg-5mg/kg B.W. daily for 10 days i.v. It has been given intrathecally 20-100mg/m². *Adverse effects* marrow failure, liver and gastro-intestinal upsets and megaloblastosis.
Fluorouracil U.S.P. ('Adrucil' in U.S.A.) is used for inoperable gastro-intestinal cancers. *Presentation* ampoules 250mg of the sodium salt in 10ml; *dose* 12-15mg/kg B.W. up to 1g daily given i.v. in 500ml of Dextrose Injection B.P. 5% delivered over a 4 hour period daily for 4 days, then half this dose for another 4 injections. A 5% cream 'Efudix' is applied for solar keratoses and skin cancers.

Anti-aminoacid
Colaspase ('Crasnitin', 'Elspar' in U.S.A.) is an enzyme isolated from *Esch. coli* called L-asparaginase which depletes tumour cells of the aminoacid asparagine. *Uses* acute lymphatic leukaemia, reticuloses. *Presentation* vials containing 10 000u; *dose* 200-1000u/kg B.W. daily for up to 28 days. The preparation is dissolved in Sodium Chloride Injection B.P. and given as an infusion. *Adverse effects* hypersensitivity, allergy, fever, chills, anaphylaxis, thrombocytopenia, bleeding, coagulation defects, urticaria, erythema, oedema, nausea, vomiting, diarrhoea, pain, anorexia, pancreatitis, proteinuria, confusion, hyperglycaemia, abnormal liver function tests.

PLANT ALKALOIDS
Two derivatives of the periwinkle have antitumour activity by interfering with the chromosomes. They are indole alkaloids.
Vinblastine Sulphate ('Velbe') *presentation* ampoules for i.v. use containing 10mg freeze-dried powder to be diluted in Water for Injections for the B.P. Injection or in 10ml Sodium Chloride Injection (B.N.F.) with a preservative which enables the reconstituted preparation to be kept. *Dose* 100-200μg/kg

B.W. weekly i.v. *Uses* reticuloses, choriocarcinoma, breast cancer.
Vincristine Sulphate ('Oncovin') *presentation* ampoules containing 1 and 5mg
with accompanying 10ml ampoule of diluent (which keeps longer), or with
Water for Injections to make the B.P. Injection. *Dose* i.v. 50-100µg/kg B.W.
weekly. *Uses* acute lymphoblastic leukaemia and Hodgkin's disease. *Adverse
effects* vincristine — prolonged therapy causes loss of tendon reflexes, proximal muscle pain, paraesthesiae, urinary retention, constipation, hoarseness,
ophthalmoplegia, which are largely reversible on stopping therapy. Vinblastine–leucopenia, thrombocytopenia. Both are painful injected extravenously.
The control of either drug requires familiarity, care and skill.

ANTIBIOTICS
These interfere with nucleic acid (RNA or DNA inhibitors).
Daunorubicin Hydrochloride (Rubidomycin, 'Cerubidin') is used for acute
myeloid leukaemia. *Presentation* vials containing 20mg of powder which is dissolved in 10-20ml of Sodium Chloride Injection and then injected into the tubing of a fast-running saline i.v. infusion. *Dose* 500µg-3mg/kg B.W. The time
between doses is 1-14 days. *Adverse effects* pain extravenously, marrow depression, cardiotoxicity which can be serious, gastro-intestinal upsets, alopecia
and pruritus.
Doxorubicin ('Adriamycin') is a hydroxylated derivative of daunorubicin. *Presentation* vials containing 10 or 50mg of freeze-dried powder with 5ml of
Water for Injections. *Dose* 400-800µg/kg B.W. daily for 3 days or
1.2-2.4mg/kg B.W. every 3 weeks is used for solid cancers and leukaemia. It
appears less toxic than daunorubicin and is now the preferred preparation.
Actinomycin D ('Cosmegen Lyovac') has been used for kidney and muscle
tumours. **Mithramycin** ('Mithracin') is tried for testicular growths, hypercalcaemia of tumour origin and to lessen pain in Paget's disease of the bone. For
the latter 15-25µg/kg B.W. is infused i.v. in 500ml of Dextrose Injection B.P.
5% over 4-6 hours, daily for 5-10 days which can be repeated in courses. Careful control is required and transient liver and renal dysfunction occur. **Bleomycin** a peptide antibiotic has been tried for squamous cell tumours (it can cause
lung fibrosis) and **Mitomycin C** for solid cancers. Mitomycin C inhibits DNA
synthesis and has an alkylating-like action. *Dose* 1-2mg i.v. daily for 3-4
weeks. **Streptozotocin** (p. 209) is used for islet cell tumours of the pancreas.

HORMONES AND ANTIHORMONES
Corticosteroids such as prednisone are used in the multi-drug regimes of
Hodgkin's disease, lymphosarcoma, leukaemia and breast cancer. They also
make patients cheerful, improve the appetite and reduce intracranial pressure
from oedema around tumours. They may help haemolytic anaemia associated
with tumours. Before the menopause women with breast cancer may be helped
by **Non-Masculinizing Androgens** (Chapter 27) and after the menopause by
Oestrogens. In carcinoma of the prostate confined to the gland, radiotherapy is
believed best and has no operative mortality. When there are bony secondaries
orchidectomy is preferred by some to oestrogen therapy, since it has no risk of
causing vascular disease or water retention. If operation is unacceptable to
patient or physician, **Oestrogens** are given initially in high dosage until the pain
is controlled and then in small maintenance doses e.g. 1-2mg of stilboestrol
daily. Larger doses are needed in resistant cases, and for these corticosteroids
are also helpful, and for any accompanying haemolytic anaemia. Radiotherapy

to the breasts before oestrogen therapy prevents gynaecomastia. Oestrogen therapy for breast or prostatic cancer may be associated initially with hypercalcaemia. **Progestogens** have been used for inoperable endometrial and renal cancers. **Drostanolone propionate** ('Masteril') and **Tamoxifen** ('Nolvadex') are believed to compete with oestrogens at receptor sites in breast cancer tissue.

Adrenal Cortex Inhibitors have been used for inoperable adrenal cancers (p. 217).

OTHER MEDICATIONS
Procarbazine Hydrochloride ('Natulan') is a monamine oxidase inhibitor and is widely used. *Presentation* capsules 50mg as procarbazine; *dose* 50-300mg daily. *Uses* reticuloses e.g. as part of quadruple therapy. *Adverse effects* marrow damage, drowsiness, antabuse effect.
Razoxane ('Razoxin') is used to treat sarcomas (with DXT) and acute myeloid leukaemia with cytarabine since the simple regime suits the elderly, infirm or those intolerant of the anthracyclines doxorubicin and daunorubicin. *Presentation* Tablets 125mg; *dose* 125mg thrice daily.
Cisplatin or *cis*-Diammine dichloroplatinum ('Neoplatin') a heavy metal derivative is expensive but very effective for testicular teratoma and ovarian carcinoma. It causes vomiting, renal damage and exfoliation of the skin.
Drug combinations have proved very effective in pulse therapy in Hodgkin's disease: the MOPP regime as per the British Lymphoma Investigation is mustine $6mg/m^2$, 'Oncovin' or vincristine sulphate $1.4mg/m^2$ both given on days 1 and 8, prednisone $25mg/m^2$ for 14 days and procarbazine $100mg/m^2$ for 10 days. Courses (e.g 6-9) are repeated at appropriate intervals. Regimes vary slightly in different centres; some use COPP where C is cyclophosphamide $800mg/m^2$ or 100 times the nitrogen mustard dose. In myeloma, melphalan and prednisone intermittently have given some benefit and have been supplemented by procarbazine, doxorubicin and the nitrosoureas, but results do not match those in Hodgkin's disease. In lymphosarcoma cyclophosphamide $600mg/m^2$ (day 1 and 8), vincristine $1.4mg/m^2$ (day 1 and 8 max. 2mg), prednisone $50mg/m^2$ (day 1 and 8) repeated every 2 weeks for a minimum of 6 courses and 3 courses after remission may be used. Not all combination therapy is additive, some may be antagonistic. **Isotopes** are used in thyroid cancer and polycythaemia rubra vera.
Palliation. Antibiotics, anti-emetics, tranquillizers, antidepressives, analgesics and hypnotics are all required at times. At first, simple analgesics are tried, later morphine or diamorphine (heroin) in Britain. Analgesics are taken prophylactically to forestall pain. Diamorphine and Cocaine Elixir B.P.C., or the same mixture with chlorpromazine added, may be valuable. Human contact and words may be as important as drugs. **Nutrition,** adequate nutrition orally or even total parenteral nutrition improves the response to anticancer therapy.

NON-MALIGNANT DISEASE
Suppression of non-malignant disease by cytotoxic therapy is being widely used. There are many risks to this therapy such as infection, marrow depression and the emergence of tumours so only serious illness should be treated. They include auto-immune diseases like idiopathic thrombocytopenia, and haemolytic anaemia, the connective tissue disorders lupus erythematosus,

dermatomyositis, and rheumatoid arthritis; biliary cirrhosis, chronic active hepatitis, the nephrotic syndrome, Wegener's granulomatosis, ulcerative colitis, Crohn's disease, polyneuropathy, myopathy, pemphigus vulgaris and severe psoriasis; in the latter methotrexate has been widely used, but liver damage has to be watched for. Cyclophosphamide and azathioprine are usually employed, though sterility is seen more with cyclophosphamide. Their use may reduce the need for corticosteroids, or cytotoxics may be tried when steroids fail. (Immunosuppression is a feature of many other drugs.)

10 ALLERGY, INFLAMMATION AND ANTIHISTAMINES

ALLERGY

This is defined as a specifically altered state of body hypersensitivity following exposure to an allergen, or antigen, which may be carbohydrate, protein or other complex chemical found in drugs, sera, vaccines, house dust, animal and vegetable proteins, pollens, furs, bacteria, protozoa, worms, insects (stings) and snake venom as well as in industrial, cosmetic and food additive chemicals. Allergens may be eaten, inhaled, injected or contact the skin. The body in response to an antigen produces antibodies and cells become sensitized. Allergic reactions are more common with a personal or family history of asthma, allergic purpura, angioneurotic oedema, hay fever, eczema or migraine. Reactions are particularly likely if the person has previously reacted abnormally to a drug. Allergic responses may involve the liver, lungs, blood, heart or brain, or the skin. They vary from mild episodes to life-threatening or even fatal attacks.

Four abnormal responses are described.

(1) **Anaphylaxis** (see below) which may be produced by penicillin, foreign sera, insect bites and contrast media. The antibody concerned is IgE.

(2) **Antigen on cell surface** (cytotoxic reactions) as when drugs attach themselves to the blood cells or platelets causing haemolysis, thrombocytopenia or agranulocytosis. Examples are incompatible blood transfusions and the drugs quinine, phenacetin. PAS, and penicillin. The antibodies involved are IgG and IgM.

(3) **Serum sickness reaction** with complexes of antigen and antibody in varying strengths (immune complex reactions) leading to lymphadenitis, small vessel damage, fever, arthritis, urticaria and splenomegaly.

(4) **Delayed hypersensitivity** of lymphocyte cells, a reaction to heavy metals and organic chemicals and not mediated by antibody.

Anaphylactic Reactions (Type 1)

These may arise within minutes of taking drugs like penicillin or foreign proteins such as horse sera, particularly if injected, but oral medication with aspirin or even inhalation may produce them. The manifestations are flushing, urticaria, cyanosis, wheeze, chest constriction, hypotension, coma, convulsions and at times death. A minor form is pollenosis or hay fever. The chemical mediators of allergic Type 1 responses include histamine and other substances released from mast cells and tissues (serotonin, bradykinin, slow releasing substances and prostaglandins).

Treatment of Allergy

The most effective inhibitor of Type 1 reaction is adrenaline which acts by a different mechanism from the antihistamines.It is a valuable first-aid remedy for the allergic reactions in asthma, serum sickness (p. 59), drug sensitivity, angioneurotic oedema and anaphylaxis. *Presentation* Adrenaline Injection B.P. ampoules 0.5 and 1ml of a solution in Water for Injections of adrenaline acid tartrate equivalent to a concentration of 1:1000 or 1mg/ml; *dose* 0.2-1ml s.c. or i.m. and in circulatory failure i.v. or intra-cardiac. Adrenaline may also

71

be inhaled as a first-aid measure. In patients with angioneurotic oedema of tongue, pharynx and glottis, airway obstruction may need immediate relief by tracheostomy so a tube should be at hand. Intravenous adrenaline is very hazardous causing hypertension, cardiac arrhythmias and death, and so is only given for extreme anaphylaxis.

In **anaphylactic shock** other measures such as oxygen, i.v. hydrocortisone and i.v. or i.m. antihistamines such as chlorpheniramine, diphenhydramine, mepyramine or promethazine are given, but antihistamines may by their sedative action cause a patient to become drowsy, or go to sleep with decrease in ventilation. The airway must be ensured and assisted ventilation performed. Fluid is lost into capillaries so this should be replaced i.v. and if this does not restore the blood pressure a vasoconstrictor is given such as metaraminol. Immediate measures include lying the patient flat, or head down. All the necessary drugs should be available when a procedure or drug liable to cause anaphylaxis is given.

Sympathomimetic or adrenaline-like drugs such as isoprenaline or ephedrine are used as alternatives to adrenaline when there is less urgency, as in allergic asthma, hay fever or urticaria.

Corticosteroids are of value for Types 1-4 actions. In particular i.v. hydrocortisone is valuable for acute conditions such as anaphylaxis, status asthmaticus, angioneurotic oedema and the toxic effects of absorbed dead worm protein in helminthic infestation.

Prophylactic measures. If reactions to a drug have occurred once it should not be given again unless it is vital as in tuberculosis. If an allergic response is feared with blood tranfusion, preliminary sympathomimetics, antihistamines and accompanying corticosteroids can be tried. Desensitization may be employed against animal furs, pollens and house dusts. Reaginic antibody (IgE) is made by lymphoid tissue and plasma cells in the bronchial and intestinal mucosa, and is produced by contact with allergens. However, if injected in the skin allergens tend to promote IgG antibody formation which has a higher affinity than IgE for antigen and acts as a blocking antibody thereby desensitizing the patient.

Disodium Cromoglycate (p. 171) can inhibit the release of histamine from mast cells given before exposure to the antigen, so it is used as a prophylactic.

Histamine constricts smooth muscle and dilates arterioles and capillaries. The capillaries leak and the tissue fluid forms a wheal. Histamine stimulates the stomach to secrete extra acid, and the adrenal medulla to produce adrenaline and noradrenaline. Large injected doses can be harmful. Many drugs are histamine liberators e.g. morphine. *Presentation* **Histamine Acid Phosphate Injection B.P.** ampoules 1ml containing 1mg as a solution in Water for Injections; *dose* $10\mu g/kg$ B.W. usually $500\mu g$-1mg s.c. Histamine was used to measure maximum gastric acidity after an augmented dose of $40\mu g/kg$ B.W., preceded by 100mg mepyramine maleate i.m. 20 minutes beforehand, to counteract its systemic effects. *Adverse effects* can occur such as flushing, headaches, fainting, hypotension, bronchoconstriction and rarely death. Safer and more effective tests are now available. **Ametazole Hydrochloride** (Betazole) is an histamine analogue. The solution keeps well unrefrigerated. *Dose* $500\mu g$-2mg/kg B.W. i.m., or s.c. *Adverse effects* flushing and headache are common. The synthetic pentapeptide **Pentagastrin** ('Peptavlon') is made up of 5 aminoacids which are part of the natural hormone gastrin and act like it. *Presentation* Pentagastrin Injection B.P. ampoules 2ml containing in solution

$500\mu g$; *dose* $6\mu g/kg$ B.W. as a single dose s.c., or i.m. *Adverse effects* nausea, retching, faintness and hypotension.

Since histamine stimulates receptors in the stomach which cannot be blocked by conventional antihistamines, receptors have been divided into H_1 and H_2 (in stomach) and recently substances which prevent histamine-induced gastric acid secretion such as **Cimetidine** have been introduced (H_2 blockers).

Anti-inflammatory drugs such as salicylates, phenylbutazone, indomethacin and chloroquine, some phenothiazines and gold have a mild suppressive effect in Type 1-4 reactions, antilymphocyte serum in Types 3 and 4, and cytotoxic agents in Type 4. Antihistamines are Type 1 inhibitors.

ANTIHISTAMINES (H_1 Blockers)

These are varied chemically but can be regarded as amine derivatives such as ethylamine, benzylamine, amino-alkyl ethers, ethylenediamines and certain phenothiazines. The research in France on antihistamines led to the discovery of the phenothiazines. In addition to opposing the harmful systemic actions of histamine,

(1) they *cause CNS depression* and hence are hypnotics making the subject drowsy. Some are less soporific than others;

(2) they are *anticholinergic* and produce dryness of mouth like atropine;

(3) they are *anti-adrenaline* and lower the blood pressure;

(4) they act *against serotonin.*

Uses. They are most helpful for allergic skin ailments like urticaria, and angioneurotic oedema. They are also prescribed as anti-emetics and some for Parkinsonism, including the control of acute drug-induced dystonia. They may help in drug skin reactions, insect bites, allergic asthma, vasomotor rhinitis, hay fever and nocturnal cough in children. Because of sedation they are useful sedatives, hypnotics, antipruritics, premedicants, and ingredients of chemical 'cocktails' for inducing sleep or anaesthesia during operative procedures.

Antihistamines are best avoided in pilots, car drivers, those in charge of machinery and when drinking alcohol. Injectable antihistamines are used for allergic emergencies, anaesthetic purposes and premedication. A few are listed in Table 1 (p. 74).

Oral Antihistamines

Many are available as syrups or elixirs e.g. the B.P.C. Elixirs of Chlorpheniramine, Diphenhydramine, Promethazine and Trimeprazine, tablets or capsules, both in short and long-acting forms. There is little to choose between the varieties, some of which are included in Table 2. **Diphenhydramine Hydrochloride B.P.** is soporific which at times is advantageous if insomnia exists, at other times, a less sedative form such as **Phenindamine Tartrate** is tried. For children **Brompheniramine Maleate U.S.N.F.** as the Elixir 2mg/5ml at a dose of 2-4mg at night is suitable for the treatment of pruritus. A widely used long-acting preparation is **Promethazine Hydrochloride Ph. Eur., B.P.** but **chemically it is a phenothiazine** and is capable, though rarely, of causing a similar type of jaundice to chlorpromazine and it should not be the antihistamine (nor should trimeprazine tartrate) used for itching in phenothiazine-induced liver disease. Here corticosteroids and cholestyramine should be tried if itching persists after withdrawal of the phenothiazine. *Adverse effects* rashes, blurred vision, drowsiness, dizziness, nausea, dry mouth, convulsions in children.

Application of antihistamines on the skin is not advised because of sensitivity: for itching calamine lotion and liquor picis carb 2% in emulsifying ointments or 'Eurax', with or without hydrocortisone, are better.

TABLE 1
SOME INJECTABLE ANTIHISTAMINES (I.M. OR I.V.)

Name Approved	Proprietary	Container	Strength mg/ml	Dose (mg)
Chlorpheniramine Maleate B.P.	'Piriton'	ampoule 1 ml	10	10-20
Cyclizine Lactate	'Valoid'	,, ,,	50	50
Dimenhydrinate B.P.	'Dramamine'	,, ,,	50	50-100
Mepyramine Maleate B.P.	'Anthisan'	2ml	25	25-100
Promethazine Hydrochloride B.P.	'Phenergan'	,, 1 and 2ml	25	25-50

TABLE 2
ORAL ANTIHISTAMINES

Name		
Approved	Proprietary	Tablets (mg)
Short-acting given three or more times daily		
Brompheniramine Maleate U.S.N.F.	'Dimotane'	4
Chlorpheniramine Maleate B.P.	'Haynon'	4
	'Piriton'	
Cinnarizine	'Stugeron'	15
Cyclizine Hydrochloride B.P.	'Valoid'	50
	'Marzine'	
Cyproheptadine Hydrochloride B.P.	'Periactin'	4
Dimenhydrinate B.P.	'Dramamine'	50
Diphenhydramine Hydrochloride B.P.	'Benadryl'	Capsules 25
	'Histergan'	25 and 50
Mebhydrolin Napadisylate B.P.C.	'Fabahistin'	50
Mepyramine Maleate B.P.	'Anthisan'	50 and 100
Phenindamine Tartrate B.P.	'Thephorin'	25
Trimeprazine Tartrate B.P.	'Vallergan'	10
		(premedication in children)
Triprolidine Hydrochloride B.P.	'Actidil'	2.5
Long-acting given once or twice daily		
Clemastine Fumarate	'Tavegil'	1
Diphenylpyraline Hydrochloride B.P.	'Histryl'	5 and Capsule
	'Lergoban'	2.5 and 5mg
Meclozine Hydrochloride B.P.	'Ancoloxin'	25
		(anti-emetic)
Pheniramine Maleate	'Daneral-S.A.'	75
Promethazine Hydrochloride B.P.	'Phenergan'	10 and 25
Promethazine Theoclate B.P.	'Avomine'	25
		(anti-emetic) travel sickness

11   CORTICOSTEROIDS

The steroid hormones of the adrenal cortex comprise:
(1) **Glucocorticoids** which are largely concerned with carbohydrate and protein metabolism, but also with sodium and water metabolism. The natural hormone is hydrocortisone. The resting adrenals produce 30mg daily, but after stress (trauma, infection) as much as 300mg.
(2) **Mineralocorticoids** which are concerned mainly with electrolyte balance. The natural hormone is aldosterone.
(3) **Sex-hormones** androgens and oestrogens present in both sexes.

GLUCOCORTICOIDS IN CLINICAL USE
These are listed in Table 3. They constitute one of the greatest advances in recent times. Commercially they may be made from vegetable steroids such as hecogenin derived from East African sisal waste. The choice of the natural, and of the synthetic, steroids is influenced by cost, safety, adverse effects, effectiveness and how familiar the doctor is with their individual actions.

TABLE 3
CURRENT GLUCOCORTICOIDS

	Oral Equivalents	Route				
		Oral	i.m.	i.v.	Joints	Topical
Cortisone	25	+	+			+
Hydrocortisone	20	+	+	+	+	+
Prednisone	5	+				
Prednisolone	5	+	+	+	+	+
Methyl-prednisolone	4	+	+	+	+	+
Triamcinolone	4	+	+		+	+
Dexamethasone	0.75	+	+	+	+	+
Betamethasone	0.75	+	+	+	+	+
Paramethasone	2	+				

Dosage
(1) *Small or physiological doses* are effective in Addison's disease and hypopituitarism, in amounts equal to that normally produced. The amount and timing should allow for the diurnal swings in plasma levels (high in the morning, low at midnight). Similar doses are given to suppress congenital adrenal hyperplasia.
(2) *Large or pharmacological doses* are used to suppress non-endocrine disease. In fatal disease there is no limit to the dose. For persistent, crippling, illnesses the smallest amount which makes life tolerable is given. Corticosteroids in these amounts benefit the patient by:
 (i) suppressing inflammatory and allergic reactions. They are the most powerful anti-inflammatory agents known,
 (ii) reducing antibody formation. Corticosteroids modify all four types of immune response especially Type III (see p. 71),
 (iii) atrophying, or lympholytic action on lymphatic tissue,
 (iv) stabilizing membrane permeability.

Before giving corticosteroids several questions have to be posed:
(1) Have less dangerous drugs failed?
(2) Are there any contra-indications to their use?
(3) Will the patient die without them?

Administration can be oral, i.m., i.v., intra-articular and topical on skin, eyes, mouth, rectum, colon and respiratory tract. Intra-articular and oral preparations are usually prepared as acetates. For quick emergency use the water soluble phosphate and succinate compounds are given.

Current Glucocorticoids
Hydrocortisone Ph. Eur., U.S.P. (Cortisol) is available for oral use in U.K. as 10 and 20mg tablets ('Hydrocortistab', 'Hydrocortone') and is used mainly instead of cortisone in Addison's disease as it is absorbed better (which can be checked by measuring plasma levels) although its half-life is less. *Dose* orally 20-80mg daily. Injections i.v. or i.m. are given before and after operations in patients taking, or who recently have taken oral steroids. When speed is essential the route is i.v. as in the hypoadrenalism of Addison's disease, in myxoedema coma, and in hypopituitary failure and also when large pharmacological amounts are needed as in status asthmaticus, allergic emergencies, shock and certain overwhelming infections. In the post-operative patient i.m. hydrocortisone is preferable as it lasts longer than i.v. injection. Hydrocortisone is also injected into joints. *Presentation* **Hydrocortisone Acetate Injection B.P.** a suspension in Water for Injections (and other stabilizers 'Hydrocortistab') for intra-articular use vials 5ml 25mg/ml; *dose* 5-50mg. **Hydrocortisone Sodium Succinate Injection B.P.** vials equivalent to 100mg hydrocortisone ('Efcortelan', 'Solu-Cortef') the contents of which are dissolved in Water for Injections, or the ready-prepared **Hydrocortisone Sodium Phosphate Injection B.P.C.** equivalent to 100mg of hydrocortisone in 1 and 5ml ampoules ('Efcortisol'); *dose* 100-500mg i.m., or i.v. Injected i.v. paraesthesiae may occasionally occur. For topical use lozenges, ointments, creams, solution tablets for enemas, suppositories 25mg B.P.C., lotions and eye drops 1% are available.
Prednisolone and **Prednisone Ph. Eur.** which is hydroxylated in the body to prednisolone are popular, cheap and interfere little with sodium and water

metabolism, but gastro-intestinal symptoms do occur. They are usually taken orally. *Presentation* Tablets B.P. 1 and 5mg as prednisone, prednisolone or their acetate compounds in many proprietary forms and also enteric coated tablets 2.5 and 5mg of prednisolone ('Deltacortril Enteric'). *Dose* 10-100mg orally in divided amounts. Injections Prednisolone Sodium Phosphate B.P. ('Codelsol') vials 2ml 16mg/ml for i.v. or i.m. use; *dose* 16-80mg. Preparations for intra-articular use are prednisolone butylacetate Prednisolone Pivalate B.P. ('Ultracortenol') and Prednisolone Acetate (B.P. 1963; 'Deltastab'). Prednisolone Sodium Phosphate Enema B.P.C. is a buffered solution ('Predsol') containing 20mg in 100ml; 'Predsol' eye drops and suppositories are also available.

Prednisolone Steaglate ('Sintisone') *presentation* tablets 6.65mg is claimed to cause less carbohydrate and electrolyte disturbance than the parent base.

Cortisone Acetate Ph. Eur. is used mainly for replacement therapy in Addison's disease and hypopituitarism. It has to be changed in the liver to hydrocortisone to work. Injected i.m. it has been used to cover operations in patients previously on corticosteroids especially as it was economical. It causes sodium retention and potassium excretion. *Presentation* Tablets B.P. 5 and 25mg, Injection B.P. suspension in Water for Injections vials 10ml 25mg/ml ('Cortelan', 'Cortistab', 'Cortisyl'). *Dose* 37.5-500mg daily in 3 divided amounts orally, or i.m. Eye drops 1% and eye ointment 1% ('Cortistab') are also available.

Methylprednisolone ('Medrone') *presentation* Tablets B.P. 2, 4 and 16mg, capsules 4mg; *dose* 12-40mg daily initially then reduced to a maintenance dose. As the **Acetate B.P.** and 'Depot-Medrone' vials are available 1, 2 and 5ml, and 2ml disposable syringes 40mg/ml for i.m. and intra-articular use. **Methylprednisolone Sodium Succinate** ('Solu-Medrone') vials 40, 125, 500 and 1000mg as powder with accompanying solvent for i.m. or i.v. use. *Dose* according to severity of illness 0.5-30mg/kg B.W. daily. The larger doses are best given slowly (at least over 10 min) i.v., or by i.v. infusion in dextrose or saline.

Fluorinated Corticosteroids

Triamcinolone ('Adcortyl', 'Aristocort', 'Ledercort') has the advantage that it causes no salt retention nor weight gain since it suppresses appetite. *Presentation* Tablets B.P.C. 1, 2 and 4mg; *dose* 8-20mg in divided amounts reduced to a maintenance dose. Injectable forms for intra-articular use are triamcinolone acetonide sterile aqueous suspension 10mg/ml 5ml vials ('Adcortyl') and 'Lederspan' which is a suspension of triamcinolone hexacetonide relatively insoluble in vials 1 and 5ml 20mg/ml (and 5mg/ml for intradermal use). For systemic use 1 and 2ml disposable syringes 40mg/ml of triamcinolone acetonide ('Kenalog') are available; *dose* 40-100mg deeply i.m. for adults. *Adverse effects* headache, flushing after food, muscle weakness are features of fluorinated compounds. Triamcinolone Acetonide B.P. is also used on the skin (avoid the face).

Dexamethasone Ph. Eur. ('Decadron', 'Deronil', 'DexaCortisyl', Millicorten', 'Oradexon') *presentation* Tablets B.P. 500 and 750µg and 2mg; *dose* 500µg-10mg averaging 1-3mg initially and maintaining at 500-750µg daily. This steroid has a long half-life and is potent in small amounts. It is used for ACTH suppression tests as it does not affect the estimation of urinary steroids and also for some patients with Addison's disease who are excessively pigmented from high ACTH levels during the night and which may be suppressed by a midnight dose (e.g. 250-500µg). Injections: Dexamethasone Sodium Phosphate B.P vials 2ml 4mg/ml ('Decadron Injection') given i.v. or i.m. 4-20mg, or intra-articular 1-4mg ampoules 1ml 5mg/ml ('Oradexon'), and vials 5ml 20mg/ml ('Decadron Shock-Pak'); *dose* 2-6mg/kg B.W. as a single injection. Intraven-ous dexamethasone is widely used in hospital practice for cerebral oedema associated with coma in cerebral or malignant malaria, trauma, tumours and after neurosurgical operations. For tumours oral administration is given for long-term use. The massive i.v. doses are used for cardiogenic and bacteraemic shock, along with other measures. Massive doses cause vasodilatation, diuresis and potassium loss. Conventional doses may stimulate the appetite.

Betamethasone Ph. Eur. ('Betnelan') is poorly soluble, in contrast to betamethasone sodium phosphate ('Betnesol'). Betamethasone is given once or twice daily, is quickly absorbed and is reasonably priced. *Presentation* Tab-lets Betamethasone B.P. 500μg and Betamethasone Sodium Phosphate B.P. 500μg and Betamethasone Sodium Phosphate Injection B.P. ampoules 1ml 4mg/ml as betamethasone for i.v. and i.m. use. Betamethasone 100μg pellets are available for buccal use as are drops for local application and Betamethasone Valerate B.P. for suppositories and skin creams, lotions and ointments 0.1%. *Dose* orally 3-5mg initially in divided doses decreasing to 500μg-1.5mg daily; i.v. 4-20mg 6 or 8 hourly for the treatment of acute aller-gic reactions, asthma and shock.

Paramethasone Acetate U.S.N.F. ('Metilar') *presentation* tablets 2mg; *dose* 2-12mg initially then 1.5-4mg daily. This finds little or no use in the U.K.

Diseases for which glucocorticoids have been prescribed though they may not be the first or best measures are listed in Table 4 (p. 80).

Supervision
Patients should have a card naming the preparation and dose and be told not to stop therapy suddenly on their own. At times of 'stress' (trauma, infection, operation, hot weather) the dose may need increasing. Infection is a common cause of death in patients on long-term steroids and overdosage leads to iatrogenic Cushing's syndrome. Withdrawal of steroids: when the course has been short the drug can be stopped forthwith, or by reducing prednisone by 2.5mg (or the equivalent for other steroids) every third day. For those who have taken steroids for months or years a suggested regime is to reduce by 1mg every month. If adrenal atrophy is suspected ACTH injections may be given. If afterwards the ability of the adrenals to respond to 'stress' is in doubt, oral or injected corticosteroids may be required at such times.

Surgery For minor operations a single i.v. dose of hydrocortisone may suffice. For major surgery 100mg 6 hourly for 48 hours is needed. Given i.v. hydrocor-tisone has an action of an hour or so and therefore i.m. injections which last 6 hours are better. There are no simple screening tests which can tell whether a patient who has had steroids in the past will have normally reacting adrenal glands. *Adverse effects* are likely with any glucocorticoid listed and at any age. Pre-existing disease such as malabsorption may make patients relatively resis-tant to their action and hypoalbuminaemia by reducing corticosteroid binding, may lead to high levels of free or unbound steroids with greater risk of toxicity and adverse effects. Since they potentiate catecholamines they may cause increased hypertension in patients with phaeochromocytoma.

TABLE 4
INDICATIONS FOR GLUCOCORTICOIDS

System	Diseases
Alimentary	Ulcerative colitis, chronic active hepatitis, prolonged cholestatic jaundice after viral hepatitis, gluten unresponsive coeliac disease, Crohn's disease.
Blood	Acute haemolytic anaemia, idiopathic thrombocytopenia, acute leukaemia, allergic purpura.
Cardiovascular	Severe rheumatic pancarditis, heart block after cardiac infarction, benign pericarditis, shock.
Connective Tissue	Lupus erythematosus, polyarteritis nodosa, temporal arteritis, polymyalgia rheumatica, scleroderma.
Endocrine	Adrenalectomy, Addison's disease, hypopituitarism, adrenal hyperplasia, acute thyroiditis, severe exophthalmic Grave's disease.
Eyes	Iritis.
Infections	Occasionally in severe typhoid, tuberculosis, influenza, meningococcal and other Gram-negative bacteraemias, anginose infectious mononucleosis.
Malignancy	Reticuloses, certain cancers e.g. breast.
Metabolic	Sarcoid and drug-induced hypercalcaemia.
Nervous	Acute polyneuritis, encephalopathy, Bell's palsy, demyelinating disorders, cerebral oedema, myasthenia gravis, petit mal status, hypsarrhythmia, intracranial metastases.
Renal	Nephrotic syndrome, retroperitoneal fibrosis, transplantation.
Respiratory	Bronchial asthma, status asthmaticus, sarcoidosis, histiocytosis, farmer's lung, diffuse fibrosis, pulmonary eosinophilia, chemical and toxic inhalations, radiation pneumonitis, stomach acid inhalation, allergic obstruction of airway.
Sensitivity reactions	Allergies to drugs, serum, worms, anaphylaxis, angioneurotic oedema, to prevent Herxheimer reactions.
Skin	Pemphigus, sarcoidosis, dermatomyositis, Stevens-Johnson syndrome, widespread lichen planus, severe eczema, exfoliative dermatitis, erythema multiforme.

MAJOR COMPLICATIONS OF SYSTEMIC STEROID THERAPY

Adrenal suppression or insufficiency

This varies with dose and duration of therapy, and is due to depression of the hypothalmic-pituitary-adrenal axis. Accurate documentation of steroid used, doses and dates is important. In therapy short courses at the lowest dose feasible are employed. Morning doses and alternate day therapy have been tried. Long-term therapy with ACTH may cause less adrenal suppression on withdrawal than corticosteroids. While there is a theoretical risk for a number of years of an inadequate adrenal response in practice this is only a problem for 6 months after ceasing therapy. In patients on corticosteroids undergoing operations, or unable to swallow, parenteral therapy is prescribed.

Gastro-intestinal

Dyspepsia, haemorrhage and perforation of peptic ulcer or intestines can occur. The risk is reduced by avoiding high doses when possible and by not giving other ulcerogenic drugs concurrently (e.g. aspirin). Enteric-coated corticosteroids and antacid therapy have been tried. If symptoms occur a barium meal is performed. Should a peptic ulcer be present and steroid therapy is essential then gastric surgery may have to be performed though nowadays reduction of acid by cimetidine would be tried.

Infection

It has been said that a quarter of patients on long-term therapy die of infection which may be by exotic organisms such as fungi. Tuberculosis may be reactivated so a chest X-ray should be performed before and during therapy every 6 months. Anti-tuberculosis therapy is advised if old lesions are present. Other infections are bacteraemia, candidosis and septic arthritis. In immigrants strongyloides and amoebic infections can become severe and invasive. Vaccination is contra-indicated with living viruses and patients should be kept away from those with chickenpox or herpes zoster.

Masking of Diagnosis

Symptoms and signs may be suppressed so diagnosis can be difficult. Peptic ulcers, or diverticulitis may perforate in a silent manner and pyogenic infections may occur with the patient feeling deceptively well and afebrile.

Iatrogenic Cushing's syndrome

The skin becomes atrophic, paper thin, transparent, easily bruised, with fluid retention, striae, buffalo hump, hypertension, and an increased risk of arterial and venous thrombosis.

Skeletal

Spinal osteoporosis, vertebral collapse, crush fractures, kyphosis and height loss can occur. A lateral X-ray of the spine during and before therapy (for control of bone density) is helpful. A high calcium diet and anabolic steroids may give marginal benefit. Osteoporosis is more likely in the elderly, the immobilized and those with rheumatoid arthritis. Suppression of growth in children occurs with corticosteroids, but not with ACTH. Charcot's neurogenic arthropathy can occur, particularly in the hips with systemic therapy or after local injection and avascular necrosis with systemic steroids.

Metabolic
Fluid and sodium retention and potassium loss is less common with modern steroids and potassium supplements are rarely necessary. Hyperlipidaemia, with increase in cholesterol, triglycerides and phospholipids, and xanthelasma, can occur as well as diabetes mellitus. Therefore urine and blood analyses at intervals are indicated, and dietary control supplemented at times by oral hypoglycaemic agents. The frequency of hypertension increases so the pressure should be taken before and during therapy.

Mental
Mental disturbances, psychosis, mania, depression, paranoia and suicide may occur. When practicable, steroid therapy is stopped, but in life-threatening situations it may have to be continued. Moreover, in mental hospitals steroids are prescribed but under close medical control.

Ocular
While a raised ocular pressure occurs mainly with drops, it can occur after systemic therapy. Ocular hypertension can be due to an irreversible open-angle glaucoma, or can in some be controlled with miotic eye drops, or possibly by a change in steroid. There may be a genetic or familial predisposition. Posterior polar cataracts are noted after long-term therapy so the rule should be to examine ophthalmologically all patients in this category.

Minor Complications
Amenorrhoea, moon face, bruising (half the patients), striae, acne, hypertrichosis, insomnia, nocturia, increased appetite and weight gain are common. Triamcinolone does not cause increased appetite.

Rarer Complications
Muscle weakness or myopathy is seen with the fluorinated steroids triamcinolone and dexamethasone. Raised intracranial pressure, convulsions, withdrawal symptoms (anorexia, fever, tiredness, muscle pain, arthralgia and arthropathy which may be lessened by gradual reduction after long use), self-prescription and addiction to steroids which are euphoric to some; pancreatitis and hypothermia are occasionally noted.

TOPICAL CORTICOSTEROIDS
These are thinly applied 6-8 hourly. Suitable amounts are 15g for hand eczema, 100g for widespread eczema and 30ml for scalp lotions. For the hair and moist lesions, lotions, creams or gels are appropriate, but for dry lesions ointments are preferred. Topical steroids are widely used and are only contraindicated in the presence of undiagnosed lesions or infection, or when a more suitable alternative is available. For infective conditions antibiotics or antiseptics are added. Corticosteroids in lotions and creams are well absorbed and penetrate the skin even when there is oozing. Sprays have no special advantage. Steroid potency is increased by fluorination, or the formation of esters or acetonides.

Indications
(1) Eczema, dermatitis, neurodermatitis. Hydrocortisone 0.5-2.5% is suitable and fluorinated steroids should be avoided on the face and in children.
(2) Psoriasis. Here diluted fluorinated steroids sparingly applied with occlu-

sion (Haelan tape occlusion) are prescribed. Relapse may be rapid and severe with pustular and exfoliative lesions. Results are best on the palms and soles.
(3) Localized pruritus ani and vulvae and lichen simplex.
(4) Very potent steroids such as fluocinolone acetonide are used in discoid lupus erythematosus, granuloma annulare, and necrobiosis lipoidica.
B.P.C. Preparations are:
Betamethasone Valerate Ointment, Cream, Lotion 0.1%,
Hydrocortisone Cream, Lotion and Ointment all 1%,
Hydrocortisone Acetate Cream, Lotion and Ointment all 1%,
Fluocinolone Acetonide Ointment and Cream 0.01 and 0.025% and 0.2% ('Synalar', 'Synandone'),
Triamcinolone Acetonide Cream and Ointment 0.01, 0.025 and 0.1% and Lotion 0.1%.

There are many brands of ointments and creams usually in 5, 10 or 15g amounts. Newer preparations are:
Beclomethasone Dipropionate B.P. 0.025% as a Cream, Lotion and Ointment or 0.5% Cream ('Propaderm'), and Fluocortolone Hexanoate and Pivalate B.P. ('Ultralanum'), and hydrocortisone butyrate ('Locoid') cream and ointment. 'Alphaderm' is 1% hydrocortisone with urea. The urea facilitates steroid absorption. Hydrocortisone Ointment B.P. is available as 0.5, 1 and 2.5% strengths. 'Dioderm' is a cream containing hydrocortisone 0.1%.

Adverse effects
With increasing use the disadvantages of topical steroids have become apparent.
(1) Sensitivity to constituents which may be antibiotics neomycin, framycetin, kanamycin, polymyxin, gentamicin, clioquinol, chloramphenicol, or lanolin, local anaesthetics or paraben.
(2) Local application leading to dermal atrophy, striae, purpura, poor scars, telangiectasia, glossy skin appearance.
(3) Potentiation of lesions such as gravitational ulcers.
(4) Lowered resistance to infections — folliculitis, *Candida albicans*, scabies.
(5) Potentiation and masking — ringworm infection 'Tinea incognito', Herpes simplex and impetigo.
(6) Rebound reactions in rosacea and psoriasis.
(7) Local hirsuties.
(8) Suppression of pituitary-adrenal axis in children. This is of no significance in adults. Hydrocortisone 1% or diluted to 0.5% causes little suppression and is best for routine maintenance. Fluorinated compounds should be avoided on the face, or used only in small amounts or for a short time. Polythene occlusion is a potent method of increasing absorption through the skin. Inhaled corticosteroids can cause pituitary-adrenal suppression.

STEROIDS AND THE EYE
Steroids suppress disease and can be used topically in allergic reactions from cosmetics, drugs, pollens, non-infective conjunctivitis, and certain forms of keratitis, iritis and iridocyclitis. They are not used in infective disorders alone, nor for dendritic ulcers or glaucoma. Antibiotics may be combined. Corticosteroid drops used continually may induce glaucoma and cataracts.

12 DIURETICS

The glomeruli filter the plasma, and the tubules under enzyme and hormonal control extract fluid and sodium and excrete potassium and hydrogen ions. Thereby the body fluids are kept at near constant osmotic, hydrogen ion, electrolyte and water levels. In oedematous states there is an excess of body sodium and salt-retaining hormone. Fluid retention is a feature of cardiac, renal, hepatic and endocrine disease, pregnancy and some drug therapies including i.v. sodium chloride and sodium bicarbonate.

Diuretics help the kidneys dispose of surplus sodium and water. They act in different ways and at different parts of the nephron. In 1938 sulphanilamide was found to have diuretic actions and in 1950 acetazolamide, a sulphonamide and one of the first orally active diuretics, was introduced, followed shortly by dichlorphenamide. These inhibited the enzyme carbonic acid anhydrase which combines carbon dioxide with water. The thiazides were found in a search for stronger carbonic acid anhydrase inhibitors. The first, chlorothiazide, was introduced in 1957. Since then the organomercurials have become virtually obsolete. Further sulphonamide derivatives — other thiazides, bumetanide and metolazone — have been introduced.

Diuresis, or increased urinary flow, can be achieved by
(1) *sodium diuretics* (natriuretics) which prevent the resorption of sodium and water or by interfering with chloride transport (and not sodium primarily as previously thought) in the cortical diluting segment like the thiazides, or the ascending loop of Henle like frusemide, bumetanide and ethacrynic acid (Figure 2).

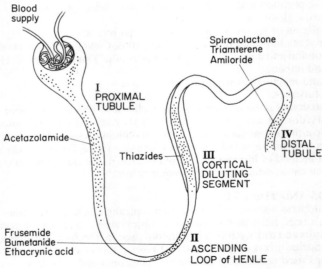

Fig.2
The nephron and four sites of action of diuretics

(2) by blocking the action of aldosterone on the distal renal tubule as with spironolactone, or preventing the same potassium for sodium exchange by direct tubular action using triamterene or amiloride;
(3) sodium excretion can also be achieved indirectly by improving cardiac function and hence glomerular flow with digitalis glycosides.

Osmotic diuretics take with them on renal excretion a corresponding amount of fluid in which they are dissolved (e.g. mannitol). Water, or other fluid, causes an increased urinary flow, but not of sodium. *Water therapy* is used to promote drug excretion, to dilute urinary crystal concentration in gout, sulphonamide therapy and cystinuria, or to reduce chemical irritation with cyclophosphamide in the bladder and analgesic levels in the renal pelves.

The control of oedema is helped by bed rest which increases glomerular flow and helps congestive failure and pregnancy toxaemia. Strict sodium restriction is only of major importance when treating unresponsive ascites in cirrhosis, refractory cardiac failure or acute glomerular nephritis. Low sodium diets are tasteless, unpopular, unappetizing and since the advent of diuretics are infrequently prescribed. Diuretics have reduced the need to remove fluid mechanically, but in severe breathlessness aspiration of a pleural effusion is helpful.

Choosing a Diuretic
Factors involved include potency, cost, duration of activity, and incidence of adverse effects. Mild diuretics are suitable for the control of blood pressure and the long-acting forms such as hydrochlorothiazide are convenient. Short-acting diuretics do not interfere with sleep at night if given in the morning. Potent 'loop' diuretics such as frusemide and ethacrynic acid are valuable for treating left ventricular failure. They should not be given at the same time as aminoglycosides or cephalosporins such as cephaloridine.

All the diuretics can cause *adverse effects* in the long-term producing biochemical disturbances such as hyponatraemia, hypokalaemia, hyperuricaemia, hyperglycaemia, hyperlipidaemia and the promotion of excessive sodium loss which may be unphysiological and associated with unwanted disturbances of acid-base and electrolyte balance. In the short term too vigorous therapy may cause sudden, profound loss of body fluid which leads to apathy, weakness, cramps, hypotension, and thrombosis of arteries and veins. Patients often feel better if allowed a little ankle oedema and are not dried out excessively (like a prune). Gentle removal, controlled by daily weighing of the patient and urine volume measurement, is desirable especially in the aged. A massive urine flow can induce prostatic symptoms and acute retention of urine in later life. Many diuretics worsen diabetes mellitus and induce gout.

POTENT DIURETICS
These are prescribed orally, or by injection when oedema is severe, the patient is ill and speed is essential, or when milder diuretics have failed. The most widely used of this group is frusemide; the least used are the organomercurials. When renal failure exists and the glomerular filtration rate is reduced (15-20ml/min) the organomercurials are ineffective, whereas frusemide, bumetanide and ethacrynic acid are useful. All but the mercurials are 'loop diuretics'.

Frusemide Ph. Eur (Furosemide U.S.P., 'Dryptal', 'Frusid', 'Lasix') given orally produces a prompt, powerful diuresis lasting 4 hours. *Presentation* Tablets B.P. 20, 40 and 500mg, Injection B.P. a solution in ampoules 2, 5 and 25ml

10mg/ml for i.m. and i.v. use. Packs with 'Lasix' and Potassium tablets separately are available. *Dose* 40-120mg orally, but if renal failure exists up to 4g doses may be necessary hence the large 500mg tablet; by injection the usual dose is 20-40mg, but in renal failure several grams have been given; up to 1000mg/24h is recommended and the infusion rate should be no more than 4mg/min. By the i.v. route diuresis is immediate and lasts 2 hours so it is excellent for acute emergencies like pulmonary oedema. Sudden deaths following i.v. injections have occasionally been reported. With massive i.v. doses especially if given quickly transient deafness has occurred, whereas up to 4g has been taken orally without this risk. Nausea, tinnitus, hyperglycaemia and hyperuricaemia may also occur. In pulmonary oedema it reduces pulmonary blood volume, by diverting blood to the leg veins ('medical venesection'). The oxygenation of the blood may not improve and it is advised that with i.v. frusemide a high mask concentration of oxygen should be given concurrently to the patient. *Drug interactions* nephrotoxicity with cephalosporins, otherwise as with thiazides.

Ethacrynic Acid Ph. Eur. ('Edecrin') is a phenoxyacetic acid derivative and is chemically distinct from the others. *Presentation* Tablets B.P. 50mg and vials U.S.P. of **Sodium Ethacrynate** ('Edecrin Injection') containing 50mg of freeze-dried powder which is dissolved and diluted in Water for Injections, Dextrose or Sodium Chloride Injections B.P. before use to 50ml. *Dose* orally 25-50mg initially to avoid excessive response and subsequently 150-400mg; i.v. 500μg-1mg/kg B.W. e.g. 50-100mg. *Adverse reactions* deafness may occur after both large oral and i.v. doses and may be permanent. Occasional gastrointestinal bleeding occurs and anorexia, nausea, vomiting with large doses.

Bumetanide ('Burinex') is a diuretic comparable in potency with frusemide but cheaper and has a peak action in 1-2 hours and duration of 4-6 hours. *Presentation* tablets 1 and 5mg; dose 1-5mg daily orally occasionally up to 15mg. For injection ampoules 4 and 25ml 250μg/ml and 4ml 500μg (0.5mg)/ml are available; *dose* usually 500-1000μg (1mg i.v. or i.m. and by infusion in 500ml of fluid 2-5mg can be given over 30-60 minutes. 'Burinex K' is a compound tablet comprising bumetanide 0.5mg and potassium 573mg (7.7mmol of K^+).

Organic Mercurials prevent the resorption of sodium and chloride by the proximal tubule. They are quick, cheap and effective and can be given up to 3 times weekly. Their action is enhanced by Ammonium Chloride B.P.C. 4 enteric coated tablets 450mg each, 2 hours before the injection. They are obsolete, contra-indicated in renal failure and used with caution if proteinuria exists. Some are injected i.m., others s.c. **Mersalyl Injection B.P.** contains mersalyl with theophylline. *Presentation* ampoules 1 and 2ml; *dose* 0.5-2ml i.m. It works in a few hours and lasts most of the day. Others are **Meralluride U.S.P.** ('Mercuhydrin'); *dose* 1-2ml, s.c., or i.m. and **Mercuderamide** ('Neptal'). *Adverse effects* are uncommon; dermatitis, stomatitis, colitis, rigors, salt depletion and occasional fatalities after i.v. injection.

MODERATE DIURETICS

These are used for the control and prevention of heart failure and the treatment of hypertension. The **Benzothiadiazines** or thiazides are orally effective substances which have largely superseded the mercurials. They act on the cortical diluting segment and cause an increased excretion of sodium, chloride, potassium and bicarbonate plus water, so reducing the plasma volume. Paradoxically, they reduce the excretion of water in *diabetes insipidus* and also the excretion of calcium in *idiopathic hypercalciuria*.

All types have similar actions, though some are longer lasting than others and the cost varies. Chlorothiazide was the first to be used, but cyclopenthiazide and bendrofluazide are cheaper and more widely used. As a group they are usually tried first unless there is renal failure when frusemide is better.

Chlorothiazide ('Chlotride', 'Diuril', 'Saluric') *presentation* Tablets B.P. 500mg; *dose* initially 1-2g daily then 1g on alternate days. The action lasts 12 hours with a peak effect at 4 hours. One gram of chlorothiazide has the same effect as 100mg of hydrochlorothiazide, hydroflumethiazide or benzthiazide, 10mg bendrofluazide or methyclothiazide, or 1mg of cyclopenthiazide.

Hydrochlorothiazide ('Dichlotride', 'Direma', 'Esidrex', 'HydroDiuril', 'HydroSaluric')*presentation* Tablets B.P. 25 and 50mg; *dose* 200mg daily then 25-100mg daily or alternate days. 'Esidrex K' has the potassium chloride in the slow release form.

Cyclopenthiazide ('Navidrex') *presentation* Tablets B.P. 500µg; *dose* 500µg-1mg daily, maintenance dose 250-500µg. It lasts 8-12 hours. 'Navidrex K' is 250µg cyclopenthiazide and 600mg potassium chloride in slow release form.

Bendrofluazide (Bendroflumethiazide, 'Aprinox', 'Berkozide', 'Neo-Naclex') *presentation* Tablets B.P. 2.5 and 5mg; *dose* 5-10mg, maintenance dose 2.5-10mg daily, or every other day. The action lasts 12-18 hours, so it should be taken early in the morning. Centyl-K and Neo-Naclex-K contain bendrofluazide and slow release potassium chloride.

Other thiazides are **Cyclothiazide** U.S.N.F. ('Anhydron') 1-6mg; **Benzthiazide U.S.N.F.** 50-200mg; **Methyclothiazide U.S.N.F.** ('Enduron') 2.5-10mg; **Polythiazide Ph. Eur.** ('Nephril', 'Renese') Tablets B.P. 1mg; *dose* 1-4mg daily and **Hydroflumethiazide B.P.** ('Hydrenox') Tablets 50mg; *dose* 25-200mg daily. *Adverse effects* all thiazides can cause potassium depletion especially if the patient has generalized oedema or liver disease, is elderly, is taking a poor diet, corticosteroids or purgatives. If thiazides are taken every other day or in small amounts there may not be a need for potassium supplements. Most people receiving daily therapy do need 24mmol of added potassium daily, more so if they have severe heart failure, or are on large amounts of digitalis. Patients taking thiazides for hypertension do not usually require supplements. Alternatively, the serum potassium can be measured and if it is more than 3.5mmol/1 no supplements need be given. Other patients in spite of added potassium still have low serum levels and require 'potassium sparers' such as spironolactone. There is also the possibility that magnesium depletion can coexist with, or exacerbate hypokalaemia. Hypokalaemia can occur with normal total body potassium levels.

Potassium Supplements available are:

Potassium Chloride Slow Tablets ('K-Kontin', 'Leo-K', 'Slow K') 600mg tablets contain 8mmol (mEq) and **Potassium Chloride Effervescent Tablets** ('Kloref', 'Sando K') which are dissolved before swallowing. *Dose* 2-6 tablets daily. 'Kloref S' is supplied in sachets containing 20mmol of potassium and 20mmol of chloride. The solid forms can cause oesophageal pain and ulceration if transit is slow and occasionally small intestinal ulceration and strictures from the solid potassium salts dissolving at high concentration. Effervescent tablets and liquid forms ('Kay-Cee-L' in U.K., 'Kaochlor', 'Kay Ciel', 'Klorvoss', 'Rum K') do not have this disadvantage. In cardiac failure supplementation by equimolar amounts of K^+ and Cl^- is best. All forms are not without risk if unsupervised since occasionally fatal hyperkalaemia can occur. Thiazides may induce hepatic coma in cirrhosis by causing hypokalaemia, occasionally marrow suppression, thrombocytopenia, pancreatitis, vomiting, diarrhoea, rashes, nausea, hypotension, hypercalcaemia, hyperglycaemia (including hyperosmolar diabetic coma), hyperlipidaemia, hyponatraemia, hypochloraemic alkalosis, azotaemia and hyperuricaemia. Loss of libido can occur. Digitoxin and lithium toxicity can be induced.

The uses, adverse effects and contra-indications of the following 'non thiazides' resemble those of the thiazides for chemically, like them, they are also related to the sulphonamides and they act at similar sites. Potassium supplements may be needed too.

Phthalimidines
Chlorthalidone ('Hygroton') acts for 48-72 hours preventing resorption of sodium, chloride and water. It is suitable for long-term use as a diuretic and in hypertension. Some patients complain of sleep disturbance due to the nocturia induced by the long action of the diuretic. *Presentation* Tablets B.P. 50 and 100mg; *dose* 100-200mg after breakfast 2-3 times weekly.

Quinazolinones
Quinethazone ('Aquamox') has maximum action at 6 hours, but lasts 18-24 hours. *Presentation* Tablets U.S.P. 50mg; *dose* 50-200mg daily initially and a maintenance dose of 50-100mg 3 or 4 times weekly. It is an expensive drug with no special advantages. **Metolazone** ('Metenix 5', 'Duilo' in U.S.A.) *presentation* tablets 5mg; *dose* 2.5-20mg daily usually with a maximum of 80mg. It inhibits sodium resorption in the proximal and distal segments of the nephron. The action starts in 1 hour, is maximum at 2 hours and total duration is 12-24 hours. It is strongly bound to the serum proteins. The drug undergoes enterohepatic recycling (excreted via the bile and then reabsorbed) and therefore remains in the body for a long time. It is capable of causing diuresis in patients with impaired renal function unlike other thiazides.

Chlorobenzamides
Clopamide ('Brinaldix') *presentation* tablets 20mg; *dose* 40-60mg daily at first, reducing to 20-40mg daily or on alternate days. **Indapamide** ('Natrilix') is a chlorobenzamide used for hypertension; *dose* 2.5mg daily.

Chlorobenzene Disulphonamides

Mefruside ('Baycaron') a benzene disulphonamide is a mild diuretic whose salt excreting properties are used as a hypotensive. *Presentation* tablets 25mg; *dose* for hypertension 12.5-50mg initially then 25-50mg every second or third day. For oedema the intitial dose is 25-100mg daily then as above.

POTASSIUM SPARERS
These are minor diuretics but they have the power to conserve potassium while enhancing the more potent diuretics and they may be useful hypotensives. They should be restricted to patients with normal renal function.
Amiloride Hydrochloride ('Midamor') *presentation* tablets 5mg is given in a dose up to 20mg daily but it is more usually prescribed combined with hydrochlorothiazide 50mg in 'Moduretic'; *dose* 1-4 tablets daily. It is more potent in retaining potassium than triamterene and less expensive than spironolactone.

Contra-indications are renal impairment, metabolic or respiratory acidosis and, since 'Moduretic' can induce hyperglycaemia because of the thiazide component, care is needed in diabetics.

Triamterene ('Dytac') acts on the distal tubule like amiloride and lasts 6-8 hours. *Presentation* Capsules B.P. 50mg; *dose* 150-250mg daily, or alternate days in divided doses. 'Dyazide' contains 25mg hydrochlorothiazide and 50mg triamterene and 'Dytide' contains 50mg triamterene and 25mg benzthiazide. *Adverse effects* nausea, vomiting, diarrhoea, and occasionally a raised blood urea and hyperkalaemia.

Aldosterone Antagonists. Aldosterone, an adrenal cortex hormone, promotes sodium resorption and potassium excretion by the distal tubule. Excess hormone is formed in heart, or liver failure, the hormonal action may be blocked by antagonists which structurally are steroids like aldosterone. **Spironolactone** ('Aldactone') is an example. *Presentation* Tablets B.P. 100 and 25mg; *dose* 100-400mg once daily or in divided doses 6 hourly. Clinically it is most useful in cirrhosis with ascites, the nephrotic syndrome and for non-surgically treated Conn's syndrome. It may also be part of the hypotensive regime when thiazides cause hypokalaemia either alone, or in combination as in 'Aldactide 25' which contains 25mg spironolactone and 25mg hydroflumethiazide and 'Aldactide 50' which contains 50mg of each. If there has been any history of liver coma it is best prescribed alone. It acts slowly and a response may take 24-48 hours. *Adverse effects* rashes, hyperkalaemia, drowsiness, nausea, vomiting, diarrhoea and because it is also an androgen antagonist gynaecomastia, impotence and amenorrhoea.

WEAK DIURETICS

Acetazolamide ('Diamox') is a non-bacteriostatic heterocyclic sulphonamide and a carbonic acid anhydrase inhibitor. It produces renal excretion of bicarbonate with an alkaline urine, loss of water, sodium and potassium. The bicarbonate loss reduces intra-ocular pressure and its major use is not as a diuretic, but in the treatment of open angle glaucoma. It finds occasional use to suppress epilepsy. *Presentation* Tablets B.P. 250mg, capsules 500mg (long-acting); vials Sodium Acetazolamide U.S.P. containing 500mg. *Dose* orally 250mg-1g daily. *Adverse effects* drowsiness, headache, excitement, depression, paraesthesiae, metabolic-hyperchloraemic acidosis, hypokalaemia; there is a low incidence of polydipsia, polyuria, rashes, marrow depression and renal stones. The drug increases urinary calcium and reduces citrate excretion both favouring deposition of calcium stones.

Xanthine Derivatives
Caffeine, theobromine and aminophylline find little medical use as diuretics.

Dehydrating or Osmotic Diuretics
These are used after cardiac arrest and in certain types of renal failure or post-operatively in obstructive jaundice to prevent renal failure. Urea i.v. has been used to reduce cerebral oedema, but rebound oedema occurs and **Mannitol Injection B.P.** in 5, 10, 20 and 25% strengths (also as 'Osmitrol') is widely used as a dehydrating agent or to promote polyuria. It is slower to act than urea, but lasts longer and has less adverse effects. As the solution is hyperosmolar it must not be allowed to escape into the tissues. A dose up to 50g is given usually as the 20% solution. In the management of cerebral oedema i.v.

glycerol has been used but the dose and concentration must be carefully judged to avoid haemolysis.

NEW DRUGS

Tienilic Acid (Ticrynafen, 'Selacryn') is a recently introduced uricosuric non-sulphonamide diuretic which has the interesting and valuable property of producing hypouricaemia. Structurally it is related to ethacrynic acid a phenoxy acetic acid derivative. Hence it is a suitable diuretic or hypotensive agent for patients with gout or hyperuricaemia. Diuresis occurs from interference with the reabsorption of sodium in the cortical diluting segment of the distal tubule. It is comparable in hypotensive activity to the thiazides; 500mg of tienilic acid exerts an hypotensive effect comparable to 50 or 100mg of hydrochlorothiazide. The hypouricaemic action is due to the inhibition of urates by the tubules in a similar manner to probenecid. The dose is 250 or 500mg once daily. *Adverse effects* electrolyte changes such as hypokalaemia occur and anti-coagulant therapy can be potentiated. Tienilic acid has been temporarily withdrawn in all countries, except France, for re-evaluation of toxicity.

Xipamide ('Diurexan')

This also has been introduced for diuretic and hypotensive purposes. The diuretic activity lasts 12 hours and the hypotensive action for 24 hours or more. *Presentation* tablets 20mg; *dose* for hypertension 20 or 40mg once daily taken in the morning when used as sole therapy. For diuresis the usual dose is 40mg daily, but the range is 20-80mg daily. The precautions are similar to those of other diuretics .

13 ANALGESICS

The treatment of pain depends on the cause since it is only a symptom of under-lying disease. Analgesics are not necessarily best. Psychogenic pain is helped more by sedatives, antidepressants, or tranquillizers; angina by vasodilators; peptic ulcer by antacids, gout by colchicine and infections by antibiotics. Persistent pain leads to depression and this secondary effect may need treatment.

Indications for analgesics are: (1) to give relief until the underlying condition is treated e.g. pleurisy, pneumonia and cardiac infarction; (2) to give relief when no cure is possible e.g. arthritis, headaches, inoperable cancers.

Types
Narcotic or potentially addictive analgesics include morphine, diamorphine and pethidine. Ideally these centrally acting analgesics should not cause mental dulling, sickness, dizziness, vomiting, constipation or sweating i.e. they should be purely analgesic and cause no respiratory depression or drug dependence.

Simple analgesics comprise paracetamol, codeine, dihydrocodeine and dextropropoxyphene.

Analgesics with **anti-inflammatory** and antipyretic actions include aspirin, the pyrazoles phenylbutazone, oxyphenbutazone and nifenazone, the anthranilic compounds flufenamic and mefenamic acids, indomethacin and propionic acid derivatives e.g. ibuprofen.

CENTRALLY ACTIVE ANALGESICS
Narcotics are used for severe pain, e.g. cardiac infarction, after surgery, accidents or with terminal cancer. Subsidiary uses are to suppress cough and diarrhoea. Some induce sleep at night, but make the patient drowsy by day. They should be avoided in head injuries. Their use is covered by the Misuse of Drugs Act (Chapter 32).

OPIUM ALKALOID DERIVATIVES (Opiates)
Opium is a brown powder obtained from the juice of the seed capsules of the opium poppy. It contains alkaloids, the most important being morphine, others are codeine and papaverine. The analgesic alkaloids are phenanthrene derivatives.

Opium Preparations
Powder Opium B.P. *dose* 30-200mg which contains 1/10th its weight of morphine; **Tincture Opium B.P.** (laudanum) is prepared to contain 10mg/ml of anhydrous morphine; *dose* 0.3-1ml (3-10mg anhydrous morphine); **Camphorated Opium Tincture B.P.** or Paregoric contains 5mg of anhydrous morphine in 10ml; *dose* 2-10ml. These are used for diarrhoea and cough. **Chalk and Opium Mixture** contains in each 10ml 5mg of anhydrous morphine. **Ipecacuanha and Opium Tablets B.P.C.** are Dover's Powder Tablets; the *dose* is 300-600mg. 'Nepenthe' is a liquid preparation of opium; *dose* by mouth, or injection adults up to 2ml and children 0.06ml for each year of life. *The prescription must only be in metric doses.*

91

Papaveretum ('Omnopon') is a mixture of soluble alkaloids as the hydrochlorides, about half anhydrous morphine. The B.P.C. Injection is a 2% solution (20mg/ml) in water, 1ml ampoules contain 10mg of anhydrous morphine; *dose* 10-20mg i.v., i.m. or s.c. Tablets 10mg containing 5mg of morphine are available, and the dose is 1 or 2 tablets. 'Omnopon and Scopolamine' injection contains 20mg of papaveretum and 400µg of hyoscine hydrobromide per 1ml ampoule. An effervescent tablet containing soluble aspirin 500mg and papaveretum 10mg is available and exempt from D.D.A. control. The *dose* is 1-2 tablets 4-6 hourly and is suitable for post-operative pain.

Morphine acts slowly by mouth as it is poorly absorbed, in 15 minutes s.c. and at once i.v. The usual route s.c. lasts 6 hours. Chemically it is a 5-ring structure. A long-acting microcrystalline form 'Duromorph' in ampoules 70.4mg/1.1ml is suitable for 12-hourly use in terminal malignancy.

Morphine Sulphate Injection B.P. is a solution in Water for Injections supplied in ampoules 1ml containing 10, 15, 20 and 30mg and in multidose bottles. *Dose* 10-20mg s.c., i.m., or i.v. though larger amounts are needed in terminal malignancy. Morphine hydrochloride Ph. Eur. or morphine sulphate is available in suppositories containing 10, 15, 20, 30 or 60mg.

Morphine and Hyoscine Injection B.P.C. contains 10mg of morphine sulphate with 400µg of hyoscine hydrobromide in 1ml ampoules.

Morphine and Atropine Injection B.P.C. contains in 1ml ampoules 10mg of morphine sulphate and 600µg of atropine sulphate. Both are given s.c. or i.m. at a dose of 0.5-1ml for premedication. 'Cyclimorph 10' contains morphine tartrate 10mg and cyclizine tartrate 50mg in each 1ml ampoule and 'Cyclimorph 15' contains 15mg of morphine tartrate and 50mg cyclizine tartrate in each 1ml. The cyclizine is an anti-emetic. It is given s.c., i.m., or i.v.

Kaolin and Morphine Mixture B.P.C. contains 700µg of anhydrous morphine in each 10ml; **Tincture of Chloroform B.P.C.** ('Chlorodyne') contains 1.37mg of anhydrous morphine in a 0.6ml dose. *Uses* diarrhoea.

Clinical and Pharmacological Actions of Morphine

(1) *Medullary centres:* inhibition of the respiratory nuclei causes depression of cough and of respiratory rate, vagal stimulation leads to nausea, vomiting, sweating and bradycardia. Morphine should not be given to asthmatic or emphysematous patients. Vomiting is a disadvantage in cardiac infarction and haematemesis and may be diminished by giving an anti-emetic. Morphine constricts the pupils and this may be a clue to poisoning.

(2) The *cardiac output* and the *blood pressure* may be lowered due to vasodilatation and the effect on the blood pressure is worse if the patient sits up.

(3) *Gastro-intestinal:* the decrease of peristalsis causes constipation, which is helpful in diarrhoea, but an added misery in the dying patient.

(4) The *skin* blood vessels are dilated and sweating may occur.

(5) *Smooth muscle:* the urethral sphincter contracts, predisposing to urinary retention. The muscle of the biliary tract, and ureter constrict so worsening biliary or ureteric colic.

(6) *Liver disease:* morphine is metabolized by the liver so it is dangerous in cirrhotics. Patients with *hypothyroidism* and *Addison's disease* as well as the *aged* are very sensitive to morphine.

(7) Morphine raises the *intracranial pressure* so it is dangerous in delirium tremens, alcoholism and head injury.

(8) Morphine is a *histamine liberator* and allergic reactions with urticaria, itching and anaphylaxis can occur.

(9) Morphine and other opium derivatives lead to *addiction* and *tolerance*. *Sudden withdrawal* can cause restlessness, tremor, and confusion, and over-dosage to coma, slow respiration, pin-point pupils, hypotension, loss of reflexes and cardiac arrhythmia.

(10) Alcohol, barbiturates, phenothiazines and monoamine oxidase inhibitors increase the action of morphine which may itself summate the effects of hypotensives.

Codeine Phosphate Ph. Eur. (chemically methylmorphine) is derived from morphine although it is naturally occurring, but it is not narcotic and addiction is uncommon. The analgesic action is 1/4-1/6th of morphine. *Presentation* Tablets B.P. 15, 30 and 60mg, syrup 25mg/5ml; *dose* 10-60mg. Codeine is included in many official and proprietary remedies. Those which contain phenacetin will be withdrawn e.g. Compound Codeine Tablets B.P. 'Codis' is 500mg aspirin and 8mg codeine phosphate. *Adverse effects* headache, constipation, dizziness, sleepiness, and in overdose respiratory depression, twitching and convulsions. The chemical modification of morphine has led to some cortical excitant qualities (convulsant action).

SYNTHETIC NARCOTIC DRUGS
Morphine Derivatives (5-ring structures)

Dihydrocodeine Tartrate ('DF 118') is chemically closely related to codeine, having as its name suggests 2 extra hydrogen atoms, but is stronger and hence more suitable for the pain of malignancy and of dental and skeletal origin. The injection is a Controlled Drug (Chapter 32). *Presentation* Tablets B.P. 30mg, syrup 10mg/5ml, Injection B.P. contained in ampoules 50mg/ml. *Dose* orally 30mg 4-6 hourly; injection s.c., or i.m. 30-60mg. It is best avoided in liver disease and asthma. Dihydrocodeinone and pholcodine are described in Chapter 20.

Diamorphine Hydrochloride (Heroin and chemically diacetylmorphine) acts like morphine, but is a stronger analgesic, respiratory depressant and euphoriant. Owing to the high risk of addiction it is banned in many countries, but not in Britain where many still favour its use in terminal malignancy and in cardiac infarction since it is said to cause less hypotension. *Presentation* Injection B.P. vials containing 5, 10 and 30mg of powder to be dissolved in Water for Injections; *dose* 5-10mg s.c., i.m., or i.v. B.P.C. Elixirs are used for terminal disease namely Diamorphine and Cocaine and Diamorphine, Cocaine and Chlorpromazine. Similar formulations exist with morphine, instead of diamorphine, which may hydrolyse with time and lose its effect. *Adverse effects* vomiting and constipation are less frequent than with morphine. In heroin addicts infections are likely and acute pulmonary oedema can occur.

Other derivatives either more potent, or more effective than morphine orally are **Hydromorphone Hydrochloride** U.S.N.F. (Dihydromorphinone Hydrochloride) *presentation* tablets 2.5mg, ampoules 1ml 2mg/ml; *dose* orally 2.5-5mg, s.c. 2mg. **Methyldihydromorphinone Hydrochloride** or Metopon *dose* 3-6mg orally and **Oxymorphone Hydrochloride** ('Numorphan') *dose* 5-10mg orally, 1.5mg s.c., or i.m. Although they may be more potent, respiratory depression may be more marked and dependency is still a problem. Narcotic derivatives of this group with low abuse potential are codeine, dihydrocodeinone, oxycodone and pholcodine.

Further derivatives are in wide use in which the morphine 5-ring structure has been chemically 'dissected'.

Morphinans
Here one ring of the morphine structure has been disrupted and 4 rings are left.
Levorphanol Tartrate ('Dromoran') is an example. *Presentation* Tablets B.P.
1.5mg, Injection B.P. a solution in ampoules 1ml 2mg/ml; *dose* 2-4mg s.c. and
i.m., 1-1.5mg i.v. and orally 1.5-4.5mg. This is more potent than morphine,
but has similar drawbacks, although it may be less constipating and emetic.

Benzomorphans
In this group a further ring has been opened and 3 rings of the morphine nucleus remain.
Phenazocine Hydrobromide ('Narphen') is several times stronger than morphine with less respiratory depression or constipation. It acts quickly, does not
contract the bile duct sphincter (unlike morphine) and nausea and vomiting
are uncommon. It is claimed that addiction develops slowly and withdrawal
effects are less frequent. *Presentation* Tablets B.P. 5mg; *dose* orally 5mg 4-6
hourly.
Pentazocine is a narcotic antagonist found to have analgesic properties and
now in wide use ('Fortral', 'Talwin'). *Presentation* Pentazocine Hydrochloride
Tablets B.P. 25mg, capsules 50 mg; Pentazocine Lactate suppositories 50mg
as base, and for parenteral use Pentazocine Lactate Injection B.P. a solution in
ampoules 1 and 2ml 30mg/ml as the base. *Dose* orally after food 25-100mg 4-6
hourly; i.m., or i.v. 30-60mg once or 3-6 hourly or by suppository up to 4 daily.
It is used for moderately severe pain, but does not replace the narcotics.
Contra-indications raised intracranial pressure, convulsive disorders, concurrent therapy with monoamine oxidase inhibitors, narcotic addicts. *Adverse
effects* dizziness, hallucinations and curious mental symptoms, nausea,
respiratory depression, sweating, vertigo and sleepiness. Precautions should
be taken if liver, renal or lung disease exist or in pregnancy. Pentazocine crosses the placenta more slowly than pethidine. Although it is not a 'Controlled
Drug' dependence and abuse have been recorded. 'Fortagesic' is pentazocine
15mg as the base with 500mg paracetamol.

  During a search for antispasmodics related to cocaine and atropine 2-ringed
structures with analgesic actions were synthesized and only later was it realized
that they were identical to two of the rings of the morphine nucleus, the other
three having been opened. These were pethidine and its congeners (derivatives).
Pethidine Hydrochloride Ph. Eur. (Meperidine Hydrochloride U.S.P.,
'Demerol', 'Dolantin') has analgesic and sedative actions, but is less hypnotic
than morphine and shorter in action. It is less depressing on the medullary
respiratory and cough centres than morphine. There is no constipation and it
usually relaxes muscle and is used in renal (but not biliary) colic. Addiction is
common. *Uses* (1) to relieve severe pain as in coronary thrombosis; (2) in obstetrics to relieve painful uterine contractions in labour, but it crosses the
placenta and may cause foetal respiratory depression; (3) premedication,
often with promethazine and chlorpromazine and this combination may also
be helpful for procedures such as cardiac catheterization. *Presentation* Tablets
B.P. 25 and 50mg, Injection B.P. a solution in Water for Injections ampoules 1
and 2ml 50mg/ml for i.m. and i.v. injection. Pethidine i.m. acts in 15min and
lasts 2-5 hours. *Dose* 25-100mg orally, s.c., i.m., or i.v. *Adverse effects* dizziness, sweating, tremor, ataxia, nausea, vomiting, tachycardia, convulsions and

respiratory depression. To counteract respiratory depression pethidine 50mg is combined with 625µg of levallorphan tartrate per 1ml as 'Pethilorfan' supplied in 1 and 2ml ampoules.
Pethidine Congeners include **Fentanyl Citrate B.P.** ('Sublimaze') used in anaesthesia and neuroleptanalgesia. *Presentation* ampoules 2 and 10ml 50µg/ml; *dose* 100-600µg i.v. Its action lasts 30 minutes. *Adverse effects* respiratory depression, hypotension. **Phenoperidine Hydrochloride** ('Operidine') *presentation* ampoules 2ml, 1mg/ml; *dose* 500µg-5mg i.v. is used to calm patients to tolerate intubation while undergoing ventilation. It is often combined with **Droperidol** ('Droleptan') a butyrophenone (p. 115) *presentation* tablets 10mg, ampoules 2ml 5mg/ml; *dose* 5-20mg orally, 10mg i.m. and 5-15mg i.v.

Methadone and Congeners
Although their action is similar their chemical relation to morphine is remote.
Methadone Hydrochloride Ph. Eur. (Amidone, 'Physeptone') has strong analgesic actions by mouth and is less soporific than morphine. *Uses* analgesia; to ease the withdrawal symptoms of morphine, and as an oral alternative, administered by clinics in the U.S.A. to heroin addicts; and to suppress cough. *Presentation* Tablets B.P. 5mg, Injection B.P. a solution in ampoules 1ml 10mg/ml, Linctus B.P.C. 2mg/5ml for adults which is diluted 1 part with 7 parts for children. *Dose* 5-10mg orally, or s.c. for adults linctus 5ml for adults; children 5ml of diluted linctus. Methadone dependence occurs, especially in women in the childbearing age. Withdrawal symptoms occur at birth in the infants who have a low birth weight, irritability, sneezing, tremor and a high pitched cry. Treatment is with chlorpromazine. **Dipipanone Hydrochloride** has strong analgesic, sedative and hypnotic effects. Chemically like methadone and dextromoramide it has a weak atropine-like action. Its rapid action lasts 4-6 hours with less respiratory depression than morphine. *Presentation* Injection B.P. contained in ampoules 1ml 25mg/ml; *dose* 25-50mg s.c., or i.m. Dipipanone Hydrochloride 10mg is combined with Cyclizine Hydrochloride B.P. 30mg (an anti-emetic) in 'Diconal' for oral use. **Dextromoramide Tartrate** ('Jetrium', 'Palfium') *presentation* Tablets B.P. 5 and 10mg, ampoules 1ml 5 and 10mg/ml, suppositories containing 10mg. *Dose* orally 5-20mg 4 hourly, 5-15mg s.c., or i.m.
Piritramide ('Dipidolor') is used for post-operative pain. It has structural relationships to diphenoxylate. *Presentation* ampoules 2ml 10mg/ml; *dose* 20mg i.m. 6 hourly for 4 doses only. It causes little vomiting and can be reversed by narcotic antagonists.
Dextropropoxyphene (see page 98).

NARCOTIC ANTAGONISTS
Chemically these are minor modifications of morphine, levorphanol and oxymorphone (an allyl group replaces one of the methyl groups) to form nalorphine, levallorphan or naloxone respectively. Being similar in structure they are able to block the action of narcotics, especially in accidental or deliberate overdose, including codeine and also dextropropoxyphene.
Nalorphine Hydrobromide is not a pure antagonist for, by itself, like levallorphan it can cause respiratory depression, drowsiness and small pupils. In obstetrics it has been used 10 minutes before delivery to protect the baby against narcotics which can cross the placental barrier. It is no longer available.

Levallorphan Tartrate ('Lorfan') *presentation* Injection B.P. ampoules 1ml containing in solution 1mg/ml; *dose* 200µg-2mg i.v. for adults and 50µg for neonates. It lasts longer than nalorphine.

Naloxone Hydrochloride ('Narcan') is a pure antagonist. With this advantage it is becoming first choice as it does not cause, given alone, respiratory depression. *Presentation* ampoules 1ml 400µg/ml; *dose* 10-20µg/kg i.v., s.c., or i.m. (0.4-1.2mg). It is also effective against pentazocine unlike the others; because of its short action it may need to be repeated every few hours. 'Narcan Neonatal' is available 20µg/ml in 2ml ampoules at a dose of 5-10µg/kg B.W. for neonates s.c., i.m., or i.v.

Naltrexone is a newer antagonist. **Buprenorphine** ('Temgesic') has partial antagonist activity and is used as an analgesic with less respiratory depression claimed than morphine. *Presentation* ampoules 1 and 2ml 0.3mg/ml; *dose* 0.3-0.6mg i.v. or i.m.

NON-NARCOTIC ANALGESICS

These are used for most of the aches and pains of life. Some of the anti-inflammatory analgesics are discussed in Chapter 29. In comparing their virtues these points should be considered: (1) short-term occasional use, (2) long-term use, and (3) the dangers of acute overdosage.

Acetylsalicylic Acid or **Aspirin Ph. Eur.** introduced in 1899 is cheap and widely used. It is far from ideal, though comparatively safe, and the best of a far from outstanding group. Also, unlike the simple analgesics it has, particularly in high dosage, anti-inflammatory actions. It is disintegrated in the stomach and rapidly absorbed in the small intestine when taken orally, but it is quickly excreted and needs to be taken 4-6 hourly and, for comfort, with food. **Plain Aspirin** Aspirin Ph. Eur. is available as Aspirin Tablets B.P. 300mg and Soluble Aspirin Tablets B.P.; the latter resemble 'Claradin', 'Disprin' and 'Solprin'. Aspirin Soluble Tablets Paediatric contain 75mg. **Enteric Coated** and delayed release aspirin modifications have been tried to avoid gastric symptoms e.g. 'Breoprin' 648mg strength 'Caprin' (324mg), 'Levius' (500mg) and 'Nu-Seals' (300 and 600mg). An alternative is to try **Buffered Aspirin** by adding glycine ('Paynocil') or aluminium oxide as with Aloxiprin ('Palaprin Forte') each 600mg tablet of which contains 500mg aspirin. 'Alka-Seltzer' is a buffered aspirin solution. *Dose* for adults is 300-1000mg per dose up to 4-15g daily in divided amounts according to the condition and tolerance. Dosage is best controlled by blood levels which should be 20-40mg/dl.

Adverse effects are common—direct local effects of gastro-intestinal intolerance, dyspepsia, vomiting, nausea, and epigastric pain (no aspirin preparation should be taken for indigestion or alcoholic hang-over), gastro-intestinal bleeding which can be massive even after 1 or 2 tablets by causing acute gastric erosions, or by causing iron deficiency anaemia from slow intestinal blood loss, or re-activation of peptic ulcers. It is possible to reduce these complications by changing the formulation and by taking each tablet with a glass of water or milk. *Hypersensitivity* (idiosyncratic or allergic) is rare but more likely in asthmatics, in those with nasal polyps, chronic rhinitis and in young people. It can be serious leading to fatal anaphylaxis, allergic purpura, thrombocytopenia, angioneurotic oedema, urticaria. Lyell's syndrome, and asthma. Rarely serum sickness and marrow suppression can occur. (Hypersensitivity is not seen with the simple analgesics like paracetamol.) *Toxicity* is dose related; moderate overdosage causes vertigo, tinnitus, deafness, nausea, vomiting and sweating. Aspirin is often taken suicidally; large doses cause restlessness, stupor, convulsions, coma, bleeding, rapid breathing and proteinuria. Problems are complex for there may be visual disturbances, hyper- or hypoglycaemia, acid-base upsets, haemorrhagic gastritis, hyperpyrexia, acute tubular necrosis, pulmonary oedema, metabolic acidosis, respiratory alkalosis and salt and water retention.

Salicylates potentiate and should not be given with anticoagulants, oral hypoglycaemic agents, or methotrexate and they antagonize uricosuric drugs and indomethacin. Aspirin affects haemostasis, alters platelet function, increases fibrinolysis and lengthens the bleeding time. Continuous consumption causes hypoprothrombinaemia. Therefore aspirin *should be avoided* in haemophilia, von Willebrand's disease, thrombocytopenia and familial telangiectasia. Chronic administration causes urinary excretion of renal tubular cells and red blood cells. Aspirin, like indomethacin, blocks prostaglandins E_2 and $F_2\alpha$, whose inhibition may be responsible for the anti-inflammatory and antipyretic actions.

Sodium Salicylate Ph. Eur. causes less gastro-intestinal bleeding than aspirin, but is a weaker analgesic. Given with plenty of water there is little gastric irritation. *Presentation* Tablets B.P.C. 500mg and B.P.C. Mixture 500mg or 1g/10ml.

Salicylamide ('Salimed') *presentation* tablets 500mg; *dose* 500mg-1g thrice daily is a safer, but weaker analgesic with sedative properties.

Paracetamol Ph. Eur. (Acetaminophen U.S.P.) has found increasing use in those who cannot tolerate aspirin, have peptic ulcers, anaemia, or are taking uricosuric agents or warfarin. *Presentation* Tablets B.P. 500mg, Paediatric Elixir B.P.C. 120mg/5ml; *dose* for adults 500-1000mg, children 0-1 years 5ml; 1-5 years 10ml. Proprietary forms include 'Calpol', 'Febrilix', 'Panadol'. 'Panadeine Co' is paracetamol 500mg with 8mg codeine phosphate, and 'Paramol 118' is paracetamol 500mg with 10mg dihydrocodeine tartrate. 'Safapryn' contains 250mg paracetamol with 300mg enteric-coated aspirin. 'Safapryn Co' has 8mg of codeine phosphate as well. The dose of paracetamol is up to 4g daily. For long-term use it may not be without risk, renal damage is a possibility. The major notorious hazard is its marked *danger when it is taken suicidally, or accidentally, in overdose.* As little as 30 tablets may be fatal; liver coma, acute hepatic necrosis, hypokalaemia, hypoglycaemia, clotting disturbances and renal failure can occur. The liver necrosis may be delayed several days.

Benorylate ('Benoral') is an aspirin-paracetamol chemical union (ester) which splits into its component parts after absorption. The object is to avoid local aspirin effects on the gut. *Presentation* tablets 750mg, suspension 400mg/ml in 150 and 300ml bottles; *dose* 10ml b.d. or 5ml q.d.s. or equivalent as tablets 4-8g daily. *Contra-indications* aspirin sensitivity, peptic ulceration; *precautions* are needed in those taking anticoagulants (adjust dose and strict laboratory control.

Phenacetin Ph. Eur. (Acetophenetidin) is converted *in vivo* to paracetamol. In Britain it is only available on prescription and its use everywhere is decreasing. However, occasional use is safe, and it does not potentiate anticoagulants or bleeding states. *Presentation* Tablets B.P. 300mg; *dose* 300-600mg. *Adverse effects* habitual ingestion leads to methaemoglobinaemia, sulphaemoglobinaemia from oxidative injury to red cells as well as haemolytic anaemia, or to renal damage from pyelonephritis and papillary necrosis (has been epidemic in Switzerland, Sweden and Australia). The term *analgesic nephropathy* is applied to kidney damage and failure following the daily and prolonged consumption of aspirin, paracetamol, phenacetin and the pyrazolones. *Abuse of analgesics* is likely in those with neuralgia, period pain, headaches, rheumatism and arthritis, frequent colds, and, curiously in inadequate personalities who take them as 'stimulants' or as 'sedatives'. Any person with chronic pain can be a candidate and gastric ulceration, anaemia and odd personalities may co-exist. Many compound analgesics are now deliberately formulated without phenacetin e.g., 'Veganin' is aspirin 250mg, paracetamol 250mg and codeine 9.58mg. **Tabs. Codeine Co B.P.** still, however, contains phenacetin, but official alternatives are now available. **Aspirin and Codeine Tablet B.P.** contains 400mg of acetylsalicylic acid and 8mg of codeine phosphate. The **Soluble Aspirin and Codeine Tablet B.P.** contains calcium carbonate 130mg, anhydrous citric acid 40mg and saccharin sodium 4mg as well. **Aspirin and Caffeine Tablet B.P.** contains 350mg and 30mg of each respectively. However, increasing the dose of aspirin (on its own) is a better analgesic and cheaper. Phenacetin has been banned from medical products in the U.K. from March 1980. It may still be prescribed for individual named patients.

Dextropropoxyphene Hydrochloride ('Darvon', 'Doloxene') chemically is similar to methadone, but it is not classed as a narcotic. It is dearer, but no better than aspirin. *Presentation* Capsules B.P. 65mg; *dose* 3 or 4 capsules daily. *Adverse effects* dizziness, headache, sedation, nausea, vomiting, abdominal pain, constipation, euphoria. Tolerance, physical or psychological dependence, or abuse can occur as with codeine. Overdosage causes pulmonary oedema, respiratory depression, convulsions, hypotension and diabetes insipidus. 'Distalgesic' a widely prescribed analgesic is dextropropoxyphene hydrochloride 32.5mg and paracetamol 325mg; *dose* 6-8 tablets daily. A soluble form is dextropropoxyphene napsylate 50mg with 325mg paracetamol. Deliberate overdose can be dangerous. Liver damage co-exists with convulsions and respiratory depression.

Diflunisal ('Dolobid') is a salicylate derivative without the acetyl group which is believed to be harmful. Its main advantage is its prolonged action. No alteration in platelet aggregation, bleeding or clotting is claimed. *Presentation* Tablets 250mg; *dose* 125-375mg twice daily. *Contra-indications* aspirin hypersensitivity. **Salsalate** ('Disalcid') is another salicylate derivative.

Nefopam Hydrochloride ('Acupan') is a non-narcotic analgesic. *Presentation* Tablets 30mg; ampoules 1ml 20mg/ml; *dose* orally 30-90mg thrice daily; 20mg by i.m. or slow i.v. injection which can be repeated after 6 hours if needed. It is used in similar circumstances to aspirin.

The search for non-steroidal alternatives to aspirin with similar anti-inflammatory actions (which codeine, paracetamol, pentazocine dextropropoxyphene and dihydrocodeine lack) has led to the introduction of many substances particularly for use in rheumatoid arthritis. (See chapter 29.)

14 DRUGS AFFECTING NEURONAL FUNCTION AND THE AUTONOMIC NERVOUS SYSTEM

The autonomic nervous system is comprised of the sympathetic and parasympathetic divisions (Figure 3). They innervate the internal secretory organs, the smooth involuntary muscle of the viscera, eyes, blood vessels, heart, bronchi and sweat glands. They thereby control digestion, excretion, sexual activity, vessel tone, sweating, heart and respiratory rate and bronchial size. The divisions in general oppose each other and are controlled themselves by medullary, hypothalmic and cortical higher centres. Two neurones are involved in the passage of impulses from the cell stations or nuclei within the brain and spinal cord to the organ supplied (Figure 4). First, a pre-ganglionic fibre ending in a distributing nerve centre or ganglion and second, a post-ganglionic fibre running from the ganglion to the organ, gland or muscle.

When a nerve impulse reaches a synapse—the region where the neurone tendrils interlock — a *neurohormone* is liberated which conveys the impulse to the adjoining neurone. The chemical transmitter for pre-ganglionic fibres is *acetylcholine*. It has a short action and is destroyed by an enzyme cholinesterase. The post-ganglionic fibres liberate either acetylcholine, or adrenaline or noradrenaline. Post-ganglionic sympathetic nerve fibres (except those supplying sweat glands) secrete from intra-neuronal stores noradrenaline or adrenaline ('adrenergic fibres'). The adrenal medulla likewise secretes these hormones. **Adrenaline** naturally released, or injected, increases heart rate and cardiac output, constricts skin blood vessels and dilates muscle and coronary arterioles, dilates the pupils, relaxes bronchial, intestinal and bladder wall muscles and contracts the bladder sphincter. *Noradrenaline* slows the heart, raises the blood pressure and constricts blood vessels. Cardiac output is unaffected or decreased. Differently responding adrenergic receptors alpha and beta were postulated by Ahlquist in 1948 to explain these responses and those to isoprenaline. The beta receptors were further subdivided in 1966 by Lands and co-workers into B_1 which mediate stimulation of cardiac muscle, inhibition of smooth intestinal muscle and stimulation of lipolysis (fat breakdown) and B_2 receptors which mediate inhibition of smooth muscle in the bronchi, in skeletal muscle arteries and uterus and promote glycogen breakdown. Adrenaline stimulates both alpha and beta receptors, noradrenaline is mainly an alpha receptor stimulator and isoprenaline a mainly beta stimulator.

Post-ganglionic parasympathetic nerve fibres release acetylcholine which slows the heart, dilates blood vessels, increases gut activity and contracts the bladder. Adrenaline-like drugs which act like the sympathetic nervous system are called *sympathomimetic* or *adrenergic*. Drugs which oppose are called *sympatholytic* or *adrenolytic*. Similarly, *parasympathomimetic* or *cholinergic* drugs are parasympathetic-like and those which oppose, *parasympatholytics*. Ganglion blocking or *ganglioplegic* drugs prevent the transmission of impulses from pre-ganglionic to post-ganglionic fibres. *Adrenergic neurone blocking* drugs interfere with the transmission of impulses in the sympathetic nerves.

SYMPATHOMIMETIC DRUGS
Adrenaline (Epinephrine U.S.P.) was extracted from the adrenal medulla, but

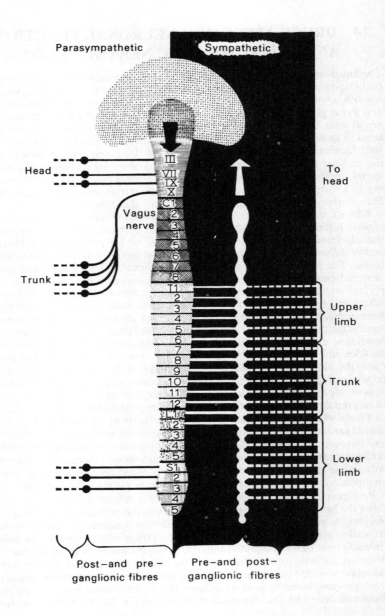

Fig. 3
Organization of the autonomic nervous system

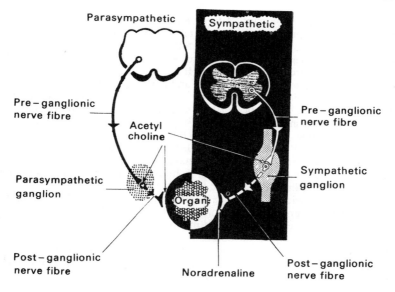

Fig. 4
Diagram showing nerve impulse transmission
in the autonomic nervous system

is now synthetically made. The B.P. Injection of Adrenaline Acid Tartrate Ph. Eur. is equivalent to a 1:1000 solution (1mg/ml) of adrenaline and usually is given s.c.; *dose* 100μg-1mg. *Uses* bronchodilator in asthma, to control angioneurotic oedema, anaphylactic shock (Chapter 10), ventricular arrest (Chapter 19), and to release glucose from the liver in hypoglycaemia (Chapter 25). A neutral solution (pH 7.4) of laevo adrenaline ('Eppy') is used as drops for the treatment of chronic glaucoma.

Blood pressure raising drugs (vasopressors or alpha receptor constrictors) have been given for hypotension following cardiac infarction, drug overdose or anaesthesia. They raise the arterial pressure by constricting arterioles and increasing the peripheral resistance. In assessing the dose frequent blood pressure recordings are necessary. When hypotension follows blood, plasma, or other fluid loss, replacement of what is lost is the correct measure. Vasoconstrictors have greatly lost popularity, including in cardiogenic shock, where alpha receptor blockers which improve tissue flow (e.g. phenoxybenzamine, phentolamine) combined with central venous pressure controlled fluid infusion are preferred or inotropic acting dopamine and dobutamine.

Noradrenaline Acid Tartrate Ph. Eur. (Levarterenol Bitartrate U.S.P., 'Levophed') *presentation* ampoules 2 and 4ml, 1mg/ml or a weaker solution 100μg/ml in 2ml ampoules. These strengths are as noradrenaline base. (If considered as noradrenaline acid tartrate the concentrations are 2mg/ml, or 200μg/ml respectively). *Administration* i.v. for circulatory failure and cardiogenic shock is usually in a concentration of 1-2mg/litre but occasionally is up to 16mg/litre in Dextrose Injection B.P. 5%, or Sodium Chloride Injection B.P. 0.9%. The correct drip rate is one which maintains a systolic blood pressure at 100-120mm of mercury. *Adverse effects* ulceration of the vein and skii at the site of venepuncture due to extreme vasoconstriction. **Phenylephrin** **Hydrochloride** 5mg s.c., or i.m. and 500μg i.v. acts like noradrenaline **Metaraminol Tartrate** ('Aramine') is quick acting, lasts longer than norad renaline and is more easily controlled. It has both alpha and beta stimulan activity and is said to improve coronary and perhaps cerebral and renal flow *Presentation* Infection B.P. ampoules 1ml and vials 10ml of a solutior 10mg/ml; *dose* s.c. and i.m. 2-10mg working in a few minutes and i.v 500μg-5mg acting immediately and lasting 30 minutes. The undiluted injec tion is for extreme urgency only. It is best added 15-100mg to 500ml oi Sodium Chloride 0.9% or Dextrose 5% Injections and infused slowly. **Mexth oxamine Hydrochloride** ('Vasoxine') is mainly used for hypotension in anaes thesia. *Presentation* Injection B.P.C. solution in ampoules 1ml strengtf 20mg/ml; 5-20mg i.v., or i.m.

Local vasoconstrictors of sympathomimetic substances such as methox amine and **Phenylpropanolamine** may counteract the effect of hypotensive therapy and cause interactions with monoamine oxidase inhibitors. Drugs which oppose the alpha or beta stimulating effects of *catecholamines* (adrenaline and noradrenaline) on receptors, and adrenergic neurone block ers are discussed in Chapter 19. The sympathomimetics acting as broncho dilators are dealt with in Chapter 20.

PARASYMPATHOMIMETICS
The cholinergic acting drugs are of two types: (1)*acetylcholine-like,* but unlike acetylcholine they are not rapidly destroyed; (2)*anticholinesterases* which stop the destruction of acetylcholine by the enzyme cholinesterase and so enhance its action.

Acetylcholine-like drugs
These drugs are choline derivatives. **Pilocarpine** is a plant alkaloid and as the sulphate or hydrochloride is available in 0.5-4% strengths (usually 1%) eye drops to constrict the pupils (miotic) and to treat glaucoma (along with neutral adrenaline drops, 5% guanethidine eye drops and timolol). **Carbachol U.S.P.** increases peristalsis and combats drug-induced constipation and urinary reten tion from non-obstructive causes. *Dose* 250-500μg s.c.
Bethanechol Chloride U.S.N.F. ('Mechothane', 'Myotonine Chloride', 'Ure choline Chloride') has similar uses to carbachol, as well as being employed in gastro-oesophageal reflux. *Presentation* ampoules 1ml containing 5mg and tablets 5, 10 and 25mg; *dose* 5-25mg orally, 2-5mg s.c.
Methacholine Chloride B.P.C. has been used 20mg s.c. for paroxysmal tachycardia. Injections of cholinergic drugs should be avoided in the elderly and those with suspected or known coronary artery disease for coronary ischaemia, angina, hypotension, dyspnoea and wheeze can occur. Airway obstruction is also worsened. In urinary retention in later life catheterization is safer than using cholinergic drugs to empty the bladder.

Anticholinesterases
Physostigmine (Eserine) is a plant alkaloid containing an indole ring used as various salts in 0.25, 0.5 and 2% solution and 0.125 and 0.25% ointment as a miotic.
Neostigmine Ph. Eur. ('Prostigmin') is used for post-operative paralytic ileus urinary retention, to counteract the muscle relaxants tubocurarine and gal

lamine and to correct glaucoma and myasthenia gravis. It acts on both voluntary and involuntary muscle. *Presentation* Tablets B.P. Neostigmine Bromide
15mg, Injection B.P. ampoules 1ml containing in solution Neostigmine
Methylsulphate 500µg and 2.5mg and eye drops 3% in 7.5ml bottles. *Dose*
orally 15-30mg, s.c., or i.m. 500µg-2mg, i.v. 1-5mg. It is often given with
atropine. The duration of action 2-5 hours depends on the dose, route given
and the severity of myasthenia gravis. In mild myasthenia gravis 15mg thrice
daily may suffice. In severe forms from 10 to 100 tablets may be necessary
divided into 2-hourly doses, supplemented by pyridostigmine. *Adverse effects*
colic, sweating, muscle weakness, muscle fasciculation, flushing, salivation,
lacrimation, diarrhoea, nausea, miosis and bradycardia, from parasympathetic
overactivity.

Pyridostigmine Bromide ('Mestinon') is weaker and slower than neostigmine
but lasts longer and is often used first as the drug of choice. *Uses* myasthenia
gravis and to counteract curare-like muscle relaxants. *Presentation* Tablets
B.P. 60mg, Injection B.P. ampoules 1ml 1mg/ml; *dose* 60-300mg orally,
2-5mg s.c., i.m., or i.v.

Ambenonium Chloride U.S.N.F. ('Mytelase') *presentation* tablets 10mg; *dose*
5-25mg orally daily in 3 or 4 divided amounts. *Uses* and *Adverse effects* as for
neostigmine.

Distigmine Bromide ('Ubretid') lasts 12-24 hours; *dose* orally one tablet of
5mg once or twice daily, or 500µg (ampoule 1ml) i.m. *Uses* as for neostigmine.
Adverse effects are prolonged.

Edrophonium Chloride ('Tensilon') has a rapid short action which is used to
diagnose myasthenia gravis (and also to terminate paroxysmal tachycardia).
After injection weak myasthenic muscles become stronger within minutes and
the effect lasts 5-30 minutes. *Presentation* Injection B.P. ampoules 1ml containing 10mg in solution; *dose* 2mg i.v. at first, repeated up to a total of 20mg.

Myasthenia gravis
This muscle disorder results from damage to the acetylcholine muscle receptors by circulating antibodies. The acetylcholine levels may be normal or
increased. Corticosteroids are helpful in unresponsive cases. Initially patients
may get worse so full ventilatory facilities should be available. Corticosteroids
can eventually be given on alternate days without the need for anticholinesterases. Immunosuppressants such as azathioprine can reduce antibody
formation and temporary relief can be had by plasmapheresis which 'skims off'
antibodies.

Myasthenic Crisis
Both over, or under dosage, with neostigmine or pyridostigmine can cause
muscle weakness. To distinguish between the two i.v. edrophonium is given. In
underdosage the injection causes rapid improvement in power whereas in the
overtreated patient in cholinergic crisis the muscle weakness temporarily
increases.

Anticholinesterase Poisons
Certain organophosphorus compounds made industrially and used in agricul-
ture as insecticides can by accident be absorbed via the skin. Death can occur in
seconds; here immediate injection of **Atropine** and **Pralidoxime** which chelates
the poison is the only cure. In industry those at risk take preventative meas-

ures, work in pairs and a charged syringe of antidote is nearby. These 'nerve gases' and sprays cause vomiting, diarrhoea, bradycardia, convulsions and nerve damage in those not killed immediately.

ANTIPARASYMPATHETIC AGENTS
Acetylcholine antagonists or parasympatholytics prevent acetylcholine liberated at nerve endings from transmitting its action to the receptors on the smooth involuntary muscle and glands. Important sources of these drugs are the solanaceous plants which contain alkaloids such as atropine, hyoscyamine and hyoscine.

Solanaceous Plants and their Alkaloids (Tropane Alkaloids)
Belladonna is derived from the leaf of the deadly nightshade (*Atropa belladonna*) and contains atropine and some hyoscine. **Hyoscyamus** from henbane and **Stramonium** from another plant contain atropine, hyoscine and hyoscyamine. All are available (Ph. Eur.) as Tinctures or alcoholic extracts. The daily doses of B.P. Tinctures of Belladonna are 0.5-2ml, Hyoscyamus 2-5ml and Stramonium up to 6ml in divided doses. Potassium Citrate and Hyoscyamus Mixture B.P.C. is used to ease painful micturition and stramonium aids sputum expectoration.
Atropine Sulphate Ph. Eur. reduces muscle tone in the intestine, bladder and eye and also reduces the secretion of the bronchial and salivary glands. *Uses* as an antispasmodic in peptic ulcer, and intestinal colic, for pre-medication to dry mouth and bronchial secretions, to speed the heart rate in sinus and nodal bradycardia after cardiac infarction, and to counteract the bradycardia and other side effects produced by choline derivatives, anticholinesterases and mushroom poisoning. Atropine is no longer advised for routine premedication by many anaesthetists in adults because of dry mouth and tachycardia it causes. When required it can be given i.v. just before anaesthetizing. Scopolamine (hyoscine) is often preferred since it has useful anti-emetic and amnesic properties. *Presentation* Tablets B.P. 500μg, Injection ampoules containing in 1ml 400, 600 and 800μg; 1 and 1.25mg as a solution in water. *Dose* 250μg-2mg orally, s.c. or i.m. A 1 or 2% solution is a mydriatic or pupil dilator. *Adverse effects* of these alkaloids are dry mouth, blurred vision, retention of urine and difficulty of micturition. Similar symptoms arise from overdosage and include mental excitability with agitation, delirium, fever and rapid pulse.
Atropine Methonitrate ('Eumydrin') as oral drops 0.6% in alcoholic solution in a dose of 0.1-0.2ml has been used for congenital pyloric stenosis, but surgery is in practice preferable.
Homatropine Hydrobromide Ph. Eur. is a short-acting mydriatic employed in 2% solution as eye drops, often with 1% cocaine. **Cyclopentolate Hydrochloride B.P.C.** ('Cyclogyl', 'Mydrilate') 0.5 and 1% is an alternative to atropine and homatropine and is shorter acting. **Tropicamide** ('Midriacyl') 0.5 and 1% is probably the best mydriatic as it is rapid and short acting and has less systemic effects. It must be followed by pilocarpine drops.
Hyoscine Hydrobromide Ph. Eur. or **Scopolamine** is used to calm restless patients, to induce sleep and to prevent sea-sickness. *Presentation* Tablets B.P. 300, 400 and 600μg. Injection ampoules 1ml containing in solution 400 or 600μg. *Dose* 300-900μg orally or by injection 300-600μg s.c.

Synthetic atropine-like drugs used in gastro-intestinal disease are discussed in Chapter 21.

15 HYPNOTICS, SEDATIVES, TRANQUILLIZERS AND ANTIDEPRESSIVES

There are now many drugs acting on the brain which affect feeling, perception, behaviour, mood, the level of consciousness and states of psychosis. The traditional distinction between sedatives and hypnotics is no longer justified in most instances for the difference is largely one of dosage since small amounts sedate and larger amounts induce sleep. Nor is there any major difference between 'minor tranquillizers' and sedatives. Ideally a minor tranquillizer should allay anxiety, fear or panic without causing drowsiness, or excessive sedation. All these types of drugs are cerebral depressants with a range from mild sedation to unconsciousness (like alcohol) and most may also be used as anticonvulsants.

HYPNO-SEDATIVES

Insomnia
With advancing age the ability to sleep is normally impaired and the duration of sleep needed decreases. Insomnia is a complaint with many causes for only a proportion of which are hypnotics really needed. For instance, if insomnia results from noise (e.g. in hospital), hunger (physical or sexual), pain, itch, cramp, nocturia, fever, diarrhoea, breathlessness, mental stimulation from drugs, depression, emotion (loss, stress, change), grief, anxiety or hallucinations these should be treated. There is currently an increasing reluctance to start patients on hypnotics (other than for short term or crisis situations e.g. bereavement), or to maintain the habit of chemically induced sleep. However, patients with hypertension irrespective of primary treatment, benefit from sleep which is associated with lowered pressure and hypnotics may be helpful. There has also been a change in prescribing habits. At present the benzodiazepines are fashionable and after 70 years the barbiturates are on the wane. Nevertheless even the benzodiazepines distort brain function and E.E.G. studies show that the sleep is not natural.
The choice of an hypnotic depends on numerous factors
(1) The fitness of the patient since some hypnotics are dangerous if the patient is anoxic, has obstructive airway disease, hypoventilation with carbon dioxide narcosis (e.g. the barbiturates and even the benzodiazepines), severe liver disease or poor renal function. The use of hypnotics rises steeply with age.
(2) The possibility of harmful drug inter-actions with oral anticoagulants and with alcohol the latter potentiating all hypnotics.
(3) The character of the drug-induced sleep pattern. Dreaming is essential to healthy mental life. Most hypnotics in sufficient dosage depress the quality of sleep (proportion of dreaming and rapid eye movement 'REM' sleep) as well as the quantity. On stopping hypnotics rebound insomnia and nightmares can occur with sympathetic nervous overactivity.
(4) The known dangers of overdosage, self-poisoning (high with barbiturates) and dependence.
(5) A rational consideration of the pharmacology including efficacy, duration of action, the way the drug is metabolized and handled by liver or kidney, the

question of liver enzyme induction, accumulation and toxicity.
(6) Cost—this should be a minor factor in comparison with safety.
(7) Quick induction of sleep and absence of hangover on waking.

Barbiturates and Related Drugs
Authorities in hospital (e.g. those in charge of poison centres) and many in
general practice no longer believe it is justified to start any patient on barbiturates (other than for epilepsy), but it seems reasonable to many doctors to
allow patients who have become well adjusted to them over the years to continue. However, increasingly doctors are showing that patients can be weaned
off them, by substituting a benzodiazepine which often may later be stopped.
Since barbiturates are still widely prescribed, in spite of their disadvantages,
they are mentioned for information purposes since they account for over 8
million prescriptions yearly in the U.K. Chemically they are derivatives of urea
and malonic acid (cyclic ureides). In Britain their names end in -one, in the
U.S.A. -al. They are used as sedatives, to allay anxiety, induce sleep, prevent
and control epilepsy and in certain metabolic diseases (e.g. Gilbert's disease)
to increase metabolic processes by stimulating or inducing liver enzymes. Barbiturates may still be used in pre-eclampsia since some paediatricians dislike
the benzodiazepines because of the risk of neonatal respiratory depression.
The ultra-short-acting barbiturates are widely and beneficially used for i.v.
anaesthesia. The liver metabolizes most forms although a proportion of
phenobarbitone is excreted unchanged by the kidneys. *Administration* is
usually orally, but can be i.m., or i.v. As sedatives the dose is divided equally in
3 amounts through the day. While their use in the control of epilepsy is unques-
tioned they are probably no longer the treatment of choice. Because of the risk
of overdose, habituation, dependence and abuse it is expected that over the
coming years their consumption as hypnotics and sedatives will be severely
reduced and indeed total prescriptions are now falling by 10% annually.
Long-Acting. Their main use is for epilepsy.
Phenobarbitone Ph. Eur. ('Luminal') *presentation* Tablets B.P. 15, 30, 60 and
100mg, Elixir B.P.C. 15mg/ml; *dose* 90-200mg for sedation; as an anticonvulsant up to 180mg daily. Phenobarbitone has a low lipid solubility and so
enters the brain slowly. It is a sedative rather than an hypnotic. **Phenobarbitone
Sodium** (Soluble Phenobarbitone,) *presentation* Tablets B.P. 15, 30, 60 and
100mg; Phenobarbitone Injection B.P. ampoules 1ml containing 200mg
('Gardenal Sodium'). *Oral dose* as for phenobarbitone; i.m. for sedation and
status epilepticus 50-200mg. **Barbitone Sodium** ('Soluble Barbitone') *presentation* Tablets B.P. 300mg; *dose* 300-600mg daily is obsolete. This group is
excreted renally and the amount excreted may be increased if desired by
forced diuresis and alkalinization of the urine (see p. 135).
Shorter Acting
Butobarbitone Ph. Eur. (Butethal, 'Soneryl') *presentation* Tablets B.P.
100mg. *Dose* as hypnotic 100-200mg orally. **Amylobarbitone** (Amobarbital
U.S.P., 'Amytal') *presentation* Tablets B.P. 15, 30, 50, 100 and 200mg; *dose* as
sedative 90-400mg. **Amylobarbitone Sodium Ph. Eur.** ('Sodium Amytal') is
more quickly absorbed than amylobarbitone. *Presentation* Tablets and Capsules B.P. 60 and 200mg; *dose* as for amylobarbitone. Ampoules are available
for injection. **Pentobarbitone Sodium Ph. Eur.** ('Nembutal') *presentation* Capsules B.P. 50 and 100mg, Tablets B.P. 100mg; *dose* 90-200mg as an hypnotic. **Heptabarbitone** ('Medomin') *presentation* capsules and tablets 200mg;

dose as an hypnotic 200-400mg. **Quinalbarbitone Sodium Ph. Eur.** (Sodium Secobarbital U.S.P., 'Seconal') *presentation* Capsules B.P. 50 and 100mg; *dose* as hypnotic 200-400mg. 'Tuinal' is quinalbarbitone and amylobarbitone; *dose* 100-200mg as an hypnotic. **Cyclobarbitone Calcium Ph. Eur.** ('Phanodorm', 'Rapidal') *presentation* Tablets B.P. 200mg; *dose* as hypnotic 200-400mg. *Dangers* barbiturates may be taken accidentally by children and deliberately for suicide by adults. Barbiturate coma is a common hospital emergency and is especially dangerous with the quicker acting forms which achieve high levels. Respiratory depression, hypotension and hypothermia are features. These drugs should be avoided in those with depression or mental illness, and not given to alcoholics nor taken with alcohol. Dependence, tolerance and withdrawal fits are common. The young are increasingly abusing them by injecting the contents of capsules i.v. Chronic intake can cause impaired mental function, slurred speech, nystagmus and ataxia. The elderly may be made confused by them and children paradoxically may become excited and restless. Barbiturates suppress REM sleep, cause dream deprivation and, when stopped, rebound insomnia and nightmares. Abrupt withdrawal of barbiturates in those used to large doses can be dangerous causing anxiety, tremor, distortion of visual perception, insomnia, postural hypotension, nausea, delirium, psychosis and convulsions (abstinence syndrome) in 2-3 days. Since they precipitate porphyria patients should not be given barbiturates in any form (including i.v. anaesthesia) if they have this disease nor if they have uncompensated cirrhosis of the liver. Chronic intake stimulates liver enzymes and this increases the metabolic breakdown and lowers the efficacy of warfarin, oral contraceptives, corticosteroids, vitamin D and possibly chlorpromazine and amitriptyline.

Carbromal like the barbiturates is a urea derivative and is a mild sedative and hypnotic. *Presentation* Tablets B.P. 300mg; *dose* 300mg-1g. *Adverse effects* it contains bromine and rashes including purpura are possible as well as other manifestations of bromism.

Piperidinedione derivatives are structurally similar to the barbiturates with similar actions and adverse effects. **Glutethimide** ('Doriden') *presentation* Tablets B.P. 250mg; *dose* 250-500mg. *Adverse effects* purpura, nausea, addiction, toxic psychosis, cerebellar ataxia, convulsions while taking the tablets in large amounts as well as on withdrawal (this is unlike the barbiturates). It is used for suicide, is an enzyme inducer and can also precipitate porphyria. **Methyprylone** ('Noludar') *presentation* Tablets B.P. 200mg; *dose* 200-400mg 15min before bedtime.

ALCOHOLS

Ethanol or **ethyl alcohol** as brandy, whisky or gin is taken as a nightcap by the elderly and is contained in euphoric preparations such as the Brompton Cocktail to reduce the distress of the dying. Alcohol potentiates the cerebral depressants.

Ethchlorvynol U.S.N.F. ('Placidyl' U.S.A.) a chlorinated carbinol is a colourless aromatic liquid. *Presentation* Capsules 100, 200, 500 and 750mg; *dose* as hypnotic 500-750mg which acts in 30 min and lasts 5 hours. It is dangerous in overdosage. This preparation is no longer available in the U.K. Similarly Methylpentynol has been withdrawn.

Chloral and related drugs are converted into trichloroethanol (an alcohol) by the body.

Chloral Hydrate Ph. Eur. is a crystalline compound and when dissolved a readily absorbed and quick acting hypnotic with a duration of 6-8 hours. The solution needs to be well diluted since it tastes unpleasant and irritates the stomach producing flatulence, distension and nausea. Trichloroethanol is metabolized by the liver and kidneys. Chloral is the safest hypnotic for infants and is suitable for the elderly. Chloral Mixture B.P.C. contains 1g/10ml and 'Noctec' capsules contain 500mg in solution. *Dose* for adults is 500mg-2g. Chloral Elixir Paediatric B.P.C. contains 200mg/5ml and children under one year of age take 2.5-7.5ml. Chloral hydrate can also be taken by enema or suppository.

Chloral derivatives aim to liberate trichloroethanol with less gastric irritation than chloral.

Dichloralphenazone ('Welldorm') contains phenazone which acts as a binder. *Presentation* Tablets B.P. 650mg, Elixir B.P.C. 225mg/5ml; *dose* 650-1300mg taken in water.

Triclofos Sodium is trichloroethyl dihydrogen phosphate which changes in the body to trichloroethanol. It is palatable, induces sleep quickly, lasts 5-8 hours and is likewise suitable for the elderly. *Presentation* Triclofos Elixir B.P.C. 500mg/5ml; *dose* adults 10-20ml (two-four 5ml spoonfuls) equal to 1-2g, infants 2.5-5ml (250-500mg), children 5-10ml (500-1000mg). Triclofos Tablets B.P. are no longer commercially available. *Precautions* chloral-type drugs should be avoided in patients with kidney, gastric or liver disorders. They potentiate alcohol and interact with coumarin anticoagulants (e.g. warfarin). *Overdosage* causes coma, hypotension, hypothermia, cardiac arrhythmias, cardiac arrest and respiratory depression. **Paraldehyde Ph. Eur.** is a cyclical ether, a simple hydrocarbon which is a colourless, volatile liquid with an unpleasant taste and smell. Solutions are given orally, parenterally or by enema. It quickly absorbed and excretion is by the liver and lungs and action is prolonged. Paraldehyde on storage decomposes on exposure to light and air and is therefore kept airtight in dark bottles. Oral paraldehyde is flavoured with iced orange; *dose* 5-10ml. For i.m. use there are ampoules 2, 5 and 10ml of Paraldehyde Injection B.P.C.; *dose* 2-10ml with no more than 4ml given in any one site to reduce the risk of abscess formation. Plastic syringes may be incompatible with paraldehyde and should not be used unless stated to be safe. Because of its safety paraldehyde can be given for confused, restless and elderly patients (but major tranquillizers are preferred) and for epilepsy where it is safer than diazepam in children. Paraldehyde Enema B.P.C. consists of paraldehyde freshly made up with 100ml sodium chloride solution; *dose* 5ml/kg B.W. to a maximum of 300ml. Paraldehyde is less effective in alcoholics and can lead to addiction. *Care should be taken to distinguish undiluted paraldehyde from dilutions in water ready for administration.* In view of possible and actual accidents and deaths there is little use for paraldehyde and diazepam is replacing it for epilepsy in adults and haloperidol and the phenothiazines in psychotic, disturbed states. **Methaqualone** is a quinazolone. *Presentation* Tablets B.P., U.S.N.F. 150 and 300mg, ('Quaalude' in the U.S.A.) and 'Mandrax' contains 250mg with 25mg of the antihistamine diphenhydramine. They are undoubtedly effective, but because of medicolegal problems they are Controlled Drugs subject to legal control and are not advised. *Adverse effects* paraesthesiae of limbs, dry mouth, headache, dizziness, anorexia, nausea, emesis, epigastric discomfort, diarrhoea, sweating, urticaria and in overdosage coma, pyramidal signs, spasticity and pulmonary oedema. Abuse and dependence are common with 'Mandrax', although some patients sleep happily taking 1 or 2 tablets as law-abiding citizens and when changed to other hypnotics have become discontented insomniacs.

Ethinamate U.S.N.F. is an hypnotic belonging to the carbamates. *Presentation* Tablets 500mg; *dose* 500-1000mg. Dependence can occur.

Chlormethiazole Edisylate ('Heminevrin') *presentation* syrup 50mg/ml; *dose* 10ml as a sedative; for hypnotic use tablets 500mg or capsules 192mg of the equivalent chlormethiazole base; *dose* 2-4 tablets or capsules. It is widely used in geriatric practice as it does not cause confusion, whereas barbiturates may cause, or increase, confusion. The plasma half-life is about 1 hour so that less hang-over and cumulative effects in the elderly are claimed than with the barbiturates. It is effective but the taste is unpleasant and needs masking with lime or orange. Dependence is possible, but to date overdosage appears less dangerous than with the barbiturates. Long-term use is not advised in those dependent on alcohol or barbiturates. Chemically it is derived from the thiazole part of thiamine or vitamin B_1.

Antihistamines such as diphenhydramine hydrochloride 50-100mg can be useful hypnotics in patients with liver or renal disease although the benzodiazepines are better. In depressed patients with early morning waking a sedative type tricyclic drug such as amitriptyline is often effective, but can cause ataxia in the morning and is dangerous in overdosage.

The most widely used sedatives and hypnotics are the benzodiazepines e.g. nitrazepam, diazepam and flurazepam and they are dealt with later.

DRUGS AND PSYCHIATRIC ILLNESS
Psychotropic drugs are correctly given only after proper evaluation of the mental state and discussion of relevant problems. Some patients need a period of time on medication to enable them to be calm enough to talk about their problems. It has often been said that human problems do not always require chemical solutions. Other drugs including alcohol, and the patient's occupation (e.g. drivers, pilots, machine operators) are taken into consideration.

ANXIETY AND TENSION (ANXIOLYTIC DRUGS)
The chemical control of symptoms such as anxiety, fear, restlessness, worry, tension and panic should be achieved by drugs influencing emotion by selective activity on the sites concerned with emotion (limbic system, amygdala) and yet have minimal effects on the cerebral cortex. The barbiturate-alcohol group performs badly on this score since they depress the cerebral cortex and cause mental dullness, impaired cognitive functions, faulty judgement and inco-ordination and at times irritability, restlessness, paradoxical excitement and insomnia, the latter especially in children who are mentally subnormal or brain damaged by cerebral palsy. Anxiety can be allayed by barbiturates e.g. amylobarbitone with the advantage of cheapness, but with the disadvantages discussed above such as dependence. Many barbiturate-containing compounds e.g. 'Bellergal' are still widely prescribed in general practice. Another drug used is **Oxypertine** ('Integrin') a major tranquilliser given in small doses and of particular value when there has been dependence on alcohol or barbiturates previously. Haloperidol, and reserpine have also been used in appropriate dosage. Beta blockers have a special place when symptoms of sympathetic nervous system overactivity are prominent such as tremor, palpitation, gastric upsets and diarrhoea. They have to be combined with a centrally active drug like diazepam.

Meprobamate Ph. Eur. ('Equanil', 'Miltown', 'Milonorm') has been used for anxiety and muscle tension and chemically it is a dicarbamate. Prolonged usage can lead to habituation. *Presentation* Tablets B.P. 200 and 400mg; *dose* 400-1200mg daily in divided amounts. It is little used.

BENZODIAZEPINES

These are claimed to act selectively inhibiting the limbic system, notably the hippocampus. Their proponents believe they are the nearest to the ideal of "tranquillization without sedation". Others hold that they act similarly to barbiturates, but with greater safety. All are structurally and pharmacologically similar and many (e.g. diazepam, chlordiazepoxide, medazepam and clorazepate) share the same intermediate active metabolites (e.g. desmethyldiazepam which has a long half-life and lasting action in the body). Introduced to treat anxiety, depending on the dose they are used for anxiety, sedation, muscle relaxation, as hypnotics (nitrazepam, flurazepam, diazepam), premedication for endoscopy, as anticonvulsants (nitrazepam, diazepam, clonazepam) and i.v. for brief anaesthesia before electrical deconversion of arrhythmias. They also stimulate the appetite and cause weight gain. Acute withdrawal syndromes due to barbiturates and alcohol can be suppressed either by oral or systemic therapy and chlordiazepoxide has been used for delirium tremens. The benzodiazepines may be combined with the monoamine oxidase inhibitors like phenelzine for severe phobias. To avoid the same mistakes as made with earlier compounds such as the barbiturates, long-continued therapy should be avoided and care is needed in prescribing them to alcoholics. In the U.S.A. the benzodiazepines are because of misuse, becoming a major problem.

There are many benzodiazepines; some are shown in Table 5. They are among the most widely prescribed drugs; chlordiazepoxide, diazepam, nitrazepam and flurazepam are especially popular. **Chlordiazepoxide Hydrochloride Ph. Eur., B.P.** is used for anxiety, muscle relaxation, sedation and alcohol withdrawal. The oral dose is 5-10mg t.d.s. up to 60mg daily and 50-100mg is given i.m. for delirium tremens. **Diazepam B.P.** is given orally in a dose of 6-30mg daily in divided doses although 5mg may be sufficient to aid sleep at night and many people cannot tolerate more than 15mg daily on a long-term basis. For status epilepticus 5-20mg is given i.v. as a bolus, or 40mg is added to 500ml of dextrose solution or saline and infused slowly. To aid endoscopy, manipulation of joints and for short anaesthesia for ECT and DC conversion of arrhythmias 5-30mg i.v., or 0.2mg/kg B.W. is injected. **Nitrazepam Ph. Eur., B.P.;** *dose* 2.5-10mg is one of the most popular hypnotics and can be given safely concurrently with anticoagulants. It is not as cheap as diazepam. It can cause confusion and dementia in the elderly so a smaller dose of 2.5-5mg may be all that is needed. It is not a safe hypnotic for patients with chronic airway obstruction. Nitrazepam is also given for infantile spasms. **Flurazepam** is a popular hypnotic in the U.S.A.; *dose* 15-30mg. Nitrazepam has not been introduced in the U.S.A.

Adverse effects because of their wide use these are given in detail: hypotension, occasional syncope, sleepiness, drowsiness, headache, muzziness, slurred speech, muddled thoughts, unsteadiness, blurred vision, diplopia, tremor, vertigo, nausea and potentiation of alcohol, dry mouth, salivation. Paradoxically they may occasionally excite, release aggression and cause hallucinations. The elderly can become disoriented, euphoric or muddled. Reduced libido, mens-

TABLE 5
THE BENZODIAZEPINES

Name Approved	Proprietary	Presentation (mg)	Dose (daily)	Action
Chlordiazepoxide Hydrochloride B.P.	'Calmoden' 'Librium' 'Tropium'	tablets 5, 10, 25 capsules 5, 10 ampoules 100mg with 2ml solvent	10-60mg	Anxiety Alcoholism
Diazepam B.P.	'Atensine' 'Valium'	tablets 2, 5, 10 capsules 2, 5 elixir 2mg/5ml ampoules 5mg/ml 2ml and 4ml	6-40mg orally 5-30mg i.v. or 0.1-0.2mg /kg B.W.	Anxiety Hypnotic Muscle relaxant Anaesthesia
Oxazepam	'Serenid D' 'Serenid Forte'	tablets 10, 15 capsules 30	30-180mg orally	Anxiety
Medazepam	'Nobrium'	capsules 5, 10	15-30mg	Anxiety
Lorazepam	'Ativan'	tablets 1, 2.5 ampoules 1ml 4mg/ml	3-10mg orally 0.025-0.05 mg/kg B.W. or 1-4mg i.m. or i.v.	Anxiety Premedication Anticonvulsant
Prazepam	'Verstran'	tablets 10	10-60mg	Anxiety
Temazepam	'Euhypnos' 'Normison'	capsules 10 and 20	5-60mg	Hypnotic
Flunitrazepam	'Rohypnol'	tablets 2	0.5-6mg	Hypnotic
Nitrazepam Ph. Eur., B.P.	'Mogadon' 'Remnos' 'Nitrados' 'Somnite' 'Somnased'	tablets 5 capsules 5	2.5-10mg	Hypnotic
Triazolam	'Halcion'	tablets 0.125, 0.25	0.125-0.25mg	Hypnotic
Flurazepam	'Dalmane'	capsules 5 and 10	15-30mg	Hypnotic
Clobazepam	'Frisium'	capsules 10	45mg	Anxiety
Clonazepam	'Rivotril'	tablets 0.5 and 2mg; injection 1mg/ml with diluent	4-8mg orally 1 mg i.v.	Anticonvulsant
Potassium Clorazepate	'Tranxene'	capsules 15	15 mg at night	Anxiety

trual irregularity, rashes, oedema and jaundice are rare complications. Generally they are safe drugs for patients with liver disease. In patients with CO_2 retention from lung disease death can occasionally occur from hypnotic doses; respiratory depression can follow i.v. injection. Dependency and withdrawal syndromes are recorded. The slow clearance of the benzodiazepines from the body avoids the disadvantages seen with abrupt cessation of other cerebral depressants with seemingly less severe withdrawal syndromes. Deliberate self-poisoning is rarely fatal in adults. Obstetricians have noted that their use in pregnant women at term is associated with floppy babies, hypothermia and poor feeders. Intravenous injection of diazepam causes phlebitis.

MAJOR TRANQUILLIZERS
Unlike the hypno-sedatives and so-called 'minor tranquillizers' the major tranquillizers (antipsychotics) do not cause dependence and their indications and pharmacological properties are different. They include the phenothiazines, thioxanthenes and the butyrophenones. Reserpine is a member of this class, but is little used in psychiatric practice.

Phenothiazines
These are strong central nervous system depressants which control aggression and psychomotor activity without impairing consciousness. They were developed from research on the antihistamines. They are used:
(1) to reduce excessive motor activity in schizophrenia, senile agitation, hypomania, toxic confusion states;
(2) to calm anxiety and suppress hallucinations, delusions, excitement and restlessness, so making the patient more manageable and co-operative;
(3) to increase appetite and weight in schizophrenia and anorexia nervosa.

Non-psychiatric Uses:
(4) to suppress sickness and vomiting in uraemia, terminal cancer, alcoholism and after irradiation;
(5) to reduce body temperature in surgery, after cardiac arrest where brain damage has occurred, in heat stroke and in thyrotoxic crisis;
(6) to control persistent hiccoughs;
(7) to facilitate premedication since they potentiate analgesics and sedatives;
(8) for terminal care since patients may become indifferent to pain and they may be combined with narcotics (see p. 93);
(9) as labyrinthine sedatives in vertigo (see p. 131).

Phenothiazines can be given orally, rectally or parenterally and are metabolized by the liver. Currently available preparations are listed in Table 6. The phenothiazines' most important action is dopamine receptor blockade. They have anticatecholamine actions (being alpha-blockers and causing peripheral vasodilation and hypotension), they are anticholinergic (causing tachycardia) and they also possess antiserotonin and antihistaminic activities. All are modifications of the same tricyclic structure containing a sulphur atom (unlike the very similar tricyclic antidepressives). It is the phenothiazine side chain which differs being aliphatic (a simple hydrocarbon structure) as with chlorpromazine, piperidine (thioridazine, pericyazine), or piperazine (trifluoperazine, perphenazine, fluphenazine). These side chains alter the pharmacological actions and the types of adverse reactions seen. The phenothiazines vary in potency, some are more sedative and others can be used as antihistamines or anti-emetics.

Chlorpromazine Hydrochloride Ph. Eur. ('Largactil') was the first major tranquillizer introduced in 1952 and is the prototype of the phenothiazines. The chlorine atom it contains makes liver damage possible for it is not a feature of promazine. *Presentation* Tablets B.P. 10, 25, 50 and 100mg, Elixir B.P.C. and U.S.P. 25mg/5ml, 'Largactil Forte' suspension 100mg/5ml, Suppositories B.P.C. containing 100mg, Chlorpromazine Injection B.P. a solution in ampoules 5ml 10mg/ml, 1 and 2ml 25mg/ml. *Dose* initially 25mg t.d.s. orally to 800mg or even more in acute schizophrenia when 2000mg daily has been given. For prolonged therapy one third to one half is given at night. For i.m. use 25-100mg is given to control acutely disturbed patients; the solution may also be injected i.v. with great care. (*Beware marked hypotension.*)

Promazine Hydrochloride ('Sparine') is not as effective as chlorpromazine and has been classed as an *intermediate* rather than a major tranquillizer, and is widely used as a sedative in elderly patients. *Presentation* Tablets B.P. 25, 50 and 100mg, suspension 50mg/5ml, Promazine Injection B.P. a solution in ampoules 1 and 2ml 50mg/ml. *Dose* orally 25-50mg thrice daily or more; parenterally 25-50mg as a single dose or 6-8 hourly.

Perphenazine Hydrochloride tablet strengths are shown in Table 6.

Thioridazine ('Melleril') is also available in syrup form and a suspension and at a dose of 25mg t.d.s. and 50mg at night is used as a tranquillizer for the elderly.

Schizophrenia is common (0.9% of the population) and relapse is likely. It is considered desirable for treatment to continue for years after apparent recovery. To prevent drug defaulting ("non-compliance") long-acting depot injections are available. **Fluphenazine Enanthate B.P.** ('Moditen Enanthate') was the first injection to be given although nowadays the decanoate is preferred. The initial test dose of 12.5mg i.m. is given, and observed, in hospital and if there is no ill-effect is followed after an interval of 4-7 days by 25mg i.m. and thereafter usually every 10-14 days. **Fluphenazine Decanoate Injection B.P.** ('Modecate') *presentation* a solution contained in ampoules 0.5, 1 and 2ml, disposable syringes 1ml, vials 10ml, 25mg/ml and Concentrate injection ampoules 1ml 100mg/ml. The decanoate is a long-chain fatty acid derivative which dissolves easily in Sesame Oil B.P. *Dose* 12.5mg initially as a test dose then 12.5-25mg i.m. every 2-5 weeks. Half doses are advised in the aged. Extra-pyramidal side-effects are very common with the injections.

Adverse effects of the phenothiazines collectively are common. They include liver damage, cholestatic jaundice and agranulocytosis which are rare, Parkinsonism which is common (controlled by orphenadrine, benzhexol, procyclidine or benztropine), dystonic reactions and abnormal postures of neck, head and limbs. These abnormal movements can continue after stopping the drugs. These rarer dystonic reactions result from tonic and often sustained contractions of localized groups of muscles. Breathing and swallowing may be affected. Akathisia is common and is an unpleasant restless feeling, often localized to the legs so the sufferer cannot sit still. Other untoward effects are induction of fits, drowsiness, restlessness, agitation, depression, rashes including sensitivity to sunshine, tachycardia, postural hypotension, cardiomyopathy with ECG changes and sudden death, dizziness, syncope, hypothermia, hyperthermia, breast enlargement, milk formation, mutism, priapism, tardive dyskinesia, lip smacking, grimacing, jerking and chewing movements of face, tongue, lips and neck, lens and corneal opacities; chlorpromazine causes lens and corneal pigmentation and thioridazine causes pigmentary retinal changes (if the dose is above 900mg daily). Phenothiazines potentiate the sedative-hypnotic group including alcohol. Drug interactions; they antagonize guanidine type antihypertensives.

TABLE 6
PHENOTHIAZINES

Name Approved	Proprietary	Tablet Strength (mg)	Daily Dose (mg) Initial (usual)	Maximum
Chlorpromazine Hydrochloride B.P.	'Chloractil', 'Largactil', 'Thorazine'	10, 25, 50, 100	75	2000
Promazine Hydrochloride B.P.	'Sparine'	25, 50, 100	75	800
Fluopromazine Hydrochloride (Triflupromazine Hydrochloride U.S.N.F.)	'Vesprin'	10, 25, 50	30-75	150
Methotrimeprazine Maleate U.S.N.F.	'Veractil'	25	25-50	1000
Trimeprazine Tartrate	'Vallergan'	10	30-40	100
Trifluoperazine B.P.	'Stelazine'	1, 5 (Capsules 2, 10, 15)	2	6-30
Perphenazine B.P.	'Fentazin', 'Trilafon'	2, 4, 8	6-12	12-24
Fluphenazine Hydrochloride B.P.	'Moditen', 'Prolixin'	1, 2.5, 5	1-2	20
Thiopropazate Hydrochloride B.P.C.	'Dartalan'	5, 10	15-30	100
Thioproperazine Mesylate*	'Majeptil'	5, 10, 25	5	90
Prochlorperazine Maleate B.P.	'Compazine', 'Stemetil'	5, 25	15	100
Thioridazine Hydrochloride B.P.	'Melleril'	10, 25, 50, 100	30-100	600
Pericyazine	'Neulactil'	2.5, 10, 25	10-90	150

*Hospital use only

Thioxanthenes
In structure they closely resemble the phenothiazines and so do their actions and adverse effects.
Chlorprothixene ('Taractan') has tranquillizing and anti-depressant actions. *Presentation* tablets 15 and 50mg; *dose* orally 30-400mg daily in divided amounts. **Thiothixene** ('Navane') *presentation* tablets 10mg; *dose* 10-60mg daily in divided amounts. **Flupenthixol Decanoate** ('Depixol') has anti-depressant and anti-psychotic action. *Presentation* ampoules and syringes 1 and 2ml 20mg/ml and ampoules 1ml 100mg/ml. *Dose* 20mg i.m. initially followed in 4-5 days by a second dose of 20mg, thereafter increments of 20mg up to 40-120mg at 3 weekly intervals. Since it is an oily solution it is only given i.m. **Flupenthixol Dihydrochloride** ('Fluanxol') *presentation* tablets 500μg; *dose* 500μg b.d. up to 3mg daily. 'Depixol' tablets contain 3mg of flupenthixol dihydrochloride and are used for schizophrenia. **Clopenthixol Hydrochloride** ('Sordinol') is used on the Continent for schizophrenia and **Clopenthixol Decanoate** ('Clopixol') is a depot form available in the U.K.

Butyrophenones
Haloperidol ('Haldol', 'Serenace')*presentation* Tablets B.P. 0.5, 1.5, 5, 10 and 20mg and oral solution 2 and 10mg/ml is used for the control of mania, agitation and schizophrenia. Capsules 500μg (0.5mg) are also available for use as an alternative to the minor tranquillizers for anxiety and tension. Ampoules 1 ml 5mg/ml. 2ml 5 and 10mg/ml are for i.m. or i.v. use to control mania and are preferable to paraldehyde. The volume injected is smaller and less painful i.m. *Dose* for mania 10-15mg daily orally reducing to a maintenance dose; for tranquillization 500μg (0.5mg) b.d. or t.d.s.; parenterally for mania up to 30mg i.m. (usually 10mg) initially then 6 hourly according to needs of the patient to a total daily dose of 60mg or more. To counteract drug-induced Parkinsonism orphenadrine 100mg t.d.s. is given. **Trifluperidol** ('Triperidol') *presentation* tablets 500μg and 1 mg; *dose* 500μg increasing by 500μg every 3-4 days up to 6-8mg daily. **Benperidol** ('Anquil') is used to treat 'deviant and anti-social behaviour'. *Presentation* tablets 250μg; *dose* 250μg-1.5mg in divided doses. **Droperidol** ('Droleptan') is used for neuroleptanalgesia and for premedication with **Fentanyl** and **Phenoperidine** to enable patients to tolerate unpleasant procedures such as intubation, ventilation and neurosurgery. *Presentation* Droperidol tablets 10mg; *dose* orally 5-20mg; ampoules 2ml 5mg/ml; *dose* 10mg i.m.

Lithium Carbonate Ph. Eur., acts by possibly altering nerve conduction, synaptic transmission and amine and sodium metabolism. Quick-acting forms are 'Camcolit 250' tablets 250mg and 'Camcolit 400' tablets 400mg. Slow Lithium Carbonate Tablets B.P. are available commercially as 'Phasal' 300mg and 'Priadel' 400mg. *Dose* 1.6g initially then 200-400mg once daily as judged by serum levels which should range between 0.8-1.4mmol/l. Treatment should be started and controlled under specialist guidance. Lithium is used to control mania and hypomania and prevent cyclical manic-depressive episodes or cyclical depression. *Adverse effects* the earliest and most common sign of toxicity is tremor, others are abdominal pain, nausea, vomiting, diarrhoea, drowsiness, slurred speech, ataxia, giddiness, tinnitus, blurred vision, thirst, polyuria, diabetes insipidus, goitre, hypothyroidism, cardiac arrhythmias, epilepsy, muscle weakness, weight gain, chorea and athetotic movements. Toxicity is reversed by stopping the lithium and giving sodium chloride. Salt depleting diuretics may precipitate toxicity and should not be given concurrently. Renal function should be monitored since persistent renal damage occurs. The anti-thyroid action has been used therapeutically in thyrotoxicosis.

Other Tranquillizers
Oxypertine ('Integrin') is an indole derivative with a piperazine side chain. *Presentation* capsules 10mg (for sedative use) and tablets 40mg (for psychoses); *dose* 30mg (e.g. 10mg t.d.s. for sedation) up to 200-300mg in divided amounts for psychoses. It is also liable to extra-pyramidal side-effects.
Pimozide ('Orap') belongs to a new series of dopamine antagonists chemically diphenylbutyl piperidines and is widely used for schizophrenia and oral dys-kinesia due to phenothiazine therapy. *Presentation* tablets 2 and 4mg; *dose* 2mg b.d. or t.d.s. up to a total of 10mg daily. A once daily regimen may suffice for maintenance. *Adverse effects* extrapyramidal symptoms, glycosuria, rashes. **Fluspirilene** ('Redeptin') *presentation* ampoules 1 and 3ml and vials 6ml of a microcrystalline aqueous suspension 2mg/ml belongs to the same chemical class. *Dose* initially 2mg i.m. increasing by 2mg weekly to 20mg weekly (usually 2-8mg weekly). **Penfluridol** is also in this group.
Loxapine Succinate ('Loxitane') is a dibenzoxazepine anti-psychotic agent. *Dose* 10mg b.d. increasing to 10-100mg daily. *Adverse effects* extrapyramidal symptoms.

ANTIDEPRESSIVES
Depression is common at all ages, particularly in later life, as a feature of conflict, loss – real or imagined (friends, relatives, animals, mental and physical prowess), drugs (most hypotensives, fenfluramine), acute illness (e.g. influenza, hepatitis), disfiguring operations (mastectomy, amputation) and recent childbirth. Drugs do not cure, but they carry the patient through until natural remission. Depression is not a homogeneous disease and for the best use of drugs selection is needed. In severe depression electroconvulsive therapy is still best and quickest. Two main classes of agents are used: the tricyclics (two benzene rings usually joined by a 7-membered ring in the middle) and the monoamine oxidase inhibitors. Monoamines are normally broken down by enzymes. All antidepressives are potentiated by alcohol.

Tricyclics
These structurally have similarities with the phenothiazines (which however have a 6-membered middle ring containing a sulphur atom) and they were dis-covered by chance in a search for newer members of the phenothiazine class. The first antidepressant tricyclic was an **iminodibenzyl** derivative called imi-pramine in which one of the middle ring atoms is nitrogen; other members of this group collectively called **dibenzazepines** include clomipramine, desi-pramine and trimipramine. Later, other types of 7-membered rings were made to give potential advantages, or differences. The **dibenzocycloheptenes** have a middle ring only of carbon and they include amitriptyline, nortriptyline and protriptyline. Subsequent modifications have been the **dibenzoxepines** with an oxygen in the middle ring (e.g. doxepin), and others with a centre ring of indole (e.g. iprindole) and even the dibenzothiepin dothiepin with a sulphur atom in the middle ring.

Rapid absorption occurs and high levels are obtained in the brain. However, plasma levels in patients given the same dose and of similar weight, age and sex vary from the subtherapeutic to the toxic. Ideally, monitoring plasma levels would be very useful. The tricyclics may have anticholinergic, antiserotonin and antihistaminic actions. Several tricyclics have been shown to potentiate the pressor effects of adrenaline and noradrenaline. The standard teaching is that these drugs should not be given with, or within 2-3 weeks of, treatment by MAOI drugs, or sympathomimetics. Nevertheless, some experts do give selected tricyclics (usually trimipramine, or amitriptyline) at night and MAOI agents by day with undoubted success, starting both at the same time. However, in less experienced hands if complications were to occur there might be legal problems since the makers' recommendations do not endorse this combination. Tricyclics can be safely combined with benzodiazepines, phenothiazines and anti-Parkinsonian agents.

Clinically the tricyclics can be divided into those with predominant *sedative* action (e.g. amitriptyline, doxepin, trimipramine) suitable for agitation and anxiety and it may be beneficial to give all or two-thirds of the daily dose at night providing it does not cause unsteadiness in the morning, and the rest at midday. This promotes sleep and the side-effects mainly occur during sleep. Other tricyclics *stimulate* drive, energy or mood by preferentially inhibiting re-uptake of noradrenaline by the nervous system. They include nortriptyline, desipramine and protriptyline. Others are classed as *neutral* (imipramine, dibenzipin).

Because they interfere with the uptake of noradrenaline and many hypotensive drugs such as the guanidines (e.g. guanethidine, bethanidine) and clonidine into the neurone controlling blood vessels their hypotensive action is lessened. Methyldopa is rarely affected but it can itself cause depression. Barbiturates ought not be given concurrently since they enhance the metabolism of the tricyclics. Most adults need a minimum of 150mg daily of a tricyclic except the elderly who need smaller amounts. Depressed children can be given them and they are also prescribed for their action on the bladder to children with enuresis, but care should be taken to ensure that they do not take an accidental overdose. If started in small or half-dosage tricyclics take days or weeks to work. The newer ones are claimed to cause less confusion in the elderly. The large choice now available makes it impossible for even psychiatrists to become familiar with all of them. What evidence there is suggests that the first generation tricyclics are as good as any. Doxepin may cause less antagonism to hypotensive therapy.

Amitriptyline Hydrochloride ('Domical', 'Saroten', 'Tryptizol') *presentation* Tablets B.P. 10, 25 and 50mg, Mixture Amitriptyline Embonate B.P.C. 10mg/5ml, Injection B.P. contained in vials 10ml 10mg/ml; *dose* oral 25mg t.d.s. increasing by 25mg to 100-200mg daily taking the major part at night. The elderly are given less (e.g. half doses). A once daily long-acting form 'Lentizol' is supplied in capsules containing 25 and 50mg and is taken at night and there is a slow release capsule containing 75mg of 'Tryptizol'. Once daily regimes are convenient, but since it has been shown that amitriptyline remains in the body for long periods all forms can be given once daily. *Dose* i.m. is 20-30mg 6 hourly. 'Triptafen' is a combination of amitriptyline and perphenazine in varying strengths.

Imipramine Hydrochloride Ph. Eur. ('Berkomine', 'Tofranil') *presentation* Tablets B.P. 10 and 25mg, syrup 25mg/5ml, ampoules 25mg/2ml; *dose* 25-75mg orally 8 hourly. Imipramine 25mg and promazine 50mg are combined in a capsule made by Geigy and used for depressed and agitated patients.

Imipramine in unbranded form is inexpensive.

Nortriptyline Hydrochloride ('Allegron', 'Aventyl') *presentation* Tablets B.P. and Capsules B.P. 10 and 25mg, liquid 10mg/5ml *dose* adults 20-100mg in divided amounts, children 1.2mg/kg B.W. Other tricyclics—Clomipramine, Desipramine, Dibenzepin, Dothiepin, Doxepin, Iprindole, Opipramol and Trimipramine—are shown in Table 7. With a large choice the longer established forms are preferred ('the devil one knows'). Some such as doxepin have been advised for anxiety and depression. Dothiepin is said to cause less post-

TABLE 7

ANTIDEPRESSIVES

Name		Presentation	Dose Oral (daily) mg
Approved	Proprietary		
Butriptyline Hydrochloride	'Evadyne'	tablets 25 and 50mg	75-150
Clomipramine Hydrochloride	'Anafranil'	capsules 10, 25 and 50mg; syrup 25mg/5ml ampoules 25mg/2ml	75-150 or more
Desipramine Hydrochloride Ph. Eur., B.P.	'Pertofran'	Tablets 25mg	50-150
Dibenzepin Hydrochloride	'Noveril'	tablets 80mg	240-560
Dothiepin Hydrochloride B.P.	'Prothiaden'	Capsules 25mg Tablets 75mg	75-150
Doxepin Hydrochloride B.P.	'Sinequan'	Capsules 10, 25, 50 and 75mg as the base	30-300
Iprindole Hydrochloride	'Prondol'	tablets 15 and 30mg as the base	75-180
Opipramol Hydrochloride	'Insidon'	tablets 50mg	150-300
Protriptyline Hydrochloride B.P.	'Concordin 5' 'Concordin 10'	Tablets 5 and 10mg	15-60
Trimipramine Maleate Ph. Eur., B.P.	'Surmontil'	Tablets B.P. 10 and 25mg Capsules 50mg	50-300

ural hypotension and iprindole less anticholinergic effects than the first generation drugs. Clomipramine (like amitriptyline and imipramine) acts more against serotonin and may be preferable in retarded depression; it is also used in cataplexy.

Adverse effects are common and resemble those of atropine namely tachycardia, dry mouth, blurred vision, constipation, drowsiness, excitability, tremor, inco-ordination, insomnia, agitation (e.g. imipramine), rash, confusion, hypomania, dizziness, sweating, plus hypotension (may be postural), hypertension, arrhythmias, muscle twitching, convulsions, neuropathy, paralytic ileus, sudden death, ECG changes, Parkinsonism, urinary retention, photosensitization, marrow depression, nausea, vomiting, anorexia, diarrhoea, parotid swelling, gynaecomastia, galactorrhoea, jaundice, weight gain. They may precipitate schizophrenia, epilepsy, glaucoma, prostatic symptoms and they worsen pyloric stenosis. Thyroxine and sympathomimetics (either oral or injected as in local anaesthetics) may be dangerously potentiated. Unfortunately many cardiac patients with angina or hypertension are depressed, and tachycardia and interference with hypotensive therapy are handicaps so tricyclics must be used with care in patients with cardiac disease. Diuretics and beta-blockers are advised in hypertensive patients taking tricyclics.

Overdosage is common and may be associated with drowsiness, agitation, ataxia, with cardiac arrest, hyperthermia, hypothermia, convulsions, cardiac arrhythmias, respiratory depression and coma. General measures include removing the poison by stomach aspiration, attention to airway, ventilation, treatment of shock and arrhythmias. Even if conscious the patient should be monitored in an intensive care unit and kept quiet in bed (reduces adrenergic stimuli). Convulsions are controlled by diazepam and arrhythmias by propranolol, practolol or pyridostigmine.

Monoamine Oxidase Inhibitors (MAOI)

By interfering with enzymatic activity they increase the concentration of brain amines. They were discovered when it was noted that isoniazid, a hydrazine drug used in tuberculosis, caused euphoria. Other hydrazines were discovered which inhibited brain amine metabolism. Patients unresponsive to tricyclics and not severe enough for ECT can be given these drugs, but special precautions are needed because of interactions with other medications and certain foods so a special diet must be adhered to because of potentially fatal extracerebral adverse effects. Examples are **Nialamide B.P.** 35-300mg daily, **Phenelzine Sulphate B.P.** ('Nardil') 15-75mg daily, **Iproniazid Phosphate** ('Marsilid') 25-150mg daily, **Isocarboxazid B.P.** ('Marplan') 10-30mg daily and **Tranylcypromine Sulphate B.P.** ('Parnate') 10-30mg daily. Tranylcypromine produces more unwanted effects, acts quickly and can cause insomnia (it has some amphetamine-like actions). It is combined with trifluoperazine in 'Parstelin'. The MAOIs are advisedly prescribed by experts in hospital and general practice and in well selected patients they are very successful. Patients who respond are often phobics. Treatment may need to be for 6 weeks before any marked clinical improvement is seen. Depressed patients who are sleeping well may respond favourably too. *Precautions* patients should be warned against taking foods with a high tyramine or other amine content (which can discharge catecholamines from the nerve endings) like cheese, Marmite, Oxo, Bovril, chocolate, broad beans (the pods contain L dopa), alcoholic drinks such as Chianti, or fermented foods. Lists of foods and drugs likely to cause trouble are available from pharmacists. Local anaesthetics are said not to be hazardous. There has been a caution if they contain adrenaline, or patients have overt cardiovascular disease but adrenaline and noradrenaline with local anaesthetics have been reported as safe with MAOI drugs (*Brit. med. J.* (1975) **3**, 591). General anaesthetics can be dangerous, as can pethidine, morphine and other narcotics (which have to be given cautiously in small doses), oral and i.v. barbiturates, indirectly acting sympathomimetic amines such as amphetamines, fenfluramine, ephedrine, phenyl-propanolamine, hypotensives, tricyclic antidepressives (but see above discussion), antihistamines and oral hypoglycaemics. *Adverse effects* are of two types. First those due to the drugs themselves some of which are like atropine e.g. dry mouth, constipation, nervousness, or euphoria. Oedema, weight increase, sweating, postural hypotension, fatigue and more rarely liver damage and jaundice can occur. The second group of unwanted effects are those due to drug or food interaction, the best known of which causes hypertension, with headache, cerebral haemorrhage, and left ventricular failure, especially when tranylcypromine is taken with cheese, or an amphetamine like drug. (Tranyl-cypromine is structurally like amphetamine whereas the other MAOIs are usually hydrazines). Hypertensive episodes can be controlled by phentolamine 5-10mg i.v., chlorpromazine 50-100mg i.v. or by labetalol 50mg i.v.

Non-Tricyclic Antidepressives
Benzoctamine Hydrochloride ('Tacitin') is tetracyclic derivative. *Presentation* tablets 10mg; *dose* 10-20mg t.d.s. It has been promulgated for anxiety, tension or depression.

Maprotiline ('Ludiomil') is structurally almost identical with benzoctamine as only a side chain differs (dibenzo-bicyclo-octadiene). *Presentation* tablets 10, 25, 50, 75 and 150mg; *dose* 75-300mg daily. *Adverse effects* include liability to convulsions. **Mianserin Hydrochloride** ('Bolvidon', 'Norval'), *presentation* tablets 10, 20, 30mg daily, is another tetracyclic compound.

Tofenacin Hydrochloride ('Elamol') is a metabolite of orphenadrine, an anti-Parkinsonian drug. Its adverse effects are like atropine. *Presentation* capsules 80mg; *dose* 80mg t.d.s.

Viloxazine Hydrochloride ('Vivalan') is an oxazine derivative stated to have little anticholinergic or sympathomimetic effects. *Presentation* tablets 50mg; *dose* 150-200mg daily in divided doses 8 or 12 hourly. It may potentiate the actions of phenytoin and interact with guanidine hypotensives.

Nomifensine Hydrogen Maleate ('Merital 25 and 50') is a tetrahydroiso-quinoline derivative. *Presentation* capsules 25 and 50mg; *dose* 50-200mg daily.

L. Tryptophan ('Optimax', 'Pacitron') is an essential aminoacid which acts by supplementing dietary sources of this natural precursor of serotonin which becomes depleted in depression. Tryptophan changes in the body into 5-hydroxytryptophan, then finally into serotonin (5-hydroxytryptamine). *Presentation* tablets containing 500mg of L-tryptophan with 5mg of pyridoxine hydrochloride and 10mg of ascorbic acid, and a powder containing 1g of tryptophan/10g. *Dose* 2 tablets 3 times daily and 6 at night for 4 weeks then reducing to 4 daily or the equivalent in powder form. For those taking levodopa pyridoxine-free tablets are available.

Amphetamines have been given to the elderly depressive in whom risks of long-term addiction are small, but in Britain even legitimate prescribing of amphetamines is not encouraged.

16 THE THERAPY OF SOME COMMON NEUROLOGICAL DISORDERS

PARKINSONISM

The discovery that there were abnormally low concentrations of dopamine in the basal ganglia of patients with Parkinsonism led to the introduction of a precursor substance, levodopa, which could be absorbed and be converted in the body to dopamine so counteracting the depletion. It is now thought that idiopathic Parkinsonism is due to an imbalance of dopaminergic and cholinergic mechanisms. Treatment therefore increases levels of dopamine or reduces cholinergic activity.

Dopaminergic Receptor Stimulators

Levodopa ('Berkdopa', 'Brocadopa', 'Larodopa') was a major advance in the treatment of idiopathic Parkinsonism (less so in post-encephalitic forms). *Presentation* Capsules B.P. 125, 250 and 500mg. Tablets B.P. 500mg and slow-release tablets 500mg ('Brocadopa Temtabs'). *Dose* 250mg initially taken after meals and increased by 250mg every 3 or 4 days. A slow titration is needed to reach the correct maintenance dose which is usually between 500mg and 4g, but can be as high as 8g daily. The drug may take weeks or months to work. Walking and ability to do things improve as does rigidity, but improvement may fluctuate during the day and decrease just before the next dose is due. After a few years some loss of efficacy is apparent and this may be due to progression of the underlying disease. Sometimes intolerable *adverse reactions* occur at doses needed to control the disease. These are nausea, vomiting, occasionally with bleeding, hypotension, restlessness, agitation, confusion, anxiety, hallucinations, delusions, choreiform jerking movements of face or limbs, "on-off attacks" with temporary relapse, dyskinesia, paranoia, nightmares, suicide, increased libido, dementia, convulsions, depression, sleep disturbance and cardiac arrhythmias. *Contra-indications* concurrent administration of pyridoxine, monoamine oxidase inhibitors or hypotensive therapy. Patients with depression (often secondary to the disease) and cardiac disease need special attention.

In order to reduce dose-related effects substances have been introduced which can prevent or inhibit the extra-cerebral conversion of levodopa to dopamine (over 90%) so making more available to the brain and less to cause side effects outside the brain. They are called **dopa decarboxylase inhibitors;** one is called **Carbidopa** (or alpha methyldopa hydrazine), another **Benserazide**. Given with levodopa an effective and maintained plasma level is possible with a fraction of the dose needed with levodopa alone. The onset of action is also quicker than with levodopa alone. 'Sinemet 275' contains 25mg of carbidopa and 250mg of levodopa and 'Sinemet 110' 10mg carbidopa and 100mg levodopa. The dose for a patient previously on levodopa is reduced to a quarter or a fifth of what it was. In a new patient half a tablet of 'Sinemet' is given t.d.s. increasing by half a tablet daily. 'Madopar 125' is 100mg of levodopa with 25mg of benserazide as the base, 'Madopar 250' is twice this strength and 'Madopar 62.5' is half. Therapy is started with 2 capsules daily of 'Madopar 62.5 or 125'. Most adverse effects are reduced e:g. vomiting, but cerebral ones can be worse e.g. the choreiform, dystonic and other movements, agitation, confusion, hallucinations, insomnia and nightmares.

Bromocriptine Mesylate ('Parlodel') is a dopaminergic agonist available as tablets 2.5mg and capsules. Because of its high cost and liability to cause psychosis it is tried for late failures to levodopa or when fluctuating serum levels cause unpredictable responses. *Doses* 2.5mg once or twice daily with increments to 40-100mg daily.

Adverse effects syncope, hallucinations, dyskinesis, constipation, nausea, extrasystoles, painful ankles, eye discomfort. It is an ergot alkaloid as is lergotrile which may be more powerful.

Centrally Acting Anticholinergic Drugs
They are still used as first choice in mild cases, as side effects are less, and with levodopa in patients who cannot tolerate the full amounts, or if levodopa or amantadine is ineffective in patients with Parkinsonism . They are also used for drug-induced Parkinsonism and the acute dystonic reactions. Atropine and hyoscine were originally used but have been replaced by synthetic anticholinergics. Many exist, few with any definite superiority and they are only modestly effective. A few are available in parenteral form for the treatment of acute dystonic reactions. Those in use have less anticholinergic action than atropine, some are antihistamines and many inhibit neuronal uptake of dopamine. Their suitability varies according to the patient's tolerance. The dose needed is often close to the toxic one and their side effects resemble those of atropine. In some mental hospitals they are given prophylactically with phenothiazines and thioxanthenes, others wait and see if Parkinsonian symptoms develop. Tremor and rigidity are helped more than the paucity of movement. Concurrent use of these drugs may reduce the side effects of the phenothiazines by lowering plasma levels.

Benzhexol Hydrochloride (Trihexyphenidyl Hydrochloride U.S.P.,'Artane') reduces muscle rigidity. *Presentation* Tablets B.P. 2 and 5mg, slow release capsules 5mg; *dose* 2mg b.d. rising to 5mg t.d.s. *Adverse effects* nausea, vomiting and anticholinergic like that of atropine (dry mouth etc.). The elderly and the arteriosclerotic may become confused, excited, or have hallucinations or delusions. **Procyclidine Hydrochloride** ('Kemadrin') along with benzhexol and biperiden share a similar structure. *Presentation* Tablets B.P. 5mg; *dose* orally 5-60mg daily in divided doses after meals to avoid gastric irritation. Ampoules 2ml 5mg/ml are available; *dose* 10-20mg i.m., or i.v. **Biperiden** ('Akineton') *presentation* Tablets U.S.N.F. 2mg of **Biperiden Hydrochloride**; *dose* orally 1mg b.d. increasing to 2mg t.d.s., ampoules 1ml 5mg/ml of **Biperiden Lactate Injection B.P.** The injection by slow i.v. route or i.m. of 5mg is reputedly highly effective for acute drug-induced dystonic reactions. If not available 5-10mg i.v. of **Diazepam** can be tried or another injectable anticholinergic.

Benztropine Mesylate ('Cogentin') is a derivative of atropine and diphenhydramine and is used for tremor and rigidity. *Presentation* tablets 2mg, ampoules 2ml 1mg/ml. *Dose* orally 500μg-1mg initially, increasing gradually up to 6mg taken at night; by injection 2mg i.m. or i.v. Since it is slowly excreted it need only be given once per 24 hours. Its sedative action is helpful in the elderly. *Adverse effects* nausea, rashes.

Orphenadrine Hydrochloride ('Disipal') is a widely used methyl derivative of

diphenhydramine, an antihistamine. *Presentation* Tablets B.P. 50mg, ampoules 2ml 20mg/ml; **Orphenadrine Citrate** ('Norflex') Slow-Release Tablets B.P. 100mg, ampoules 2ml 30mg/ml. *Dose* orally 150-400mg daily in 3-4 divided amounts after meals. *Adverse effects* gastric irritation, euphoria.
Benapryzine Hydrochloride ('Brizin') is a newer anticholinergic introduced in 1974 claimed to have less side effects than benzhexol in patients taking levodopa. Structurally it is a diphenylmethane derivative with similarities to diphenhydramine. *Presentation* tablets 50mg; *dose* 50mg 3 or 4 times daily.
Ethopropazine Hydrochloride (Profenamine) is a phenothiazine yet has anti-Parkinsonian activity and which is no longer available in the U.K. *Adverse effects* drowsiness, ataxia, lassitude, paraesthesiae, muscle cramps, marrow depression. **Methixene Hydrochloride** ('Tremonil') is a thioxanthene (see p. 115) with a phenothiazine-like structure with antispasmodic and antihistaminic properties. *Presentation* tablets 5mg; *dose* 2.5-20mg t.d.s.

Substances Releasing Endogenous Dopamine
Amantadine Hydrochloride ('Symmetrel') is an amine of limited efficacy in Parkinsonism. It is a cerebral stimulant and can at times cause livedo reticularis, oedema, cardiac arrhythmias, nausea, convulsions, restlessness, insomnia, confusion and hallucinations. It has been also used to prevent influenza and to treat herpes zoster and some forms of pre-senile dementia. *Presentation* capsules 100mg, syrup 50mg/5ml; *dose* 100mg daily for a week then 100-200mg daily. It may spare the dose of levodopa and the anticholinergics, but because of its very high cost unless it is clearly effective its use should be sparing.

Stimulation of dopamine receptors by agonists related to apomorphine is under trial.

ANTICONVULSANTS AND EPILEPSY

Indications for Treatment
The number of attacks of epilepsy is important as a few each year, especially nocturnal, may not warrant treatment. Other attacks may occur with fever and with menstruation. Excessive treatment carries a risk of adverse effects. Chopping and changing of therapy should be avoided and withdrawal and introduction of new medications are best done in graded dosage. The aim should be to control attacks with the smallest dose. Drugs should be given for at least 3 years and not stopped suddenly. For children a twice daily regimen is more convenient for they often omit a mid-day dose. *Correct therapy* (until a satisfactory general purpose anticonvulsant arrives) depends on an accurate diagnosis of the type of epilepsy. The types are (1) grand mal or major epilepsy with tonic-clonic fits; (2) focal epilepsy often arising in the temporal lobe; (3) petit mal absences, a condition of children and adolescents associated with brief and frequent interruptions of consciousness and in which falling is rare; (4) rarities such as myoclonic fits and infantile spasm. Fits may be symptomatic of trauma, tumour, meningitis, and metabolic disease (e.g. hypocalcaemia, uraemia, hyperosmolar coma); and (5) patients who have had neurosurgery such as craniotomy with particularly brain excision are at risk and are given at least a year's anticonvulsant therapy.
Certain drugs may induce fits (see p. 253) such as the tricyclics, pheno-

thiazines and corticosteroids, others do so on withdrawal e.g. barbiturates and alcohol. Fits may also be brought on by drugs which lower the blood sugar, or the serum calcium, or cause water retention and brain oedema. Starvation and excessive fluid intake may provoke attacks.

Drugs Used in Major and Focal Epilepsy

The sequence usually tried is phenytoin, phenobarbitone, primidone, then sulthiame. All are usually started in full doses, except primidone. In the elderly and in children the sedation and mental dulling of the barbiturates is a disadvantage and restlessness and agitation can occur in children. Many now try phenytoin first but not in young girls. Carbamazepine finds increasing use.

Barbiturates

Phenobarbitone is given to adults in doses of 30-60mg t.d.s. **Methylphenobarbitone** ('Prominal') *presentation* tablets 30, 60 and 200mg; *dose* 400-600mg daily has no special advantages and is changed to phenobarbitone in the body. The effectiveness of therapy can be judged by measuring the blood levels (10-25µg/ml or 42-105µmol/l since 1µg = 4.2µmol/l). This is not for everyday use but is helpful for those not responding in the normal way and helps exclude underdosage (subtherapeutic levels) and overdosage (toxic levels). Barbiturates cause dose related side effects such as ataxia and dysarthria; they cause liver enzyme induction (overactivity) and idiosyncratic responses such as rashes.

Hydantoins are structurally related to the barbiturates (ureide derivatives), but are less sedative.

Phenytoin U.S.P. (Diphenylhydantoin, 'Dilantin', 'Epanutin') *presentation* Phenytoin Sodium Ph. Eur. Tablets B.P. 30, 50 and 100mg (they are composed of fine particles which are more soluble and changed into acid in the stomach and have an increased 'bioavailability'), Capsules B.P.C. 25, 50 and 100mg; 'Epanutin Infatabs' tablets 50mg of Phenytoin Acid; Phenytoin Suspension B.P.C. 30mg/5ml also as the acid and Phenytoin Injection B.P.C. a ready-mixed preparation of Phenytoin Sodium 250mg/5ml. There is probably an important difference in the bioavailability (absorption) between the acid and the sodium salt. *Dose* a loading dose of 200-1000mg is given by some according to body weight, others start with 50-400mg once daily (since the half-life is 22 hours) or in divided amounts. Children take 3-10mg/kg B.W. Blood levels should be 10-25µg/ml (40-100µmol/1). *Interactions* phenobarbitone taken concurrently often *lowers the blood levels of phenytoin* by stimulating liver enzymes (and so may carbamazepine), whereas isoniazid, disulfiram and sulthiame inhibit its metabolism with, at times, *dangerously toxic levels* occurring. Warfarin also raises the blood levels of phenytoin. Phenobarbitone and phenytoin are combined in some branded products e.g. 'Garoin' contains 100mg phenytoin and 50mg phenobarbitone sodium; possible interactions reducing efficacy should be remembered. **Ethotoin** ('Peganone') Tablets B.P. 500mg; *dose* 1-3g daily and **Methoin** (Mephenytoin, 'Mesontoin') Tablets B.P. 100mg; *dose* 100-600mg daily are occasional alternatives, but methoin is more toxic and ethotoin less effective. *Adverse effects* are those from too much therapy (intoxication), side effects at normal doses, and unexpected idiosyncratic or unpredictable reactions, namely dizziness, nausea, sedation, slurred speech, diplopia, nystagmus, tremor, incoordination and ataxia (usually reversible by lowering the dose). Lymphadenopathy, osteomalacia and hypocalcaemia (from interference with vitamin D metabolism and also seen with phenobarbitone), interference with vitamin K metabolism, folates (megaloblastic anaemia), marrow depression, an acromegalic-like facial picture, hirsuties, hyperglycaemia, and inappropriate secretion of antidiuretic hormone are rarer complications. Gum hypertrophy is very common (majority) and a correlation has been found with serum levels.

Primidone ('Mysoline') is changed in the body partly to phenobarbitone, but it is not certain whether all its actions can be explained by this, or if its actions are identical. It is used as an alternative, but because of drowsiness it is not usually combined with phenobarbitone. *Presentation* Tablets B.P. 250mg, Mixture B.P.C. 250mg/5ml in bottles of 150 and 1000ml. *Dose* 125mg to begin with at night increasing to 750mg-1.5g daily. *Adverse effects* drowsiness, vertigo, ataxia, diplopia, slurred speech.

Sulthiame ('Ospolot') is a sulphonamide derivative. *Presentation* Tablets B.P. 50 and 200mg, suspension 50mg/5ml. *Dose* 200-600mg daily in divided doses. It is used for myoclonic attacks, focal epilepsy and hyperkinetic syndromes. It is not potent alone, and inhibits phenytoin and phenobarbitone metabolism so their levels increase. *Adverse effects* hyperventilation, ataxia, agitation.

Carbamazepine (p. 132) in a dose of 200-1600mg daily orally can be used for grand mal and temporal lobe epilepsies as well as trigeminal neuralgia, tabetic lightning pains and diabetes insipidus.

Pheneturide is a urea derivative. If given concurrently it can inhibit phenytoin metabolism. *Presentation* tablets 200mg; *dose* 600-1000mg daily. *Uses* temporal lobe or psychomotor epilepsy. *Adverse effects* drowsiness, ataxia, nystagmu, rash, proteinuria.

Status Epilepticus

For this the choice is between diazepam 5-20mg i.v. (Watch B.P. and respiratory depression. For hospital use, only, and under careful observation) and **paraldehyde** 2-8ml i.m. for adults (some paediatricians still consider it as first choice), **Phenobarbitone Sodium** 100-300mg i.m., for adults (but watch for respiratory depression) and occasionally **Phenytoin Sodium** 100-250mg i.v. in the ready-mixed form given *slowly*, but it is probably ineffective alone unless one gives doses up to 1000mg. If given i.m. blood levels and absorption are unpredictable. **Chlormethiazole Edisylate** i.v. may be effective if other remedies have failed. Exceptionally, i.v. anaesthetics, or muscle relaxants with assisted respiration may be needed. Fits in the newborn can be controlled by primidone 62.5mg b.d., phenytoin 25mg b.d., or t.d.s., sulthiame 5mg/kg B.W. in 3 divided doses, or carbamazepine 50mg b.d., or t.d.s. Hypocalcaemia and hypomagnesaemia should be excluded.

Infantile spasm (hypsarrhythmia) responds to **Nitrazepam** and ACTH. Rarely, convulsions in infants are responsive to pyridoxine. For alcohol withdrawal fits and toxaemic convulsions (eclampsia) Chlormethiazole Edisylate i.v. may be effective but it causes phlebitis and may depress respiration in the foetus. A simple hydrocarbon (aliphatic) structure is **Sodium Valproate** ('Epilim') introduced from France. It increases the cerebral levels of gamma aminobutyric acid an inhibitory neuro-transmitter, and is useful in grand mal, petit mal and in myoclonic epilepsy. *Presentation* tablets 200mg, and 500mg enteric coated tablets, syrup 200mg/5ml in 200ml bottles; *dose* 200mg b.d. initially then between 600-2400mg daily in 3 divided doses. Children over 20kg start with 400mg daily in divided doses 20-30mg/kg B.W., and under 20kg 20-50mg/kg B.W. providing plasma levels do not exceed 200μg/ml. *Adverse effects* hair loss and thrombocytopenia. **Clonazepam** ('Rivotril') a benzodiazepine is also claimed to be useful against all types of epilepsy. *Presentation* tablets 500μg (0.5mg) and 2mg; ampoules containing 1mg of clonazepam in 1ml solvent, plus an ampoule of 1ml Water for Injections. *Dose* orally 500μg (0.5mg)-1mg daily for infants, 4-8mg for adults in 3 divided doses; i.v. 1mg with Water for Injections given slowly (over 30 seconds).

Petit Mal

The **succinimides** and the **oxazolidinediones** are the best established and each group possesses a basic 5-membered cyclic ring with similarities to the hydantoins. **Ethosuximide** ('Emeside', 'Zarontin') is the first choice since it is less toxic than the other succinimides and diones. *Presentation* Capsules B.P. 250mg, Elixir B.P.C. 250mg/5ml; *dose* 500mg-2g in divided doses. Other members are **Phensuximide** ('Milontin' in U.S.A.) *presentation* Capsules B.P.C. 250 and 500mg; *dose* 500mg-1g daily increased by 500mg fortnightly to 3g, and **Methsuximide** *presentation* capsules 300mg; *dose* 300mg daily rising by 300mg weekly to 1200mg daily.

The diones are used when the succinimides are unsuccessful, although Sodium Valproate or Clonazepam may now be better alternatives. **Troxidone** (Trimethadione U.S.P., 'Tridione') *presentation* Tablets U.S.P. 150mg, Capsules B.P., U.S.P. 300mg; *dose* 900-1800mg in divided doses daily for adults, children 300-900mg daily. **Paramethadione** ('Paradione') *presentation* Capsules B.P. 300mg; *dose* as for troxidone. *Adverse effects* light intolerance, nausea, hiccoughs, rashes, marrow damage, liver and kidney toxicity. Both classes of drugs can provoke the onset of grand mal and phenytoin or phenobarbitone may have to be added.

Cataplexy

These are falling attacks without loss of consciousness due to loss of muscle tone. They may respond to clomipramine or imipramine by an effect on muscle tone.

OTHER INVOLUNTARY MOVEMENTS

Tremor: essential or familial forms may be helped by diazepam, propranolol (or alcohol) and worsened by sympathomimetics such as adrenaline and orciprenaline, the tricyclic antidepressants, lithium, thyroxine and caffeine.

Tics: childhood types and Gilles de la Tourette (verbal tics) may respond to haloperidol.

Chorea and hemiballismus, oral-facial dyskinesias and generalized torsion dystonia can be helped by a phenothiazine (e.g. chlorpromazine, prochlorperazine, thiopropazate or trifluperazine), reserpine, or tetrabenazine. Drugs such as the neuroleptics, phenytoin and the contraceptive pill can cause chorea. **Tetrabenazine** ('Nitoman') depletes neuronal stores of serotonin and catecholamines in the CNS. *Presentation* tablets 25mg; *dose* 12.5mg b.d. increasing by 25mg every third day until 200mg daily is reached or toxicity occurs. Its main use is in Huntington's chorea, hemiballismus and senile chorea. *Adverse effects* drowsiness, akathisia, depression (it is chemically related to reserpine), ataxia, confusion, nausea and Parkinsonism.

Dystonia may also be induced by phenothiazines, metoclopramide, or haloperidol. If due to a piperazine-like phenothiazine a change to a piperidine-type may help, or to reserpine or tetrabenazine, or paradoxically even doubling the dose of the offending drug. Acute episodes often require parenteral anti-Parkinsonian anticholinergic drugs (see p. 122)

Autistic Hyperkinetic children may be helped by methylphenidate or dexamphetamine (two Controlled Drugs), or by sulthiame.

Muscle Disorders

Myotonia congenita can be helped by quinine and at times prednisone, procainamide (250-500mg 3 or 4 times daily) or phenytoin (100mg 3 or 4 times daily). *Periodic paralysis* in the hypokalaemic form is treated with spironolactone or amiloride plus potassium salts. Unexpectedly acetazolamide (250mg t.d.s.) and thiazide diuretics may be effective in the prophylaxis to both hypo- and hyperkalaemic attacks. Normokalaemic forms respond to sodium chloride intake, fludrocortisone and acetazolamide.

NEURO-MUSCULAR BLOCKERS

These act either by interfering with acetylcholine 'non-depolarizing' (e.g. tubocurarine, gallamine) or they cause the voluntary muscle to be no longer receptive to its action 'depolarizing' (e.g. suxamethonium). *Uses* as a muscle relaxant in surgery and to treat tetanus.

Tubocurarine Chloride Ph. Eur., B.P. ('Tubarine') is of plant origin. It acts in 3-5 minutes and lasts 20 minutes. *Presentation* Injection B.P. ampoules 1.5ml of a solution 10mg/ml; *dose* 5-20mg. This type of relaxant is counteracted by cholinergic drugs.

Suxamethonium Chloride Injection Ph. Eur., B.P. (Succinylcholine Chloride U.S.P.) is a solution in Water for Injections containing 50mg (equivalent to 36.5mg of cation per ml) in ampoules 2ml and vials 10ml. *Dose* 30-100mg as the base. It is used mainly for procedure needing brief muscle relaxation such as E.C.T. and intubation before anaesthesia. It is not counteracted by cholinergic drugs. Other uses are for tetanus 50-100µg/kg B.W. per min to prevent spasms, and after major cardiac surgery to paralyze muscles during mechanical ventilation. *Adverse effects* prolonged depression of breathing if the enzyme serum cholinesterase is lacking, post-operative muscle pain, hypotension, cardiac arrhythmias, cardiac arrest, malignant hyperpyrexia and myoglobinuria.

Alcuronium Chloride ('Alloferin') is an alkaloid from the calabash plant, stronger but shorter in action than tubocurarine and used like it. *Dose* 10-25mg i.v. initially. **Pancuronium Bromide B.P.** ('Pavulon') is a steroid derivative given in a dose of 100µg/kg B.W. It has similar uses to tubocurarine and raises the pulse, blood pressure and cardiac output.

Tetanus

In countries with advanced facilities all but the mildest cases are treated in selected intensive care units and require tracheostomy, i.v. muscle relaxants, assisted ventilation, attention to fluid and energy intakes, sedation, antibiotics and large doses of human tetanus immunoglobulin. In poor countries or in mild cases convulsions or muscle spasms are controlled by diazepam, chlorpromazine, barbiturates or morphine with little surgical interference.

Spasticity

Cortical disease (e.g. strokes) and spinal disorders (e.g. multiple sclerosis) cause considerable havoc. As yet spasticity is medically incurable. Many preparations have been claimed to reduce increased muscle tone; among them are **Mephenesin** ('Myanesin'), a glycerol ether, and the related **Chlorphenesin Carbamate** ('Maolate' Upjohn U.S.A.), tigloidine hydrobromide ('Tiglyssin') an atropine-like structure, chlorzoxazone ('Paraflex') and chlormezanone ('Trancopal'). The benzodiazepines are more effective. **Baclofen** ('Lioresal') is a newer agent of possible promise and is a semi-synthetic derivative of gamma amino butyric acid (an inhibitor in the brain of synaptic transmission). It reduces voluntary muscle spasm by an action at spinal cord level probably on the gamma fibre system. *Presentation* tablets 10mg; *dose* 5mg t.d.s. up to 40-60mg daily. *Adverse effects* hypotonia, fatigue, vomiting, vertigo, sedation and confusion. It is contra-indicated in epileptics and pregnancy. *Special precautions* as to dosage are needed during hypotensive therapy, cardiovascular disease, previous peptic ulceration and severe psychiatric disturbances. **Dantrolene Sodium** ('Dantrium') is a recently introduced furantoin derivative. *Presentation* capsules 25 and 100mg; *dose* 25mg daily increasing weekly by 25-50mg weekly up to 400-800mg daily. It is stated to work directly on the muscle and not the spinal cord. *Adverse effects* possible liver damage, sedation, weakness, diarrhoea. It is restricted to hospital use at present.

Nocturnal Cramps

Metabolic conditions (diabetes mellitus, salt depletion, iron deficiency, hypothyroidism, hypomagnesaemia, diuretic therapy and vitamin B deficiency) are excluded. **Quinine Sulphate** 200-300mg is given in idiopathic cases, before going to bed. Quinine increases (like its isomer quinidine) the refractory period of muscle and so reduces the liability to tetanic stimuli and cramps. An occasional patient may show hypersensitivity by itching, urticaria, flushing or tinnitus. An alternative medication **Mephenesin** causes muscular relaxation by a spinal cord effect and the dose is 250-1000mg.

Cerebral Stimulants

These are rarely indicated other than **caffeine** which can be taken as a beverage, or as a medication by itself, or with an analgesic such as aspirin. Chronic consumption of strong coffee may be relevant in cardiac arrhythmias, insomnia and indigestion.

Dexamphetamine Sulphate ('Dexedrine') is a 'Controlled Drug' and because of the liability to abuse is restricted in use. *Presentation* Tablets B.P. 5mg. *Dose* it is used mainly in Britain for narcolepsy; 5-10mg is given in the morning and midday, with if necessary ephedrine $500\mu g$ (0.5mg)-1mg in the afternoon and phenobarbitone 60mg at night to prevent insomnia. Occasionally it is tried in hyperkinetic children and it may be justified in the elderly depressed person in whom addiction and abuse are unlikely. Indeed, tranylcypromine an antidepressant has similar actions and structure, **Pemoline** ('Kethamed', 'Ronyl', 'Volital') an oxazolidine derivative is used as a non-amphetamine stimulant for fatigue. *Presentation* tablets 20mg; *dose* 20mg once or twice daily up to 120mg daily. *Adverse effects* insomnia, liver dysfunction, anorexia, headache, rash. Not to be given to children under six.

HEADACHES

Treatment depends on the cause (e.g. meningitis, tumour, haemorrhage, arteritis, depression or anxiety).

Vascular Headaches (migraine, migrainous neuralgia, cluster headaches). Attacks may be prevented by dealing with anxiety, anger, frustration, work, foods (e.g. chocolate, cheese, alcohol) and hypertension. The contraceptive pill may relieve or worsen them. Regular oral ergotamine tartrate, diuretics (pre-menstrually), and hormones have been tried without convincing success. For an acute attack rest in a quiet, darkened room and aspirin, codeine or a mixture e.g. dextropropoxyphene and paracetamol ('Distalgesic') are tried, or ergotamine and if necessary an anti-emetic.

Prophylactics

The aim is to reduce the frequency and severity of attacks, and prophylactics are taken daily irrespective of whether a headache is present or not.

Clonidine Hydrochloride ('Dixarit') is an indole but not an ergot derivative. Its action is complicated but it acts as a CNS noradrenaline agonist. It is available in a low-dose tablet which should not be confused with that for hypertension. *Presentation* tablets $25\mu g$; *dose* $25-75\mu g$ b.d. **Propranolol** has been said both to reduce the frequency of migraine and to precipitate it, even in non-hypertensives.

Methysergide Maleate ('Deseril') a lysergic acid derivative containing an indole ring is a vasoconstrictor with a selective action against serotonin (otherwise called 5-hydroxytryptamine itself an indole). Because of the adverse effects it is only advised for severe migraine. *Presentation* Tablets B.P. 1mg (as the base); *dose* 1-2mg b.d. or t.d.s., but the dose may have to be restricted in view of its dangers. *Adverse effects* insomnia, mental stimulation (chemically it is like lysergic acid LSD), tingling, cold limbs, nausea, vomiting, weight gain, fluid retention, oedema, tachycardia, postural hypotension and precipitation or worsening of angina. The prescription should be limited to a few months because it can cause retroperitoneal fibrosis and to detect this the renal function and ESR should be measured at intervals. The drug may also damage the aortic valve. **Dihydroergotamine Mesylate** may also be given prophylactically. **Pizotifen** ('Sanomigran') is another antiserotonin, structurally a tricyclic compound with an efficacy similar to methysergide. *Presentation* tablets $500\mu g$ (0.5mg); *dose* $500\mu g$ t.d.s. *Adverse effects* drowsiness, weight gain.

Vasoconstrictors

These are taken for the pain and are derived from the indole-containing ergot alkaloids.

Ergotamine Tartrate Ph. Eur. can be taken sublingually, orally, by suppository, inhalation or by injection. *Presentation* Tablets B.P. 1 and 2mg, Injection B.P. ampoules 1ml $500\mu g$/ml, Ergotamine Compound Suppositories 'Cafergot' suppositories (ergotamine tartrate 2mg, caffeine 100mg, belladonna alkaloids $250\mu g$ and allylbarbituric acid 100mg). *Dose* orally 1-2mg up to a total of 6mg, $250-500\mu g$ s.c. or i.m. Proprietary forms include 'Femergin' tablets and ampoules for injection, 'Cafergot' tablets (1mg ergotamine tartrate, 100mg caffeine), and 'Migril' (ergotamine tartrate 2mg, cyclizine hydrochloride 50mg, caffeine hydrate 100mg) 'Lingraine' tablets are for sublingual use and contain 2mg of ergotamine tartrate. 'Medihaler' ergotamine tartrate is

TABLE 8
VESTIBULAR SEDATIVES

| | Presentation | | | |
	Tablet	Ampoule or Vial	Single Dose	Duration (hours)
Antihistamines				
Cinnarizine ('Stugeron')	15mg	—	15mg	4-6
Cyclizine Hydro-chloride B.P. ('Marzine', 'Valoid')	50mg	1ml 50 mg	50mg	8
Dimenhydrinate B.P. ('Dramamine', 'Gravol')	50mg	5ml 50mg/ml	50mg	8
Meclozine Hydro-chloride B.P. ('Ancoloxin')	25mg (and pyridoxine 50mg)	—	50mg	12-24
Mepyramine Maleate B.P. ('Anthisan')	50,100mg Elixir 25mg/5ml	2ml 50mg	50-100mg	6-8
Promethazine Hydro-chloride B.P. ('Phenergan')	10, 25mg Elixir 5mg/5ml	1ml 25mg 2ml 50mg	25-50mg	4-6
Promethazine Theo-clate B.P. ('Avomine')	25mg	—	25mg	6-8
Histamine Analogues				
Betahistine Hydro-chloride ('Serc')	8mg	—	8mg	8
Parasympatholytics				
Hyoscine Hydro-bromide B.P.	300μg 400μg 600μg	1ml 400μg 1ml 600μg	300-600μg	8

TABLE 8 *(continued)*
VESTIBULAR SEDATIVES

	Presentation Tablet	Ampoule or Vial	Single Dose	Duration (hours)
Phenothiazines				
Prochlorperazine Maleate B.P. ('Stemetil') ('Vertigon')	5 and 25mg (suppositories 5 and 25mg) 10 and 15mg slow-release capsules	— —	5-30mg 10-15mg	4-6 12-24
Prochlorperazine Mesylate B.P. ('Stemetil')	Syrup 5mg/5ml	1ml 12.5mg 2ml 25mg	5-30mg	4-6
Thiethylperazine Maleate ('Torecan')	10mg (suppositories 10mg)	1ml 10mg	10mg	4-6

inhaled (360μg per dose) and is said to be as quick and effective as injections, but it is unsuitable for asthmatics. **Dihydroergotamine Mesylate** ('Dihydergot') the hydrogenated derivative is safer than the natural alkaloid ergotamine and the *oral form* can be given prophylactically even in pregnancy, as well as for acute attacks of pain. *Presentation* tablets 1mg (equal to 860μg of the base), an oral solution 2mg/ml, and ampoules 1ml 1mg/ml. *Dose* 1.5-3mg orally prophylactically, 1-2mg s.c. or i.m. for an attack which can be repeated, or orally 2-3mg repeated half hourly up to a total of 10mg. *Adverse effects* of ergotamine; nausea, vomiting, diarrhoea, cold limbs, tingling, burning and pain in fingers and toes, cramps, venous thrombosis, convulsions, angina and rarely gangrene. Ergotamine tartrate is contra-indicated in pregnancy, peripheral vascular disease and coronary artery disease such as angina. Ergotamine habituation can occur with daily doses of 1mg or more and para-doxically can cause persistent headaches. Ergotamine tartrate is present in 'Bellergal' and 'Bellergal Retard', so chronic administration can be dangerous in those with latent or actual vascular disease especially when infection, liver, or renal disease, anaemia or hypertension co-exist.

Trigeminal Neuralgia
Mild forms respond to analgesics such as aspirin, or Gower's mixture which contains sodium bromide, glyceryl trinitrate, gelsemium and belladonna (very old fashioned). At times, phenytoin works (as it might do also for the pain of

stump neuroma, tabetic pain and diabetic neuropathy). **Carbamazepine** ('Tegretol') is used for more severe cases and is a dibenzazepine like the tricyclic antidepressant imipramine hence it has psychotropic properties. *Presentation* Tablets B.P. 100 and 200mg, syrup 100mg/5ml: *dose* 200-1600mg daily. *Adverse effects* are common—unsteadiness, drowsiness, rashes, anorexia, diarrhoea and less frequently marrow depression. Intractable neuralgia is treated by alcohol or phenol injections, or by nerve section.

VERTIGO AND VESTIBULAR SEDATIVES
Acute vertigo is a frightening and distressing complaint immobilizing the patient who may also be vomiting. Stress and anxiety may need attention. Preparations used are mentioned in various chapters and are listed in Table 8 for convenience. They are also used for travel sickness. Cinnarizine, dimenhydrinate, hyoscine and prochlorperazine are popular. Precautions in their use should be taken in the elderly, in epileptics, and those with glaucoma or prostatic enlargement.

INFECTIONS
The most amenable to treatment are the bacterial infections, but rickettsial, fungal, protozoal and (with poor results) viral encephalitis due to herpes simplex can be treated. Complications such as fits, fluid depletion, brain oedema, bacteraemia and collections of fluid and pus need treatment. The organisms involved vary in the neonate, child and adult and in different parts of the country. For instance in the neonate Gram-negative bacilli, *Staph. pyogenes* and *Str. pyogenes* are offenders, in children *H. influenzae, N. meningitidis* and *Str. pneumoniae,* and in adults the same organisms are involved, but often debilitating disease is present which gives the infection a high mortality.

Undiagnosed Meningitis
The C.S.F. is always examined and nose and throat swabs and blood cultures taken. Diagnosis may not be obvious, or obscured by previous therapy. While awaiting diagnosis in children chloramphenicol, or ampicillin alone can be given, or some paediatricians still use chloramphenicol, penicillin and sulphonamides together—although penicillin and chloramphenicol may be an ineffective combination. The penicillins cross into the C.S.F. in meningitis in effective amounts, although some clinicians still give 10 000-20 000u of benzylpenicillin intrathecally as well.

In general i.v. therapy is advised as this gives quick and high blood levels. *Staph. pyogenes* (staphylococcus). Benzylpenicillin 1-4 million units (0.6-2.4g) 2-4 hourly i.v. then i.m. is given and for penicillinase-forming organisms flucloxacillin 250-500mg 6 hourly by injection and later by mouth and intrathecally 10-40mg for adults and 3-5mg for children. *Str. pneumoniae* (pneumococcus). Because of a high mortality and underlying, unfavourable disease large amounts of benzylpenicillin 2 million units 2 hourly are given i.v. at first then i.m. for at least a week and often supplemented by once or twice daily intrathecal penicillin. *Str. pyogenes* (streptococcus). Benzylpenicillin is given, or sulphonamides in allergic subjects. The initial dose of sulphadiazine is 1-2g slowly i.v., or i.m. of the parenteral preparation (p. 23), but if the patient is conscious and not vomiting an initial dose of 3-6g can be taken orally and then 1-1.5g 4 hourly or 2g 6 hourly. Sulphonamides are never given intrathecally.

N. meningitidis (meningococcus) is again occurring in epidemics and can kill in a matter of a few hours. Complications include circulatory failure, intravascular coagulation, hyperthermia, limb gangrene, fits and cerebral oedema and shock from adrenal haemorrhage. With the advent of sulphonamide-resistant strains benzylpenicillin is given as for pneumococcus. In allergic subjects chloramphenicol is tried. In the area south of the Sahara many thousands of cases occur annually. Here, chloramphenicol has proved cheap, effective and suitable for 'foot doctors' in doctor-less regions at a dose of 4-6g in equally divided amounts at 6 hourly intervals. Rifampicin, minocycline, and for some strains, sulphonamides have been used for pharyngeal carriers and contacts of cases of meningitis. For contacts close clinical supervision is more reliable with penicillin given at the first sign of disease.

Gram-negative rod infections such as *Esch. coli, Proteus spp.* or *Ps. aeruginosa* need specific antibiotics according to laboratory guidance. Injected ampicillin, cephalosporins, chloramphenicol, gentamicin or tobramycin may be required.

Haemophilus influenzae. Chloramphenicol 100mg/kg B.W. daily i.v. then orally in equally divided doses 6 hourly is best. Ampicillin is popular, but not as effective as some organisms are resistant; the dose is 400mg/kg B.W. daily in equally divided amounts 4 hourly. For resistant cases i.v. carbenicillin has been successful. The intrathecal dose of ampicillin for adults is 10-40mg, carbenicillin 40mg, cephaloridine 50mg, and colistin 500-1000u/kg B.W. once daily.

Listeria monocytogenes responds to ampicillin.

Mycobacterium tuberculosis. Unless the patient is unconscious or cannot swallow isoniazid 10-15mg/kg B.W. with para-aminosalicylic acid 12g both orally and streptomycin 500mg-1g daily i.m. are given and sometimes streptomycin 50-100mg intrathecally, or isoniazid, rifampicin and ethambutol. Isoniazid, rifampicin and cycloserine readily cross into the C.S.F. (see p. 31). In countries without injectable preparations isoniazid, para-aminosalicylic acid and pyrazinamide can be given via an intragastric tube.

Spirochaetal infections such as *Treponema pallidum* are treated with benzylpenicillin or procaine penicillin daily for about 2 weeks.

Viral infections such as herpes simplex have been treated with cytarabine, vidarabine or idoxuridine i.v. when they cause encephalitis. They are toxic (see p. 33). Fungi such as *Cryptococcus neoformans* are treated with amphotericin B. 20mg in an i.v. infusion and flucytosine singly or preferably together. Flucytosine ('Alcobon') is supplied in infusion bottles 2.5g in 250ml of sodium chloride. The i.v. dose is 100-200mg/kg B.W. Blood levels of 25-50µg/ml are aimed at and doses are reduced in renal impairment.

CEREBROVASCULAR DISEASE

This is a major cause of death and disability in Western Countries and interestingly in Japan, (where apoplexy ranks as the main cause). Control of hypertension, diabetes, emboli, arteritis and arteriosclerosis is imperative to reduce cerebro-cardiovascular disease.

17 DRUG OVERDOSE, POISONING AND COMA

Poisoning, deliberate and accidental, now accounts for 10-20% of acute medical admissions. Most are manipulative gestures by young women. There are over 60 000 admissions annually and a mortality of 7000 or so. Since more deaths occur outside hospital the hospital mortality is under 1%. Drugs frequently taken for suicide or self-poisoning include barbiturates, aspirin, antidepressives, tranquillizers (Benzodiazepines), paracetamol and alcohol, individually or in combination. Diagnosis is helped by examination of all drug-containers at home, clinical evidence occasionally (e.g. in narcotics and tricyclics) and by laboratory screening tests of gastric contents, blood and urine. Blood levels can verify the diagnosis, assess severity and response to treatment. In drug-induced coma the patient is kept alive by *supportive measures* (attention to airway, ventilation, circulatory failure, anoxia, electrolytes and acid-base balance). The patient recovers while the drugs are metabolized, or excreted and is treated as for coma in general, or as if anaesthetized.

Symptomatic treatment deals with the complications which frequently arise namely hypothermia, hyperthermia, respiratory failure, pulmonary oedema, arrhythmias, cardiac arrest, renal failure, dehydration, convulsions and cerebral oedema. Most poisoning is dealt with non-specifically without any *specific antidote* being available. Other measures include the *prevention of absorption* and the removal of the drug or poison, and speeding its *elimination*.

An initial assessment evaluates the patient and the priorities to be given to the supportive therapy. Initial appearances can be falsely deceptive with aspirin, paracetamol, iron, tricyclics and paraquat poisoning and conversely over-alarming with the benzodiazepines.

Conscious and Alert Patients

Inducing vomiting by Ipecacuanha Emetic Draught, Paediatric B.P.C., or the equivalent Syrup Ipecacuanha U.S.P. 10-15ml is likely to be the best measure for children, being faster in action than waiting for a stomach wash-out and is probably as effective. Saline emetics can induce hypernatraemia and deaths have occurred so that no more than 2 teaspoonfuls of salt in a glass of warm water should be taken. In children losing fluid from the bowel as well, salt should be avoided as an emetic.

Unconscious Patients

The first priority is to *maintain a clear airway*. If the cough and pharyngeal reflexes are absent *an endotracheal tube is passed*. Pharyngeal and occasionally bronchoscopic suction are required to aspirate inhaled vomit and retained secretions. If stomach contents have entered the lung corticosteroids are given i.v. (they are also helpful with irritant and poisonous fumes and gases). If there is hypoventilation, hand ventilation initially, followed by machine maintained intermittent *positive pressure ventilation* is given with air enriched by oxygen. For ventilation lasting a few days a plastic endotracheal tube is safe and few patients are unconscious long enough to require tracheostomy. Analeptics or respiratory stimulants to counteract respiratory depressants such as the barbiturates are no longer prescribed. In overdosage with narcotics (or undue susceptibility in the aged and emphysematous) naloxone 0.4-1.2mg i.v. repeated at intervals as an antidote counteracts the effects of morphine, codeine, heroin, methadone, pethidine, diphenoxylate, dextropropoxyphene, as well as pentazocine, whereas nalorphine and levallorphan do not reverse the effects of pentazocine. Naloxone is a pure antagonist with no agonist activity although costly. Its short period of action can be counteracted by giving it i.m. or by i.v. infusion. Codeine overdosage can cause both respiratory depression and convulsions.

Shock and circulatory failure are countered by restoring lost fluid (external losses from vomiting, bowel, skin, hyperventilation, or internal into capillaries). Absolute or relative hypovolaemia is treated by i.v. dextrose or electrolyte solutions, plasma expanders such as human albumin fraction, modified gelatin solutions ('Haemaccel', 'Gelofusine'), low molecular weight dextran or occasionally blood. The volume of fluid and rate of administration are judged by manometry (central venous pressure, pulmonary artery pressures as in 'shock units'), arterial blood pressure, chest radiographs to exclude pulmonary oedema, and urine flow, as well as clinical features (e.g. warmth of extremities, jugular venous pressure, auscultation of lungs). Electrolyte and acid-base balance are corrected. Vasopressors as a means of restoring the arterial blood pressures are out of favour, but isoprenaline, dopamine or dobutamine ('Dobutrex') have been used to improve the circulatory flow.

Aspiration or emptying of the stomach is often carried out in those who have digested drugs or poisons. A wide bore tube at least 1cm in diameter is used. The question of lavage is debatable; in certain circumstances some hold it may even promote absorption and the yield is small. The removal of aspirin, paracetamol, iron and possibly tricyclic antidepressives should be attempted even if several hours have elapsed. The tricyclics produce an ileus which cause them to be retained. Aspiration or lavage is carried out after the unconscious patient's airway has been safeguarded with a cuffed endotracheal tube and resuscitation has been performed. Conscious patients in particular should be in a head down position to prevent inhalation. A bronchoscope and powerful sucker should be at hand. Rarely gastric intubation by inducing vagal stimuli may invoke convulsions, cardiac arrhythmias and arrest. Because of the risks of inhalation paraffin (kerosene) should be left where it is in the stomach. With corrosives the standard advice is not to attempt aspiration, or lavage, because of the risks of perforation. Nevertheless, staff in some experienced poisons units do perform skilled, gentle lavage.

Promotion of excretion may be achieved by forced diuresis, that is deliberately increasing the urinary flow when drugs are eliminated by this route. Because of its risks it is not as popular now. Diuretics such as frusemide may be given as well as i.v. fluids to increase urine flow to 500ml/h. Only a few drugs are so treated. The urine pH may be altered, either made alkaline to increase the excretion of weak acids e.g. phenobarbitone, aspirin, and lithium salts, or made acid to hasten elimination of weak bases e.g. amphetamines, fenfluramine, narcotics and some monoamine oxidase inhibitors. Up to 12 litres of fluid can be given daily i.v. to the young, but this is risky in the elderly inducing pulmonary oedema. Hypokalaemia also occurs. The urine output is measured by catheterization. In salicylate poisoning a 'cocktail' of Sodium Chloride Injection B.P. (0.9%) 500ml, Laevulose Injection B.P. 5% 1000ml and Sodium Bicarbonate Injection B.P. 1.4% 500ml is given in rotation. The 2 litres are infused i.v. each hour for 3 hours (6 litres).

Even in special units peritoneal dialysis, haemodialysis, charcoal haemoperfusion or exchange blood transfusions are rarely required. Good results with coated charcoal haemoperfusion have been attained at the Guy's Hospital poisons unit with severe barbiturate and glutethimide poisoning, and this form of treatment may be applicable to methanol, ethchlorvynol, methaqualone, trichloroethanol and salicylates in severe overdosage.

Antidotes, although infrequently used, are of interest; some are listed in Table 9.

TABLE 9
ANTIDOTES

Toxicant	Antidote
Acid	Alkalies
Alkalies	Acid
Bromides	Chlorides
Coumarins	Vitamin K_1
Cyanide	Sodium Nitrite U.S.P.
	Sodium Thiosulfate U.S.P., Ph. Eur.
	Dicobalt Edetate ('Kelocyanor')
Fluoroacetate	Sodium Acetate
Histamine liberation	Adrenaline, Corticosteroids, Antihistamines
Lysergic Acid Diethylamide	Phenothiazines
Metals	
Mercury, Lead	Dimercaprol, Penicillamine Sodium Calciumedetate,
Iron	Desferrioxamine
Muscarine (mushrooms)	Atropine
Narcotics	Naloxone
Organophosphorus insecticides	Atropine and Pralidoxime
Toxins	
Anthrax	
Botulinus	Antitoxins
Snake	
Tetanus	

Intensive nursing care is applicable to all types of coma. This means observations on vital functions (pulse, respiration, blood pressure, central venous pressure, pupil size, depth of consciousness, colour, fluid intake and fluid loss), as well as nursing of the skin, mouth (to prevent parotitis), eyes, particularly prevention of exposure keratitis, avoidance of nerve compression (e.g. peroneal paralysis causing foot drop) and turning of the patient to forestall pulmonary complications. Care of humidifiers, tubes and monitoring machines may also be part of the nurse's duties.

Psychiatric assessment: this is advised as policy in all self-poisoning irrespective of the severity of the gesture. The psychiatrist should see the patient when the mental effects of the drugs such as confusion and drowsiness have passed off and a clear history can be given.

Fluid and energy intake: the average patient will recover before intravenous feeding with special solutions is needed. Unconscious patients in general can (as after brain damage or stroke) be fed by intragastric tube. Two to three litres of fluid are given enriched by glucose, eggs, 'Complan' and emulsified fat for calories. One thousand Calories equals 4.2 mega Joules. A 2000 Calorie diet (8.4 MJ) can be achieved by using a pint of milk (400Cal), a 2-ounce egg (90Cal), glucose 2 ounces (240Cal), half an ounce of 'Ovaltine' or 'Horlicks' (240Cal), 2 ounces of 'Complan' (250Cal), 1 ounce double cream (130Cal) and 4 ounces of orange juice (40Cal). One ounce is approximately 30g. In the unconscious person the protein content should be no more than 70g and water depletion is to be avoided. (1 Calorie = 1000 calories = 4200 Joules.)

Special Examples
Paracetamol in a dose of 10g and above can cause liver damage and necrosis and death can occur from liver, cardiac or renal disease when 15g or more have been ingested. Such patients should be admitted and observed for several days irrespective of their initial condition, and predictive tests performed such as liver function, blood sugar, prothrombin time and high paracetamol levels (e.g. >200µg/dl) which should be related to the time of taking the overdose and the time levels take to fall. Gastric emptying is worthwhile within 12 hours. Some experts advise leaving 20g of activated charcoal, or 50g of cholestyramine within the stomach, but the value is uncertain. In severe cases if available cysteamine i.v. has been tried, but it is unpleasant and toxic. Other sulphur containing aminoacids 'sulphydril donors' may perhaps also protect the liver (cysteine, methionine, acetyl cysteine, penicillamine). Cysteamine blocks the formation of toxic oxidation products of paracetamol, but is a problem to prepare and paracetamol levels need to be measured. Methionine is cheap, less toxic and easier to prepare. It acts by speeding the synthesis of glutathione which removes the toxic products formed from paracetamol. *Dose* 2.5g i.v. or orally every 4 hours until a total of 10g. In specially equipped liver failure units charcoal haemoperfusion has been tried to remove the products of liver failure. N-acetylcysteine injection ('Parvolex') is now available.

In **tricyclic antidepressive** poisoning death may (rarely) result from cardiac arrest, ventricular arrhythmias, hyperthermia, coma or convulsions. Patients should be kept quiet in bed and sedated if conscious. In severe cases physostigmine salicylate, or pyridostigmine has been claimed to lessen coma and block the peripheral atropine-like effects. Their use involves risk and is rarely necessary.

Poison Centres
With few exceptions poisonings are admitted to hospital and selected cases are dealt with in an intensive care or poisons unit, where there is close cooperation between nurses, doctors and chemical laboratories. With so many poisons of medicinal, industrial, household and agricultural origin a central reference poisons unit is invaluable. Some maintain a 24 hour service. Telephone numbers of the major British centres are given in the B.N.F. and in the U.S.A. in the Physicians Desk Reference.

18 ANTICOAGULANTS AND COAGULANTS

Pathological clotting occurs in response to vessel injury, and disease, sluggish blood flow, increase in blood platelets, red cells, serum lipids and alteration in the intrinsic clotting mechanisms induced by disease and drugs. When the vessel endothelium is injured platelets stick to the exposed collagen. The platelet permeability changes and intracellular substances such as adenosine diphosphate are released which are powerful stimuli to platelet clumping. The coagulation mechanism is activated and the fibrin formed enmeshes the platelets making a thrombus. Intravascular clotting is a major cause of death and illness blocking vital arteries in the brain, heart, gut, lungs, limbs and kidneys and obstructing limb, pelvic, brain, and hepatic veins with the risk of emboli. Subclinical fibrin deposition and fibrinolysis probably occurs all the time in healthy people.

Prevention and treatment of pathological thrombosis is

(1) **to reduce high blood lipids;** to avoid oestrogens in high risk patients; and to avoid dehydration and hypotension.

(2) **to inhibit or alter platelet function.** There are two main groups of drugs. The first are the non-steroidal anti-inflammatory drugs. **Aspirin** has been used in patients who have had transient cerebral ischaemic attacks when these were believed to be due to platelet thrombo-emboli for instance causing amaurosis fugax or transient blindness. One or two tablets weekly will alter the clotting mechanisms. **Sulphinpyrazone** ('Anturan') has similar uses and also has been given to prevent clotting in those with valve prostheses and arterio-venous shunts, but it potentiates the coumarin anticoagulants. The second group of analogues share the pyrimidopyrimidine ring structure and **Dipyridamole** ('Persantin') an example has been used to prevent thrombosis in those with cardiac valve prostheses, or associated with renal transplant rejection. Reduction of platelet formation in polycythaemia rubra vera (p. 195) and primary thrombocythaemia may lessen the risk of clotting.

(3) **to inhibit fibrin formation** using oral anticoagulants which are vitamin K antagonists and inhibit Factors II, VII, IX and X or parenterally given anticoagulants such as heparin (which is antiprothrombin, antithrombin and antithromboplastin) and ancrod (an antifibrinogen). All these can be dangerous, at times fatal, and need close monitoring and supervision.

(4) **by activating fibrinolysis with activators** which by enzymic action convert plasminogen to plasmin the enzyme which is fibrinolytic (e.g. streptokinase, urokinase).

ORAL ANTICOAGULANTS

Structurally they resemble vitamin K_1 and in some way block or displace vitamin K from an enzyme system responsible for the formation of the prothrombin-complex by the liver and also act against other factors concerned with clotting (mainly factor VII). They are hence antimetabolites. Chemically they are of two types: the **Coumarins** and the **Indanediones.**

Indications for Anticoagulation

(1) It is generally agreed that they are valuable in the treatment of *venous*

thrombosis of the legs or pelvis after operations, pregnancy and accidents, and for pulmonary embolism. They may be prescribed prophylactically to bed patients particularly at risk of venous thrombosis namely the elderly, the obese, those with fractures such as of the hip, those with varicose veins and eczema, those on the contraceptive pill, and those with blood disorders favouring blood clotting. Patients who have had previous venous thrombosis or embolus if confined to bed are also given anticoagulants.

(2) Persistent or recurrent *atrial fibrillation* is a risk because static atria can contain clots and cause emboli. If associated with mitral stenosis anticoagulation is usually prescribed (as well as valvotomy); with other causes it is desirable, but not always logistically possible. Sino-atrial disease with the bradycardia-tachycardia syndrome is another indication.

(3) Cardiovascular; surgical patients with valve prostheses, coronary artery bypass, acute peripheral arterial emboli, or who are having arterial surgery.

(4) Electrical conversion of arrhythmias is usually preceded for 10 days or so by anticoagulation.

(5) Large chambered hearts as in cardiomyopathy are liable to form clots on the ventricular wall.

(6) Carotid artery stenosis and transient ischaemic attacks such as fleeting blindness and hemiparesis.

(7) In arterial disease their use is controversial, both for short- or long-term use. Their popularity is waning, but they are still widely used for those with worsening angina and cardiac infarction. With the trend to short stay in bed in hospital they are probably not needed for 'good-risk' cardiac infarction. In the bad-risk patient they reduce the evidence of leg thrombosis (fibrinogen labelled isotope studies), but it has not been easy to show they also reduce mortality. They also prevent mural thrombosis.

(8) Other indications include idiopathic pulmonary hypertension, and some cardiologists treat all mitral stenotics even in sinus rhythm because of the possible hazard of cerebral embolus.

Administration
There is a correlation (as in all therapy) between clinical success and the close monitoring of therapy. The dose should be reviewed if there is fever, intercurrent illness, or if any other drugs which may enhance or decrease the action are added. Safety depends on frequent blood tests. For nursing mothers taking anticoagulants the risks are not great for the baby taking breast milk who can be given prophylactic oral vitamin K_1 1-2mg weekly. For the pregnant woman oral anticoagulants should be replaced by heparin a few weeks before expected delivery. Heparin does not cross the placenta. Oral anticoagulants such as warfarin after absorption are bound to plasma proteins and very little is free. However, the drug is largely confined to the small plasma intravascular compartment. Problems arise because other drugs can displace bound warfarin so that comparatively more becomes free in this small plasma compartment and pharmacologically more active. The coumarins are more widely used than the indanediones because dangerous allergic side effects are less.

Coumarins
Warfarin Sodium ('Coumadin', 'Marevan') *presentation* Tablets B.P. 1, 3, 5 and 10mg. *Dose* orally 5-15mg to start, then 2-12.5mg daily as a maintenance dose. Larger loading doses are dangerous. Other coumarins include

Cumetharol, Dicoumarol (Bishydroxycoumarin), **Ethylbiscoumacetate** ('Tromexan'), **Nicoumalone B.P.** ('Sinthrome') and **Phenprocoumon U.S.N.F.** ('Liquamar').

Indanediones
Phenindione ('Dindevan') *presentation* Tablets B.P. 10, 25 and 50mg. Absorption differs between brands: fine particle 'Dindevan' is well absorbed. *Dose* loading 100-150mg given on the morning of the first day and 100mg at night, 50mg on the second day, 25mg on the morning of the third day and thereafter 25-100mg daily in divided doses. It takes 48 hours to work, lasts 24-36 hours and is less cumulative than warfarin so it may not cause as severe and prolonged bleeding. It is wise to take the same precautions over possible drug interactions as with coumarins.

Bleeding can occur from overdosage, unrelated defects in plasma and platelet clotting factors, interactions with other drugs, pathological lesions (intestinal or renal tract bleeding may be a sign of an ulcer or tumour) or trauma; it can even take place at 'safe' or normal prothrombin times.

Oral anticoagulant activity *is increased* by heart failure causing liver congestion, primary liver disease such as cirrhosis when the prothrombin time may be raised; in ill patients with poor nutrition and fever; by a myriad of drugs e.g. phenylbutazone, indomethacin, propionic acid analgesics, alcohol, broad spectrum and non-absorbed antibiotics (reducing vitamin K_1 in gut), corticosteroids, clofibrate and sulphonamides (a fuller list is given on p. 249). All drugs given with coumarins should be viewed with caution; beta-blockers, hypotensives, digoxin, diuretics and benzodiazepines seem safe.

Factors *decreasing activity* include diuretics since they improve congestive heart failure; antithyroid drugs, rifampicin, barbiturates, glutethimide, and ethchlorvynol by the mechanism of increased liver cell metabolism. Since hypnotics are almost universally thrust on patients in hospital a drug like a barbiturate may, when stopped on leaving hospital cause warfarin to have a much stronger action—with possible fatal results. Diazepam or nitrazepam is safer. Some families have a genetic resistance to warfarin.

Failure of oral anticoagulant therapy can arise when patients do not take their drugs; when there is underlying intravascular coagulation, or an underlying cancer. Repeated venous thrombosis may then still occur.

Adverse effects minor bleeding from nose, kidneys or into the skin is not rare. More unusual is bleeding into the skin with necrosis and into fatty tissues (breasts, buttocks, omentum), muscles (from i.m. injections), pericardium, joints, peritoneum, and retroperitoneal tissues, pleural spaces, adrenals, kidneys, brain, carpal tunnel, nerve trunks, and peripheral nerves (femoral, sciatic, lumbosacral roots), epidural and subdural spaces, spinal cord, gut (with ileus), haematoma and obstruction. Bleeding, if trivial, is treated by adjustment of dose, or if major, by fresh blood, fresh frozen plasma or vitamin K_1 orally, i.m., or i.v. 5-20mg as 'Aquamephyton'.

Indanediones produce in under 1% hypersensitivity reactions—rashes, itching, diarrhoea, fever, hepatitis, proteinuria, eosinophilia, leukaemoid reaction, thrombocytopenia, agranulocytosis, pancytopenia, stomatitis, hypothyroidism, ulcerative colitis, steatorrhoea, anuria and myocarditis—some are fatal.

Long-term treatment depends on the underlying disease, the patient's age and co-operation and laboratory facilities. The hospital doctor should keep both the patient and his family doctor informed of the current dosage and prothrombin time. The patient should be given a card with his name, drug, dose, hospital doctor in charge and recent prothrombin times. Booklets provide information on drugs to avoid (either home remedies like aspirin or doctor prescribed medications). The patient's home or work telephone number should be known. The patient is told to notify any doctor or dentist who wishes to operate that he is taking anticoagulants and the patient should stop therapy if he bleeds excessively. In practice patients still die of haemorrhage unnecessarily when other doctors prescribe antibiotics (broad-spectrum or intestinal) or antirheumatics, knowing, or not knowing, the patients are taking warfarin. *Contra-indications* are recurrent haemorrhage, or a recent bleed from a peptic ulcer, or from the retina; active peptic ulceration; active ulcerative colitis; intensive salicylate therapy; malignant hypertension, polyarteritis nodosa; pericarditis and bacterial endocarditis; renal failure; bleeding disorders; recent operations on the eye, brain and spinal cord; pregnancy (except those with prosthetic valves already on anticoagulants, or who develop venous thrombosis). Breast feeding is safe when taking warfarin.

Surgery for operation on the nervous system or eye, therapy is stopped at least 2 days beforehand. For minor surgery therapy is continued, or the dose is reduced. After surgery anticoagulants can be started on the third day.

INJECTABLE ANTICOAGULANTS

Heparin ('Pularin') a mucopolysaccharide is a natural anticoagulant which delays the clotting of blood and also clears the plasma of fats. It is obtained from the lungs or intestines of animals. It acts within minutes of being given i.v. and lasts 4-6 hours. Given s.c., it lasts 8-18 hours, but is less effective. It is given for 36-48 hours before oral anticoagulants start to work, or in venous thrombosis it may be the sole therapy for 7-10 days. An important use is as prophylaxis against venous thrombosis in medical and surgical patients when it is given 5000u 8 or 12 hourly s.c. Other uses are after arterial surgery and for disseminated intravascular coagulation (consumption coagulapathy). *Presentation* Injection B.P. a solution of heparin calcium or heparin sodium in Water for Injections ampoules 1 and 5ml contain 1000 and 5000u/ml without preservative; vials with preservative 5ml contain 5000, 25 000 or 125 000u. Heparin Retard injection contains 20 000u in 2ml ampoules. For prophylactic use there are ampoules 0.2ml with 5000u of either heparin sodium ('Minihep', 'Pabyrn', 'Uniparin') or heparin calcium ('Calciparine', 'Minihep Calcium'). Also available are pre-loaded syringes containing 5000u in 0.3ml ('Heparin Immuno'). *Therapeutic dose* i.v. 10 000-12 500u initially then 5000-10 000u 4-8 hourly. The heparin can be injected as a bolus directly into a vein, or via a Gordh needle, catheter or rubber tubing of an infusion as intermittent therapy. It is common practice to add 40 000u to a bottle of Dextrose Injection B.P. 5% and to deliver this over 24 hours. Heparin should not be added to many solutions e.g. with adrenaline, benzylpenicillin, erythromycin, hydrocortisone, kanamycin, oxytetracycline, prochlorperazine, promazine, promethazine, streptomycin, tetracycline or vancomycin. Control of dosage is achieved by keeping the clotting time at 2-3 times the normal. *Adverse effects* overdosage is liable in liver and renal disease and leads to bleeding in the same sites as with oral anticoagulants. Its action can be neutralized by protamine sulphate; approximately 1mg neutralizes 100mg of heparin. It is available as **Protamine Sulphate Injection B.P.** in ampoules 5 and 10ml 10mg/ml. No more than 50mg should be given at any one time. Other reactions to heparin are urticaria, conjunctivitis, rhinitis, fever, anaphylaxis (including that to the contained chlorocresol), angioneurotic oedema, asthma, a painful blue, ischaemic vasospastic limb reaction with a burning sensation, transient alopecia, thrombocytopenia and with long-term use osteoporosis. Patients receiving heparin in therapeutic amounts should not be given i.m. injections because of the risk of bleeding into muscles. Calcium heparin is less painful than sodium heparin.

Thrombolytic and Fibrinolytic Agents (Clot Dispersing)
If heparin is ineffective in pulmonary embolus or venous thrombosis an effective, but expensive alternative is **Streptokinase** ('Kabikinase', 'Streptase') an enzyme of streptococcal origin available as a freeze-dried powder. It is antigenic and has a molecular weight of 48 000. Plasmin can break down peptides especially those containing lysine and arginine so that derivatives of lysine (see later) will counteract the action of fibrinolysins. *Presentation* vials 100 000, 250 000, 600 000 and 750 000u. Streptokinase Injection B.P. is made by dissolving the contents in Water for Injections. To suppress anaphylactic and febrile reactions prednisolone 25mg twice daily orally or i.m. is given. Previous heparin must be neutralized. *Dose* the schedule is complex and should be checked against the maker's directions. Initially 600 000u is dissolved in 5ml of Water for Injections and infused in 100ml of Dextrose Injection B.P. 5%, or Sodium Chloride Injection B.P. over a period of 30 min i.v., or directly into a pulmonary artery catheter. The same dose of 600 000u is given in 500ml sodium chloride or dextrose solution over 6 hours at a rate of 100 000u/h, and this may be repeated up to 72 hours. The action takes 12 hours. *Precautions* if possible its use should be avoided immediately after an operation, during menstruation, or in the presence of an active peptic ulcer because of the high risk of bleeding, which may also occur from venepuncture sites. Streptokinase can be followed by heparin and the oral anticoagulants. **Urokinase** is a less antigenic enzyme produced by the kidney and obtained from human urine. It acts similarly and may prove to be superior, but great quantities of urine are needed for even small amounts. The molecular weight is 55 000. The complication of severe haemorrhage can be countered by **Aminocaproic Acid** ('Epsikapron') which is an antifibrinolysin, which inhibits competitively the activation of plasminogen to plasmin. It is a derivative of the basic aminoacid lysine. *Presentation* effervescent powder 50% strength supplied in sachets each containing 3g of aminocaproic acid and as a syrup containing 300mg/ml in bottles of 250ml; *dose* 100mg/kg B.W. every 3-5h orally according to severity. It has been prescribed for menorrhagia (e.g. with the intra-uterine device) in a dose of 3g 4-6 times daily.**Tranexamic Acid** ('Cyclokapron') has similar uses but is more potent and is restricted to hospital use. It is a structural modification of aminocaproic acid of shorter length and containing a rigid cyclical ring for stability. *Presentation* ampoules 5ml 100mg/ml, tablets 500mg; *dose* 15-30mg/kg B.W. or 1-2g in an intravenous infusion every 8h, in dextrose or saline solutions, or the same daily dose orally. These preparations are not given in pregnancy and except for menorrhagia (in women using the coil) are only given in hospital. Aminocaproic acid or tranexamic acid can be used supplementary to factor VIII therapy in minor surgical procedures in haemophiliacs.
Ancrod ('Arvin') a purified fraction of the venom of the Malayan pit viper,

reduces plasma fibrinogen and has been used as a fibrinolytic. *Presentation* ampoules 1ml containing 70u. *Dose* initially 70u given over 15 min i.v. and then 40-70u 6 hourly, or 1-4u/kg B.W. per 12 hours. Heparin is probably as good and is much less expensive.

COAGULANTS

Surgical clotting agents or haemostatics are used locally in surgery and dentistry. **Human Thrombin B.P.** is made from plasma and is an enzyme which converts fibrinogen to fibrin; **Thrombin U.S.N.F.** is derived commercially from bovine plasma and is made as a powder which is dissolved in Sodium Chloride Injection and applied to the bleeding site. **Human Fibrinogen B.P.** is supplied as a powder which is dissolved in pyrogen-free Water for Injections and mixed with thrombin at the time of use topically. **Human Fibrin Foam B.P.** is formed by mixing fibrinogen with thrombin. Human-derived haemostatics carry the risk of serum hepatitis. **Russell Viper Venom** acts as a potent haemostatic. **Adrenaline** solution used locally causes vasoconstriction and is a useful haemostatic e.g. for nose bleeds. Oxidized cellulose B.P. ('Oxycel', 'Surgicel') and Gelatin Sponge B.P. are absorbable preparations which provide a synthetic matrix for clotting.

19 CARDIOVASCULAR THERAPY

DIGITALIS TYPE GLYCOSIDES

Digitalis is obtained from the white *(Digitalis lanata)* or the purple foxglove *(Digitalis purpurea)*. The active principle is a glycoside composed of a steroid-like part, combined with various sugars. Digitalis plants contain various glycosides and their precursors. They act on the vagal, medullary and parasympathetic centres, on the sino-atrial and atrioventricular nodes and on the conducting tissues of the heart. These effects slow the heart (negative chronotropic effect). Drgitalis also strengthens the force of heart muscle contraction (positive inotropic effect) and constricts the major veins. Consequently the heart acts more effectively, the circulation improves, particularly to the kidneys, and surplus body water and salt are excreted.

Uses are mainly **to treat congestive heart failure** especially when severe or refractory, whatever the rhythm disturbance. In view of the problems involved with the glycosides the tendency is to treat mild heart failure with diuretics alone. **Supraventricular arrhythmias;** both in atrial fibrillation and atrial flutter the rate is reduced to safe levels, but digitalis therapy rarely restores sinus rhythm. However, **paroxysmal atrial or nodal tachycardia** may stop under its influence, or the rate is made bearable until the paroxysm stops spontaneously. Digitalis has a debated use in **cardiac infarction,** but is given if co-existing cardiogenic shock, supraventricular arrhythmias, or heart failure are present although the doses are often smaller than usual. Digitalization, or quick saturation of the body by digitalis is less popular than it was, but can be achieved by a large loading dose, usually orally, followed by a smaller maintenance dose equal to that excreted daily. It used to be taught that once a patient was started on digitalis he must always be kept on it, but this is not so. Failure or arrhythmias may be a temporary affair and the elderly person may be helped (in life expectancy) by stopping digitalis, or reducing the amount given.

Preparations

Digitalis Folia Ph. Eur. obtained from the dried leaves of *Digitalis purpurea* contains various glycosides but the principal one is digitoxin. The leaf preparation keeps well if protected from light and moisture. Unpredictable in duration it has been largely replaced by the more potent (and dangerous) pure glycosides. *Presentation* Prepared Digitalis Tablets B.P. 30, 60 and 100mg. The initial digitalizing dose is 180mg t.d.s. on day 1, 120mg on day 2, 60mg t.d.s. on day 3 and thereafter 30-200mg daily. The action starts in 2-3 hours and is maximum at 6 hours.

Digoxin Ph. Eur. obtained from *Digitalis lanata* is the most widely used preparation, but the many brands and batches of the same brand can differ in formulation (physical state or particle size), the rate and extent of absorption and plasma levels achieved. It is wise to keep to one brand because of the variation in drug dissolution and absorption (bioavailability). *Pharmacology* it is a pure glycoside and in solution, or in small particle size, is quickly absorbed orally. The extent of absorption is 70-80% and depends little whether taken with food, or not, but is affected by gastro-intestinal motility. Absorption is also decreased in malabsorption states. In the blood only 25% is bound to plasma proteins. Digoxin is excreted unchanged by the kidneys so that blood levels depend on renal function. Digoxin is not metabolized and is relatively rapidly eliminated. Digoxin is cleared by the kidney to such an extent that it means it must also be secreted by the renal tubules. The tubular excretion may be partially blocked by spironolactone which has a similar steroidal structure and digoxin blood levels may rise. The fast excretion means that unless there is renal failure overdosage is not prolonged. The normal half-life (time for plasma levels to fall by 50%) of digoxin is 30-35 hours. *Presentation* oral Tablets, B.P. 62.5μg (0.0625mg) 'Lanoxin P.G.', 125μg (0.125mg) and 250μg (0.25mg), Digoxin Elixir Paediatric B.P.C. ('Lanoxin PG Elixir' is advertized for paediatric and geriatric use) 50μg/ml (0.05mg/ml). Care is needed over decimal points since occasionally children are unintentionally given 10 times the correct dose. *Dose* for rapid digitalization in adults is 1-1.5mg preferably in divided doses over 24 hours followed by an oral maintenance dose which must be selected according to renal function. Daily requirements usually range from 0.125-0.5mg (125-500μg) daily, but can be as low as 62.5μg. Infants are digitalized with 25μg/kg B.W. 6 hourly and maintained on 25μg/kg B.W. daily. *Parenteral* Digoxin Injection B.P. a solution contained in ampoules 2ml 250μg/ml (0.25mg/ml), and Digoxin Paediatric Injection B.P. for hospital use 25μg/0.25ml and 100μg/ml. For the (rarely necessary) urgent control of heart rate digoxin 500-1000μg(0.5-1mg) for adults can be given i.v. providing no form of digitalis has been given for at least 2 weeks before. For those who cannot swallow or who are vomiting i.m. digoxin is suitable.

Medigoxin (Betamethyldigoxin, 'Lanitop') by a slight chemical modification of digoxin has achieved almost 100% absorption and acts by mouth in 2-4h and 1-4min after i.v. injection. It is eliminated at a similar rate to digoxin. *Presentation* tablets 100μg (0.1mg), ampoules for i.v. use 2 ml 100μg/ml. *Dose* orally for digitalization 2 tablets twice daily then 200-300μg (0.2-0.3mg) daily in single or divided amounts; i.v. 200-400μg.

Occasional Alternatives

Digitoxin Ph. Eur. ('Nativelle's Digitaline') is obtained from Digitalis species and is slower acting but more potent than digoxin. It is almost completely absorbed and is metabolized by the liver and a significant proportion is excreted in the bile, which may be reabsorbed by enterohepatic cycling. The half-life is 5-7 days. Hence digitoxin accumulates in the body; also it is highly bound to the plasma proteins. In the presence of renal failure it is better to use it rather than digoxin since it is not entirely dependent on renal excretion although the non-active metabolites are eventually excreted renally. If there is toxicity this may be reduced by cholestyramine which binds to it in the gut. *Presentation* Tablets B.P. 100μg, an oral solution 1:1000 (1mg/ml) and ampoules 1ml containing 200μg/ml for i.v. use. An initial digitalizing dose is 1000-2000μg (1-2mg) in divided amounts then 50-250μg once daily.

Lanatoside C ('Cedilanid') obtained from *Digitalis lanata* is very poorly absorbed and is metabolized to digoxin; it has no advantage over digoxin and is not advised. *Presentation* tablets 250μg; *dose* 1-1.5mg initially, then 250μg 6 hourly until control occurs. **Deslanoside** is derived from lanatoside C and by alkaline hydrolysis becomes more soluble and able to be injected. Deslanoside Injection U.S.N.F. ('Cedilanid Injection')*presentation* ampoules 2ml containing 400μg/2ml is used for rapid i.v. digitalization in a *dose* of 800-1200μg i.v. **Ouabain** is the active glycoside of *Strophanthus gratus*. *Presentation* ampoules

1ml 250µg/ml; *dose* 125-250µg i.v. Tablets 2.5mg are available and the dose is 10mg b.d. orally. Ouabain is mainly used for rapid effect by parenteral injection, since the oral form is poorly and unpredictably absorbed.

Advere effects are common in spite of knowledge about digitalis glycosides action and pharmacokinetics and rapid methods of measuring blood levels. Perhaps 20-25% of those taking digitalis preparations suffer symptoms of toxicity. Overdosage occurs particularly in the aged in whom glomerular flow rate is decreased and the incidence of coronary artery and conduction system disorders is increased. Cardiotoxicity may precede other symptoms. Toxicity is related to hypokalaemia, hypercalcaemia, hypomagnesaemia, anoxia, acid-base disturbance, hypothyroidism and renal failure. The commonest symptoms are fatigue, visual disturbances and muscle weakness. Digitalis toxicity is often fatal, although it is the most diseased hearts which are likely to show ill-effects. A recent cardiac infarction makes the use of digitalis more hazardous. The symptoms of toxicity are non-specific and there is a narrow margin between therapeutic and toxic levels. They are *gastro-intestinal* (nausea, anorexia, abdominal pain, diarrhoea); *cardiac*—virtually any arrhythmia can occur (bradycardia, coupled beats, extrasystoles, rapid regular, or irregular atrial, nodal or ventricular rhythms especially complex or double arrhythmias, regularity of response in atrial fibrillation eventually with complete heart block and the association of atrial tachycardia and variable ventricular block). A fatal arrhythmia may be the first manifestation; *nervous* and *psychiatric* (delirium, hazy vision, disturbed red-green perception, blind spots, yellow vision, hallucinations, facial pain, fatigue, decreased muscle strength); *endocrine;* gynaecomastia.

Treatment consists of stopping the drug, giving potassium unless there is slow heart block, or an appropriate anti-arrhythmic such as lignocaine or phenytoin. Chelating agents and specific antibodies have been used. Blood levels may indicate whether toxicity is likely. Levels over 2ng/ml may be associated with toxicity. Levels over 3 are usually associated with manifest toxicity when taken 8 hours or so after the last dose. *Drug interactions* certain drugs influence absorption by altering gastro-intestinal motility (propantheline decreases motility and promotes digoxin absorption and metoclopramide increases motility and decreases absorption) or by sequestration decrease absorption (cholestyramine), increase potency (diuretics causing hypokalaemia), or interfere with tubular renal excretion (spironolactone competes with digoxin for excretion).

CARDIAC DEPRESSANTS USED IN DYSRHYTHMIAS

As yet there is no scientific way of predicting which anti-arrhythmics will work in spite of sophisticated electro-physiological research. Therapy is still empirical. Ideally an anti-arrhythmic drug should be quickly effective, absorbed orally, safe and long acting. No such drug exists. Any new agent should be judged by whether it is better and safer than the others.

Quinidine

This is a cardiac depressant which increases the refractory or resting period of the myocardium and its conducting tissues. Many doctors are cautious or unwilling to use it because of a small risk of sudden death even with small doses because of idiosyncrasy. However, with attention to blood levels, proper administration and the newer long-acting varieties a limited revival in interest has occurred. *Uses* to prevent or abolish atrial fibrillation, atrial tachycardia and atrial flutter, especially after electrical conversion (DC shock) has restored sinus rhythm, since its use helps to maintain a normal rhythm. If used primarily to treat fast supraventricular rhythms digoxin is given first. In ventricular tachycardia it is used alone. Because of the danger of cardiac syncope its therapeutic use should be started in hospital under careful control, preferably in a coronary care unit. However, after a test dose many doctors do give small doses necessary to prevent arrhythmias, such as extrasystoles, without referring patients to hospital. *Presentation* **Quinidine Sulphate** Tablets B.P. 60, 125, 200 ('Quinicardine') and 300mg, **Quinidine Bisulphate** is a more soluble salt which is incorporated in a slow release plastic matrix permitting safer blood levels (4-8mg/litre) and permits a more convenient twice daily regimen. *Presentation* slow release tablets ('Kinidin Durules') or capsules ('Kiditard') 250mg equivalent to 200mg of quinidine sulphate. *Dose* a test amount of quinidine sulphate is given. If there are no side effects such as sickness, hypotension, or tinnitus larger doses are prescribed namely 300mg 2 hourly for 6 doses which can be repeated the next day at twice this amount. In practice electrical conversion is preferred and afterwards quinidine sulphate 200mg 8 hourly, or better still the slow release form is given 1 or 2 'Durules' twice daily. **Quinidine Gluconate U.S.P.** sterile solution 800mg/10ml can be injected for the control of arrhythmias refractory to safer therapy. *Adverse effects* the most serious event is cardiac arrest from asystole, or circulatory failure from rapid increase in heart rate. Hypersensitivity also causes tinnitus, vertigo, headache, rashes, nausea, vomiting, diarrhoea, abdominal pain, purpura, hypotension, or fever. Accumulation leading to toxic levels causes various ECG changes hence monitoring and frequent tracings are taken. Making the urine alkaline for any reason (e.g. with antacids) may decrease excretion and lead to toxic levels in the blood. Other interactions may occur with warfarin.

Lignocaine Hydrochloride (Lidocaine)

Lignocaine is of major importance in the coronary care unit in the treatment and possibly in the prevention of ventricular fibrillation, ventricular tachycardia and extrasystoles but controlled trials have not proved this. Primary ventricular fibrillation often occurs without warning after cardiac infarction. *Presentation* ampoules and vials of varying strengths; Injection B.P. is a solution in vials 0.5, 1 and 2%. Astra make 5ml disposable syringes ('Xylocard') 20% strength (1ml=200mg, total amount=1g) which is diluted usually by adding it to a 500ml infusion of Dextrose Solution B.P. 5%, and a 2% strength in a 5ml syringe (1ml=20mg) which is given undiluted in a *bolus dose* of 70-100mg i.v. which can be repeated. A loading dose is needed to achieve a therapeutic concentration and to maintain these levels 3mg/min (range 2-4mg/min) is needed in those with normal hepatic function. The dose needs to be infused accurately with a constant infusion pump. Doses usually have to be reduced in the presence of liver, renal or cardiac failure. 'Xylocard' 10% is a pre-loaded syringe containing 3ml 100mg/ml for i.m. use for instance before sending the patient to hospital. The deltoid is used and to promote absorption the area is rubbed after the injection. *Adverse effects* excessive concentrations can cause drowsiness, convulsions, agitation, disorientation, blurred vision, speech disturbances, euphoria, tremor, respiratory depression, hypotension and bradycardia. *Contra-indications* are third degree block, severe conduction disturbances, heart failure or hypotension not due to tachyarrhythmias and hypersensitivity to the amide type of local anaesthetic. Should lignocaine fail to prevent ectopic ventricular activity procainamide, disopyramide, or mexiletine are tried. **Tocainide** is a new orally effective congener.

Mexiletine ('Mexitil') is like lignocaine in chemical structure, but is also effective orally and has been used for resistant ventricular arrhythmias and the outpatient treatment of ventricular ectopic beats. *Presentation* capsules 50 and 200mg, ampoules 250mg/10ml. *Dose* orally 400-600mg, then 150-300mg 6-8 hourly. It may also be given i.v. *Adverse effects* nausea, vomiting, ataxia, tremor, bradycardia and hypotension.

Procainamide Hydrochloride

Procainamide ('Pronestyl') is a derivative of procaine a local anaesthetic and is a cardiac depressant like quinidine and lignocaine and is like them metabolized by the liver so that in heart failure with liver congestion its action may be exaggerated, so caution is needed. *Uses* mainly for ventricular tachycardias and extrasystoles, but supraventricular rhythms may also respond. It is given i.v. in the acute control of arrhythmias, or orally on a long-term basis although the latter is not popular because of frequent adverse reactions such as lupus erythematosus. *Presentation* Procainamide Tablets B.P. 250mg, Procainamide Injection B.P. contained in vials 10ml 100mg/ml. *Dose* oral 1g then 250mg-1g 2-4 hourly. It has become apparent that the drug by mouth has only a short effect and needs to be given 3 hourly by night and day. This is impractical, even in hospital, so long-acting forms (Procainamide 'Durules') are prescribed 8 hourly. The tablets are 500mg and the daily dose is 4-5g e.g. 1.5g 8 hourly and blood levels should be 4-8μg/ml. This regimen is suitable for the treatment of chronic ventricular ectopics for a few months. By injection it may be given i.m. in amounts similar to the oral dosage, or i.v. For the latter a solution 25mg/ml is given at a rate up to 100mg/min to a total up to 1g. During injection a careful watch is made on the blood pressure. *Adverse effects* anorexia, diarrhoea, nausea, vomiting, hypersensitivity, chills, fever, rashes, flushing, confusion, systemic lupus erythematosus (chronic administration), leucopenia, agranulocytosis and conduction defects of the heart. *Precautions* are needed in renal impairment, known allergy such as asthma, heart block, digitalis toxicity and fast atrial fibrillation.

Phenytoin Sodium

Phenytoin Injection B.P.C. is a ready-mixed form in solution for parenteral use. A 5ml ampoule contains 250mg. The drug has been widely used in cardiac centres in the U.S. for the treatment of digitalis-induced arrhythmias in a dose of 125-250mg i.v. Given too quickly it can cause fatal cardiac arrest or respiratory depression. It must be injected over 5-10min with continuous ECG monitoring. Oral phenytoin has been used to suppress cardiac arrhythmias and in part it may act by a cerebral effect.

Other Anti-Arrhythmics

Adrenoceptor-Blockers (Beta-Blockers) are of great value and **Propranolol** dose up to 1mg i.v. and **Practolol** 5-20mg i.v. bolus dose at a rate of 2mg/min are used particularly for supraventricular and occasionally for ventricular arrhythmias. Other injectable forms are available if practolol is withdrawn. **Bretylium Tosylate** ('Bretylate') occasionally works against resistant ventricular arrhythmias by virtue of an anti-sympathetic activity, but is slow to act taking 20min or more. *Presentation* ampoules 2ml 50mg/ml; *dose* 0.1ml/kg B.W. (=5mg/kg B.W.) i.m. stat then 200mg i.m. 2 hourly to a total of 2g.

Verapamil Hydrochloride ('Cordilox') *should not be given with, or after beta-blockers, or after cardiac infarction, or in damaged hearts.* Its main and successful use is to terminate paroxysmal tachycardia in otherwise fit people. *Presentation* ampoules 2ml containing 5mg; *dose* 5-10mg i.v. given over 1-10min. Verapamil increases the time taken for the heart impulse to pass through the atrioventricular node (transit time) and has an action on the flux of calcium ions in the heart. *Adverse effects* asystole, hypotension.

Disopyramide ('Rythmodan') reduces calcium entry into cardiac cells, prolongs the atrioventricular refractory period and slow conduction in the myocardium and Purkinje system thereby reducing cardiac excitability. The drug reduces cardiac force (negatively inotropic) and is anticholinergic. It also has local anaesthetic actions. Peak levels occur 2-3 hours after oral administration. *Presentation* ampoules 50mg of disopyramide base/5ml, capsules 100 and 150mg and 'Norpace' disopyramide phosphate capsules 150 and 100mg as base; *dose* i.v. 50-150mg given over 5 minutes, orally 300-800mg daily in divided amounts 6 or 8 hourly. *Uses* it is being used to reduce the incidence of ventricular and supraventricular dysrhythmias after cardiac infarction, to suppress ectopic beats and to treat the Wolff-Parkinson-White syndrome. *Special precautions* are needed in partial heart block and it is not advised in complete block. Patients with glaucoma and urinary obstruction are at risk because of the drug's anticholinergic action. Dosage should be reduced in renal failure. *Adverse effects* are frequent—dry mouth, constipation, urinary hesitancy, acute retention of urine, blurred vision, increased pulse, QRS and QT widening.

Ajmaline an indole alkaloid obtained from *Rauwolfia serpentina* used in Europe and Japan has recently been tried in Britain for various arrhythmias, including the Wolff-Parkinson-White syndrome, where it prevents electrical impulse re-entry in the abnormal pathway. *Dose* orally 150-600mg daily, 50-100mg i.v. and 50-150mg i.m. *Adverse effects* nausea, vomiting, diarrhoea, liver damage, occasional agranulocytosis.

Parasympathomimetics or cholinergics such as **Neostigmine Methylsulphate** Injection B.P. 1mg s.c. or i.m. or **Edrophonium Chloride** Injection B.P. 2-10mg i.v. can be used to stop paroxysmal tachycardia, but their stimulation of bowel action makes their use unpleasant.

If drugs fail to restore fast rates to normal sinus rhythm, or if there are urgent symptoms of haemodynamic embarrassment DC conversion is tried. In ventricular fibrillation and ventricular flutter it is obligatory and in ventricular tachycardia and atrial flutter it is speedier and more efficient.

SYMPATHOMIMETICS

These chemical agents have the ability to speed heart rates (positive chronotropic action) and hence are used in bradycardia syndromes e.g. heart block and to prevent recurrent transient asystole. Examples are **Orciprenaline** and **Isoprenaline.** Nowadays, the practice is to increase the heart rate when symptoms occur in heart block by electrical pacemakers inserted pervenously, or otherwise, working at a fixed rate or on demand. It is at times necessary to give anti-arrhythmic drugs to certain patients with inserted pacemakers to prevent the occurrence of fast intermittent arrhythmias (as in the bradycardia-tachycardia syndrome). After cardiac infarction, sinus, nodal or even ventricular bradycardia may respond to 2mg of isoprenaline diluted in 500ml of Dextrose Injection 5% infused i.v. at a rate usually of 0.5-1µg/min, but occasionally up to 4µg/min by constant infusion pump. The same technique may be employed before starting oral therapy with isoprenaline for heart block to ensure no extrasystoles are induced if oral therapy is needed. Should an electrical pacemaker not be used (or refused) **Isoprenaline Slow Tablets B.N.F.** ('Saventrine') strength 30mg at a *dose* of 60-120mg 8 hourly may be tried. Anticholinergics such as **Atropine** may be given i.v. 600-1200µg (0.6-1.2mg) to speed the heart rate in sinus and nodal bradycardia associated with (usually inferiorly placed) cardiac infarction. Though widely used this has an occasional risk of inducing ventricular arrhythmias.

Two points should be made in the treatment of arrhythmias—an accurate diagnosis is essential (e.g. ventricular tachycardia from supraventricular tachycardia with aberrant conduction) and all anti-arrhythmics are hazardous. Intravenous therapy should be carried out in hospital, or in a fully-equipped ambulance. Drug-induced arrhythmias also occur (see p. 250).

CARDIAC ARREST
This emergency arises during surgical, radiological and anaesthetic procedures, i.v. drug therapy (e.g. aminophylline or phenytoin), and most commonly from cardiac disease. Apart from external cardiac massage and ventilation via a secure airway certain drugs are used and provided in an emergency kit. The proper use of medications depends on knowing the arrhythmia present e.g. ventricular fibrillation or asystole and the changes in metabolism likely to result. In asystole a thump on the chest, an intracardiac needle prick or injecting 5ml of 1:10 000 strength adrenaline i.v. directly into the left ventricle may start the heart. An alternative is 200µg of **Isoprenaline Sulphate** as a bolus dose i.v., or 2mg of **Isoprenaline Hydrochloride B.P.** ('Suscardia') infused i.v. at an appropriate rate in 500ml Dextrose Solution B.P. 5%; both measures will work if the blood is circulating (i.e. for bradycardia, but not complete asystole). **Calcium Gluconate** 10ml or Calcium Chloride 0.5-1ml of a 10% solution is also given i.v. Failing this, cardiac massage and electrical pacing are attempted in asystole. In ventricular fibrillation DC conversion is given without delay but is more likely to work if the patient is fully oxygenated and any acidosis largely corrected. Should DC conversion be unsuccessful it can be repeated after i.v. **Adrenaline, Lignocaine,** or **Propranolol** are given; the dose of the latter is 1-2mg given very slowly. Metabolic acidosis follows cardiac arrest and the severity depends on the duration. This is corrected by 50-150mmol/l of **Sodium Bicarbonate** in 4.2 or 8.4% strengths. To counter cerebral oedema 10 or 20% mannitol i.v. up to 50g, or dexamethasone 4mg i.v. can be given.

VASODILATORS
Arteriolar size (lumen) is controlled by the sympathetic nervous system and the natural muscle tone which both adjust the flow of blood to various organs and contribute to the peripheral resistance so maintaining systemic arterial blood pressure. The vasomotor nerves liberate noradrenaline and the adrenal medulla adrenaline which together constrict the vessels by their action on alpha receptors. Other receptors on vessels (beta 2) when activated dilate arterioles—a response which can be produced by adrenaline (which has therefore mixed actions) and isoprenaline. Vasoconstriction can be medically combatted by drugs:

(1) acting on the higher centres in the brain,

(2) blocking impulses across the autonomic sympathetic ganglia e.g. ganglion blockers,

(3) blocking impulses in the post-ganglionic sympathetic nerve fibres (adrenergic neurone inhibitors),

(4) depleting neuronal stores of noradrenaline, or impeding noradrenaline liberation or re-uptake of noradrenaline by nerve endings,

(5) alpha receptor blockade e.g. by phentolamine, phenoxybenzamine, and the phenothiazines, or by beta 2 receptor stimulation,

(6) direct action on arteriolar muscle 'anti-spasmodics'.

Vasodilators cause reflex tachycardia, increased cardiac output and secondary catecholamine (adrenaline, noradrenaline) release. General vasodilators are used to treat arterial hypertension, shock and heart failure and with less evident value peripheral arterial disease. So called 'coronary vasodilators' are used to treat angina, but their mode of action is complex.

ANTI-ANGINAL REMEDIES

Glyceryl Trinitrate (trinitrin, nitroglycerin, GTN) relieves angina by the nitrite ion formed directly relaxing smooth muscle and dilates coronary arteries, peripheral arterioles and capacitance venules. Cardiac output, blood pressure, cardiac work and oxygen needs transiently decrease. *Presentation* Tablets B.P. 300, 500 and 600μg; *dose* 500μg-1mg. Tablets are made with mannitol which improves their shelf life. Tablets work rapidly when dissolved sublingually and faster if crunched. The effect lasts 15-20 min. GTN works best if taken before any effort likely to induce angina since exertional angina normally ceases promptly with rest. Trinitrin also relieves emotionally caused angina and other forms at rest. There is no limit to how many tablets which can be taken daily , though repeated use may suggest lack of potency or a more serious stage of the disease. Trinitrin is also prescribed as a 2% ointment (U.S.A.), when absorbed it has a more prolonged systemic effect. *Adverse effects* burning of the tongue suggests a potent preparation—as does facial flushing—throbbing headaches, giddiness and faintness. Hypotension can occur especially with alcohol and may restrict its use. Sympathetic mediated reflex tachycardia may be prevented by beta-blockade. *Long-acting forms* of glycerol trinitrate are 'Nitrocontin', 'Sustac' 2.6 and 6.4mg tablets; *dose* 2.6-12.8mg several times daily. They are swallowed whole and their efficacy is unproven, and tolerance may develop. Intravenous GTN is also under trial.

Bigger organic nitrate molecules delay hepatic metabolic breakdown, but a greater dose is needed to be effective as they are intrinsically less active. **Sorbide Nitrate** (Isosorbide Dinitrate, 'Cedocard', 'Isordil', 'Sorbitrate', 'Vascardin') *presentation* tablets 5 and 10mg; *dose* 10-20mg orally or sublingually 2 or 3 times daily acts more slowly, but it lasts longer than glyceryl trinitrate with similar side effects. 'Sorbitrate' tablets 5mg are chewed. **Pentaerythritol Tetranitrate** ('Mycardol', 'Peritrate') tablets 10 and 30mg and a delayed action form 'Peritrate S.A.' 80mg are taken before food, but are of uncertain value. **Prenylamine Lactate** ('Segontin', 'Synadrin') has a predominantly inhibitory effect on catecholamine uptake and release by storage granules in the myocardium. It also alters calcium transport in the cell. The sympathetic drive on the heart and the oxygen needs are decreased. *Presentation* tablets 60mg; *dose* 60mg t.d.s. increased to 300mg daily. *Adverse effects* nausea, vomiting, diarrhoea, hypotension, arrhythmia (torsade de pointes), rashes. It should not be

TABLE 10

BETA ADRENORECEPTOR ANTAGONISTS (Beta-Blockers)

Name	Presentation	Daily Dose	Beta-Receptor Blockade	I.S.A.	Membrane Effect
Acebutolol Hydrochloride ('Sectral')	capsules 100, 200 and 400mg ampoules 5ml 5mg/ml	300-1200mg orally 8-12 hourly up to 25mg i.v.	cardioselective	+	+
Alprenolol Hydrochloride B.P. ('Aptin') not available in Britain	Tablets 50 and 100mg Durules 200mg Ampoules 10ml 10mg/ml	150-800mg orally in divided doses	all	+	+
Atenolol ('Tenormin')	tablets 100mg	100-200mg orally in single or divided doses	cardioselective	0	0
Metoprolol Tartrate ('Betaloc', 'Lopresor')	tablets 50 and 100mg	200-400mg orally in divided doses	cardioselective	0	0
Nadolol ('Corgard')	tablets 40 and 80mg	80-640mg daily	all	0	0
Oxprenolol Hydrochloride B.P. ('Trasicor')	Tablets 20, 40, 80 and 160mg ampoules 2mg	80-1000mg or more orally divided 8 or 12 hourly	all	+	+
Pindolol ('Visken')	tablets 5 and 15mg	7.5-45mg orally in divided doses 8 hourly	all	+	±
Practolol* B.P. ('Eraldin')	ampoules 5ml 2mg/ml	i.v. 5-20mg	cardioselective	+	0

TABLE 10 (*continued*)
BETA ADRENORECEPTOR ANTAGONISTS (Beta-Blockers)

Name	Presentation	Daily Dose	Beta-Receptor Blockade	I.S.A.	Membrane Effect
Propranolol B.P. ('Inderal', 'Berkolol')	Tablets 10, 40, 80, and 160mg Injection ampoules 1ml 1mg/ml	30-1000mg or more orally in divided dose 8 or 12 hourly	all	0	+
Sotalol Hydrochloride ('Betacardone' 'Sotacor')	tablets 40, 80, 160, and 200mg ampoules 5ml 2mg/ml	240-640mg orally divided 8 hourly up to 320mg then 12 hourly	all	0	0
Timolol Maleate ('Blocadren', 'Betim')	tablets 10mg	5-60mg orally divided 8 hourly	all	0	0

I.S.A. = stimulating or partial agonist activity.
All have hypotensive activity.
Membrane activity = local anaesthetic or quinidine-like effect.
+ = some, ± = little, 0 = none.
*Long term use not advised. Hospital prescription only for coronary care.

used with beta blockers or quinidine
Dipyridamole ('Persantin') 50-150mg daily has been used for unstable angina and coronary artery spasm and also **Verapamil Hydrochloride** ('Cordilox') is a papaverine derivative. *Presentation* tablets 40 and 80mg; *dose* 40-80mg t.d.s. A major proportion of the dose is taken up by the liver (first pass effect), so the oral dose must be large. It has a negative inotropic action and should be avoided in heart failure, bradycardia and conduction defects.
Nifedipine ('Adalat') along with verapamil and prenylamine is pharmacologically a calcium antagonist. It has both a coronary and a peripheral vasodilator action. Unlike the other two nifedipine can be safely given with beta blockers. *Presentation* capsules 10mg; *dose* 10-20mg t.d.s. swallowed or if bitten open sublingually. A special use is for Prinzmetal or variant angina. It, like perhexiline, is an alternative to or an adjunct of beta blockers. *Adverse effects* headache, flushing, angina at rest.
Perhexiline Maleate ('Pexid') well absorbed and metabolized by the liver has been introduced to prevent attacks of angina and suppress ventricular ectopic.

beats. *Presentation* tablets 100mg; *dose* 100mg twice daily to a maximum of 400mg daily. *Adverse effects* dizziness, headache, nausea, vomiting, less commonly ataxia, peripheral neuropathy, rash, flushing, liver dysfuntion, hypoglycaemia, impotence and weight loss.

Beta-Blockers

Angina occurs when the oxygen supply is less than the oxygen demands of the heart. Certain drugs called adrenoceptor blockers or **beta-blockers** lessen oxygen requirements by reducing the heart rate (negatively chronotropic), force of contraction (negatively inotropic) and by lowering blood pressure and lessening emotional and exercise-induced surges of tachycardia and hypertension. Beta-blockers also constrict coronary arteries and this may unfortunately *reduce oxygen supply* and so can occasionally induce angina. Their total action which is usually beneficial, depends on a balance of these good and harmful effects. In practice the beta-blockers have brought great benefit to angina sufferers.

The principal *beta-blockers* are listed in Table 10. Propranolol, oxprenolol, alprenolol and pindolol are the most widely used for angina and a small dose is given at first (propranolol 20mg t.d.s. or oxprenolol 40mg t.d.s.) in case undue sensitivity, as shown by bradycardia, is seen. The dose is increased until the resting or standing pulse is 50-60/min, or the post-excercise pulse is below 100, adverse effects occur, or no benefit is noted.

Alprenolol is available in S. Africa, Australia and Scandinavia. Oral practolol has been discontinued. The doses for the treatment of *angina* and *hypertension* are similar. *Other uses* for this group include functional heart disease, the hyperdynamic heart syndrome, obstructive cardiomyopathy, migraine, the tachycardia of thyrotoxicosis, phaeochromocytoma, arrhythmias, familial tremor. Parkinsonism and the alcohol-withdrawal state. *Adverse effects* patients with uncontrolled heart failure, heart block with bradycardia, or asthma should not be given a beta-blocker. All, particularly propranolol, which has no intrinsic sympathetic or stimulant agonist activity (I.S.A.) may induce heart failure in susceptible subjects and may induce or worsen asthma. Bradycardia, hypotension, insomnia, nightmares, hallucinations, depression, tiredness, worsening of angina, claudication, hypoglycaemia, Raynaud's phenomenon have all been recorded (particularly with high doses)—as have gastro-intestinal symptoms e.g. nausea. Practolol caused constipation, psoriasiform and eczema-like rashes lupus erythematosus, antinuclear, antibodies, secretory otitis media with deafness, corneal changes and dry irritating red eyes, with reduction of tear flow. Rarely, fluid retention, paradoxical rise in blood pressure (in hypertension) and deterioration in renal function can occur with any beta-blocker. Eye symptoms e.g. visual perceptual disorders, have been recorded with propranolol and other beta blockers but not as severe as with practolol. Beta-blockers are not advised in pregnancy so they should be used cautiously in women of childbearing age (see p. 216).

In pregnancy complicated by thyrotoxicosis beta blockade has been employed, and in certain forms of cardiomyopathy there may be no alternative to prescribing beta blockers during pregnancy. Before and during labour especial care is needed to monitor foetal heart rate.

Management of Angina

In addition to medication it is important to regulate the life style (if adverse) and physical activity, to ensure mental calmness by adjusting hours of work, leisure and sleep and to try to avoid provoking situations. The treatment of hyperlipidaemia, hyperuricaemia, and hyperglycaemia may have a prophylactic effect, and possibly ameliorate ischaemic disease if present. Correction of obesity, anaemia, hypertension and the wearing of lighter clothing does in fact help some. Emotionally-induced angina may be prevented by sedatives (and beta-blockers). In some patients stopping cigarettes, caffeine and alcohol is valuable for pharmacological, metabolic and other reasons. Abrupt cessation of beta-blockers must be avoided since death, arrhythmias, cardiac infarction and rebound angina have been noted. When angina is sudden in onset, repetitive or continues in bed, hospital admission, anticoagulants and analgesics may be necessary, plus diuretic therapy if there is associated left ventricular failure. Underlying infarction is possible. For medical failures aorta-coronary bypass grafting offers immediate relief and perhaps a better long-term prognosis in those with blockage of more than one vessel.

CARDIAC INFARCTION

In uncomplicated cases treatment with a narcotic analgesic (morphine, heroin, pethidine) controls the pain, though vomiting, bradycardia and postural hypotension may be unwanted side effects. In Britain heroin i.v. is often preferred to morphine except when there is left ventricular failure when the vasodilation of morphine is helpful by reducing venous return. A suitable dose of heroin is 5mg i.v. slowly and subsequently 2.5mg i.v. until the pain is relieved. An anti-emetic should be given if the patient is to be moved (e.g. 'Cyclimorph'). Narcotics also control anxiety and restlessness and ensure sleep, but co-existing emphysema or airway disease should be excluded. Later, a benzodiazepine sedative is valuable. In good risk patients, who are mobilized a few days after leaving the coronary care unit anticoagulants are now less often given. For others i.v. heparin followed by oral anticoagulants are prescribed paying regard to possible drug interactions with sedatives and hypnotics. Hypoxia is common and oxygen is given if the patient is in pain, breathless, shocked, or looks ill. The motions should be kept soft and straining at stool avoided by preventing faecal impaction, taking Bran for breakfast and using a bed-side commode and suppositories.

Complications frequently arise

(1) **Arrhythmias** of any type (abnormally fast, slow or irregular) and sinus tachycardia and ectopic beats (extrasystoles) are the most frequent. Arrhythmias are likely in the first few days in over 90% of patients. Ventricular fibrillation, always (unless it spontaneously disappears), and ventricular tachycardia and atrial flutter usually are terminated by DC conversion. Slow rates from sinus, nodal and occasionally complete heart block respond to i.v. atropine 600-1200μg or an isoprenaline infusion 2mg in 500ml of Dextrose Injection 5%. Frequent extrasystoles (e.g. 1:9) are treated by lignocaine, procainamide, practolol, mexiletine or phenytoin in the doses previously mentioned. Digoxin is given for supraventricular tachycardias such as atrial fibrillation. For atrioventricular block pervenous pacing is used if the circulation is inadequate, but with inferior infarction it is rarely needed.

(2) **Left ventricular failure** if mild responds to diuretics and if severe to a

digitalis preparation plus a diuretic, care being taken to avoid hypoxia. For resistant pulmonary oedema positive pressure ventilation or peritoneal dialysis may be effective. Congestive failure responds to medical measures.

(3) **Cardiogenic shock** has a very high mortality (about 80%). Many drugs are tried—digoxin or ouabain i.v., anti-arrhythmics, inotropic agents such as glucagon 2-5mg i.v. then 4-20mg/h, and the sympathomimetic amines isoprenaline, noradrenaline, dopamine, dobutamine and salbutamol. **Dopamine Hydrochloride** ('Intropin') improves cardiac and renal flow. *Presentation* ampoules 5ml 40mg/ml. The solution is diluted in Sodium Chloride Injection or Dextrose Injection 5% and the maker's data sheet should be consulted. The infused concentration is 400-800μg (micrograms)/ml. Fluid replacement may help a few who are hypovolaemic, and so may glucose-insulin regimes. Massive doses of i.v. corticosteroids such as 50-100mg/kg B.W. of hydrocortisone have been tried and vasodilators to improve tissue flow and reduce cardiac work e.g. sodium nitroprusside 30-150μg/min, phentolamine or phenoxybenzamine. To aid management both the central venous and the pulmonary artery wedge pressures should be measured. Assisting the circulation with intra-aortic balloons has also helped. Surgery has an occasional part to play in excising infarcts, improving blood flow with coronary artery bypass, and repairing ruptured ventricular septa and mitral valve incompetence. After bypass or open-heart surgery salbutamol 10-15 μg/min by peripheral vasodilation allows increased cardiac output by improving flow.

PERIPHERAL VASODILATORS

Uses arteriolar spasm e.g. in Raynaud's disease, or blockage by atherosclerosis or by Buerger's disease. Drugs dilate vessels by (1) blocking the catecholamine hormones adrenaline and noradrenaline which normally stimulate the alpha-receptors in the arterioles to constrict the muscle ('alpha-blockers'), (2) by direct relaxation action ('spasmolytics') or (3) by stimulating the beta-receptors in the vessel wall which normally oppose the action of the alpha-receptors ('beta 2 stimulants').

Alpha-Adrenergic Blockers

By blocking the catecholamines the vessels dilate and so tissue perfusion improves. The body responds to vasodilation particularly if there is a fall in blood pressure by releasing more catecholamines which stimulate the heart to beat faster, increase its output and this may induce or worsen angina. Alpha-blockers are chemically of two types. The **imidazolines** which resemble in structure the natural substance histamine include tolazoline and phentolamine (and also the hypotensive agent clonidine also used for migraine). The other type is phenoxybenzamine chemically related to the cytotoxic nitrogen mustards hence its potential for adverse effects.

Tolazoline Hydrochloride ('Priscol') also has some direct action. *Presentation* Tablets B.P. 25mg; *dose* orally 25-50mg q.d.s. Resembling as it does histamine it can increase gastric acidity and worsen peptic ulcers.

Phentolamine ('Rogitine') *presentation* Tablets of the Hydrochloride B.P. 20mg, Phentolamine Mesylate Injection B.P. contained in ampoules 1ml 10mg/ml. This is a short and quick acting preparation. *Dose* orally 20-100mg 4-6 hourly (it is well absorbed), or i.v. 5-10mg or 1mg/min. *Uses* as a diagnostic and therapeutic agent in phaeochromocytoma; orally (on trial) on a long-term basis with a beta-blocker to treat arterial hypertension, and i.v. like phenoxybenzamine for cardiogenic shock. It may also be combined with chlor-promazine 50mg i.m. to reduce the hypertension caused by a reaction to a monoamine oxidase inhibitor. *Adverse effects* are common; nausea, vomiting, diarrhoea and tachycardia.

Phenoxybenzamine Hydrochloride ('Dibenyline') *presentation* Capsules B.P. 10mg, powder 10g for preparing solution in ampoules 2ml 50mg/ml. *Dose* orally 10-20mg daily; in phaeochromocytoma 40-100mg every 12 hours for 10-14 days before the operation. For cardiogenic shock it is given i.v. in 500ml of Dextrose Injection 5% in a dose of 1mg/kg B.W. over 1-2 hours and with i.v. fluids and central venous pressure measurements to prevent underfilling of the circulation. By mouth it is erratically absorbed and i.v. the hypotensive effect may be difficult to reverse.

Co-Dergocrine Mesylate ('Hydergine') contains the mesylates dihyd-roergocornine, dihydroergocristine and dihydroergokryptine in equal propor-tions. It is used to treat cerebrovascular disease and is claimed to increase and improve neuronal metabolism but not by a vasodilator action. *Presentation* tablets 1.5mg. *Dose* 1.5mg t.d.s. *Adverse effects* gastro-intestinal, flushes, rashes, nasal blockage, hypotension. **Naftidrofuryl** ('Praxilene') 100mg t.d.s. also alters brain metabolism and like cyclandelate is used for those with cere-brovascular disease. An injectable form ampoules 5ml 8mg/ml and 10ml 20mg/ml is also available for acute peripheral arterial ischaemia e.g. rest pain.

TABLE 11
SOME VASODILATORS

Name		Tablet	Daily Dose
Official	Proprietary	Strength (mg)	(mg)
Bamethan Sulphate	'Vasculit'	12.5	50-125
Betahistine Hydro-chloride	'Serc'	8	24-48
Buphenine Hydro-chloride (Nylidrin Hydrochloride U.S.N.F.)	'Arlidin' (U.S.A.)	6	18-36
Cyclandelate	'Cyclospasmol' 'Cyclobral'	400 tablet and capsule suspension 400mg/5ml	800-1600
Inositol Nicotinate	'Hexopal'	500	1000-3000
Isoxsuprine Hydro-chloride (as resinate)	'Duvadilan Retard' 'Defencin'	20 and 40 (capsule)	20-80
Nicofuranose	'Bradilan'	250	750-2000
Naftidrofuryl	'Praxilene'	100 (capsule)	300
Nicotinyl Alcohol Tartrate	'Ronicol'	25 and 150 (slow release)	150-300
Thymoxamine Hydro-chloride	'Opilon'	40	160-480

Thymoxamine Hydrochloride B.P. is another alpha adrenergic blocker (see Table 11).

Direct Action On Vessel Wall

Nicotinic Acid *presentation* tablets 50mg; *dose* 50-250mg is given for chilblains and included in 'Amisyn' and 'Pernivit'. Derivatives include inositol nicotinate, nicotinyl alcohol and nicotinyl alcohol tartrate which are long-acting. Bamethan and cyclandelate are further examples (see Table 11).

A new type of approach is seen with **Oxpentifylline** ('Trental') claimed to reduce blood viscosity by an action on red cells, *dose* 100-200mg t.d.s. orally.

Sympathomimetic Beta-Stimulators

These include **Nylidrin Hydrochloride U.S.N.F.** and **Isoxsuprine Hydrochloride.** They are therefore given with caution to patients with ischaemic heart disease, thyrotoxicosis, tachycardia or hypertension since they cause trembling, nervousness and palpitation.

Value of medical measures. When arterial insufficiency is due to arteriosclerosis vasodilators and anticoagulants are of doubtful value. The development of a collateral circulation may occur naturally and improve symptoms. Smoking should be forbidden and diabetes or hyperlipidaemia corrected. Otherwise, arterial surgery has most to offer.

DRUGS WHICH LOWER BLOOD PRESSURE

The aim of treatment is to reduce the crippling consequences of hypertension such as heart failure, retinopathy, renal disease, aortic dissection and strokes. The evidence suggests that it successfully does this, and there is now suggestive evidence that coronary artery disease can be prevented by the beta blockers. Treatment is essential in malignant hypertension and hypertensive encephalopathy and usually beneficial for hypertension associated with subarachnoid haemorrhage and aortic dissection, strokes, renal failure and angina. A raised blood pressure is also treated in pregnancy with benefit to the mother and perhaps to the foetus. Judgement is needed as to how energetic treatment should be and when it should be started in the presence of certain complications. A major clinical and logistical problem is whether to treat the asymptomatic patient particularly with only marginally raised levels. A raised blood pressure alone is not an indication to treat, especially in middle-aged women and in the elderly. Some selection is desirable, for treatment is *not without cost, risk or discomfort*. There should be a balance of benefit versus nuisance value of therapy. A preliminary assessment is needed to judge severity and to detect the minority with surgically treatable hypertension. Prognosis is worse in certain families and in the young male, in Negroes, at higher levels especially if recently accelerated, and when accompanied by signs of organ damage. For a given level of blood pressure the risk of vascular disease can vary 20-fold if added factors are present (smoking, diabetes, hyperlipidaemia). Surveys also show that with progressive rise of systolic and diastolic levels even within the 'normal range' there is a decreased longevity.

Control is satisfactory when levels are normal when the person is subjected to usual life stresses. The blood pressure should be measured lying down, sitting, standing for 5 minutes and after exertion. Readings should be made in both arms and at different times of day. Patients can be taught to perform home readings. There is less error if phase V is taken for the diastolic readings.

The blood pressure has a circadian rhythm and falls during sleep and in early morning so drugs act strongly then and postural hypotension is likely. There is considerable individual variation in dosage between people since hypotensive drugs are variably absorbed (e.g. guanethidine) or metabolized (e.g. hydrallazine).

Hypertension is not a homogeneous entity and abnormalities of sympathetic nervous system control, peripheral resistance, renin-angiotensin-aldosterone secretion (or other mineralocorticoids), cardiac output and plasma volume ideally should be separately considered. Such measurements are not yet feasible in ordinary practice where the approach must be pragmatic.

The search for the ideal hypotensive continues (i.e. cheap, well tested, effective, taken once daily with a minimum of side effects). At present hypertension may be reduced by various drugs acting at different sites (Figure 5). The aim is

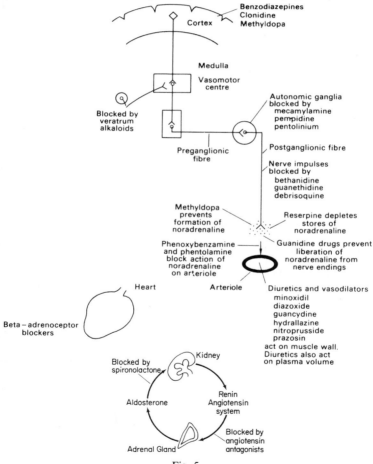

Fig. 5
Sites of action of hypotensive drugs

either to re-set the pressure control centres, or to reduce the sympathetic constrictor activity thereby relaxing their resistance (arterioles), or increasing the capacity of the venules, so reducing cardiac output. Other drugs reduce the natural (inherent) tone of the vessels. All drugs have side effects and their use is contra-indicated with recent cardiac infarction, and caution is needed with recent strokes and with severe renal failure.

(1) The *afferent impulses* from vessels can be blocked as with the little used veratrum alkaloids.

(2) *Cerebral cortical activity* can be depressed by sedatives such as the benzodiazepines and by reserpine, methyldopa and clonidine which exert a central effect. Anxiety and stress make an important neurogenic component both to labile and to fixed hypertension.

(3) The *ganglion blockers* prevent transmission of impulses across autonomic ganglia. Unfortunately although powerful they are crude and unselective for they paralyse the parasympathetic system and interfere with sympathetic transmission to organs other than vessels and so cause dry mouth, difficulty in focusing, constipation, paralytic ileus, sexual impotence and difficulty in micturition. Neostigmine reverses these effects. They lower the blood pressure only when the patient is upright and pressures are measured lying, sitting and standing. Blood pools in the capacitance venules so reducing venous return. Examples are pentolinium, mecamylamine, trimetaphan and pempidine.

(4) The sympathetic *post-ganglionic adrenergic neurone blockers* are more selective but they interfere with organs other than vessels and so may disturb sexual function. They are postural hypotensives and their activity is enhanced by exercise, warm temperatures, and by vasodilatation caused by meals and alcohol. Examples include bethanidine, guanethidine and debrisoquine. The adrenergic drugs also deplete stores of noradrenaline e.g. reserpine. Methyldopa acts as a false transmitter, but also has a central action.

(5) The neuronal *liberation and re-uptake of noradrenaline* is prevented by guanethidine type drugs.

(6) As previously mentioned *alpha-blockers* can reduce the blood pressure. Prazosin is now considered to be a post-synaptic alpha blocker. Indoramin is under trial. The phenothiazines are alpha blockers. Labetalol is both an alpha and a beta blocker.

(7) Clonidine has both central and peripheral actions. Initially there is a central reduction of sympathetic outflow and later both the vasoconstrictor and the vasodilator influences on the peripheral vessels are modified so that eventually the resistance tends to fall. It is a noradrenaline agonist.

(8) *Direct vasodilators* include diazoxide, minoxidil, guancydine, hydralazine and sodium nitroprusside. Reflex tachycardia is met and sodium and fluid retention is a common complication. The oral varieties are often combined with a beta-blocker and/or a diuretic. The diuretics e.g. thiazides also have a direct action on muscle.

(9) *Beta-blockers* lower blood pressure by means not fully understood. They reduce cardiac output, alter plasma volume, and some suppress renin levels. (The thiazide diuretics elevate renin levels.)

(10) *Plasma volume reduction* and salt excretion will lower blood pressure and this can be achieved by diuretics, anti-aldosterone agents, dietary salt restriction, weight loss and dialysis.

(11) Bed rest will lower blood pressure and may be an effective measure in pregnancy toxaemia.

(12) Methods under trial include angiotensin antagonists e.g. saralasin and captopril. Hospital experience is that many patients are still not controlled with beta blockers, diuretics and vasodilators.

RAPID CONTROL OF BLOOD PRESSURE
In acute left ventricular failure, hypertensive encephalopathy, hypertension induced rapidly by drugs, malignant hypertension, or aortic dissection injectable therapy is at times desirable.

Injectable Forms
Pentolinium Tartrate ('Ansolysen') *presentation* Pentolinium Injection B.P. a solution in vials 10ml 5mg/ml. A test dose of 1mg is given s.c. then this is increased every 12 hours by 1-2mg to 2.5-20mg each injection, s.c. or i.m. Alternatively 1-2mg i.v. in emergencies is given every 2-5 minutes. The patient is treated sitting so that any hypotension can be counteracted by lying flat (postural hypotensive).
Trimetaphan Camsylate B.P. ('Arfonad') is brief acting and used by anaesthetists to lower blood pressure and reduce bleeding. *Presentation* ampoules ready-mixed 250mg/5ml. A concentration of 1mg/ml is made by dilution in Sodium Chloride Injection or Dextrose Injection and the rate is about 3-4mg/min to achieve the desired pressure.

More widely used now are the following. **Diazoxide** ('Eudemine') *presentation* Injection B.P. a solution in Water for Injections contained in ampoules 300mg/20ml; *dose* 300mg (5mg/kg B.W.) injected rapidly in 30 seconds which allows it to fix to the vessel walls and act. Slower injections are absorbed onto the plasma proteins. The patient should be flat and venous extravasation avoided. Its action lasts up to a day, but can be repeated after 4-8 hours. Chemically it is a thiazide derivative without any diuretic action. *Adverse effects* chest pain, prolonged hypotension and an occasional fatality. **Clonidine Hydrochloride** *presentation* ampoules 150µg/ml is widely used abroad to control blood pressure. When given i.v. a transient elevation of blood pressure can occur, but this does not appear with i.m. administration. *Dose* 150µg. **Sodium Nitroprusside B.P.** ('Nipride') is cheap, non-toxic in short-term use, and a directly acting arteriolar vasodilator. It is of value if there is heart failure as it does not worsen it and acts by reducing afterload. It is given as a continuous infusion i.v. of a 0.01% (100mg/litre) solution at an approximate rate of 30-150µg/min. Injectable **Labetalol Hydrochloride** and **Hydralazine** are available in the U.K.

Oral Therapy
For mild or moderate hypertension the backbone of therapy is a diuretic, usually with a beta-blocker, or in certain countries reserpine. If this is not adequate more potent drugs are added for monotherapy is not usually sufficient.
Diuretics either thiazides such as **Chlorothiazide** 1g or **Hydrochlorothiazide** 50mg daily, or a long-acting form such as **Chlorthalidone** are prescribed. If hypokalaemia is a feature added potassium is given, or a potassium sparing diuretic such as spironolactone. The disadvantages of diuretic therapy are that biochemical control is needed to detect the unpredictable occurrence of hypokalaemia, and diabetes mellitus and gout may be precipitated. Adding a diuretic enables the dose of more potent hypotensives to be reduced and is more acceptable than curtailing salt intake. Many hypotensives e.g. vasodilators, beta-blockers and adrenergic blockers cause sodium retention and

weight gain which needs to be countered by diuretics. The diuretics are by far the cheapest form of treatment.

Beta-Blockers are popular since they do not cause postural hypotension, patients often feel less tired with them and interference with sex is unusual. The initial dose should be small since some patients are sensitive to the loss of their catecholamine drive on the myocardium. Therapy may not work quickly; results can take weeks. The doses given are **Propranolol** 20mg twice or thrice daily up to 1g or more (1-3g) but hallucinations and mental symptoms become a problem at higher doses, **Oxprenolol** 80mg daily increasing to 1000mg, **Alprenolol** 150mg daily up to 800mg and **Pindolol** 5mg daily up to 45mg (see Table 10). Many beta blockers can be given in practice once daily e.g. acebutolol (400mg tablets), sotalol, pindolol and atenolol (50-200mg). Once daily slow release forms include 'Inderal LA' 160mg capsules and 'Slow Trasicor' 160mg tablets. Beta blockers are often given with a diuretic separately or combined ('Co-Betaloc', 'Trasidrex', 'Tenoretic', 'Viskaldix') and a third drug e.g. a vasodilator such as hydrallazine (up to 200mg daily) or prazosin.

Beta blockers are particularly suitable for labile hypertension and hypertensives with angina, migraine, hyperdynamic circulations, arrhythmias and mental stress. They have been used for renal hypertension with impaired renal function. They are best avoided in pregnancy, and patients with intermittent claudication and Raynaud's disease may be made worse. In the young liable to sudden excessive exercise (e.g. children, adolescents and young people with hypertension) beta blockers interfere with physiological responses. **Labetalol Hydrochloride** has beta and alpha blocking activity. *Presentation* tablets 100, 200 and 400mg; ampoules 20ml containing 100mg. *Dose* orally 100mg t.d.s. rising to a maximum of 2.4g daily. By injection i.v. bolus 50mg over 1 min every 5 min to a total dose of 200mg. *Adverse effects* headache, nausea, lethargy, postural hypotension, hypertension in phaeochromocytoma.

Rauwolfia Derivatives

Rauwolfia Serpentina is an Indian plant containing the indole containing alkaloids reserpine, deserpidine and rescinnamine. Many preparations of rauwolfia and of the pure alkaloids exist. **Reserpine Ph. Eur.** ('Serpasil') acts centrally on the brain and locally on the nerves depleting noradrenaline. It slows the pulse, calms the mind as well as being a hypotensive. *Presentation* Tablets B.P. 100, 250, 500μg, and 1mg, elixir 50μg/ml. *Dose* 250-500μg daily. *Adverse effects* the important one is depression with a risk of suicide, lethargy, nasal stuffiness, fluid retention, diarrhoea, Parkinsonism, decreased libido, nightmares, agitation, activation of peptic ulcers, hypotension, flushing, nausea and purpura. It is still widely used abroad as it is very cheap. Reserpine is combined with diuretics e.g. 'Serpasil-Esidrex' and 'Abicol'. Whole root preparations of *R. serpentina* act largely because of the reserpine content, and are contained in 'Hypertane', 'Hypertensan', 'Rautrax' and 'Raudixin'. **Methoserpidine** ('Decaserpyl') is a synthetic derivative claimed to be less depressing. *Presentation* Tablets B.P. 5 and 10mg. *Dose* 30-60mg daily in divided amounts. Like reserpine it should be avoided in depressed patients.

Adrenergic Neurone Inhibiting Drugs (Post-Ganglion Blockers)

These are still used for severe hypertension as they are good for rapid control. Like the ganglion blockers they cause unwelcome postural and exertional hypotension.

Guanidine Derivatives are similar in action.
Guanethidine Monosulphate ('Ismelin') is given once daily and has its maximum effect in the morning. *Presentation* Tablets B.P. 10 and 25mg, ampoules 10mg/ml for i.m. use. *Dose* orally 10mg daily increasing by 10mg weekly to 300-500mg if necessary. An average dose is 30-60mg daily. *Adverse effects* diarrhoea, faintness and dizziness, muscle weakness, heaviness of limbs, fluid retention, impotence, stuffy nose, shivering and bradycardia with digitalis.
Bethanidine Sulphate ('Esbatal') *presentation* Tablets B.P. 10 and 50mg. *Dose* 20-200mg daily. It resembles guanethidine, but is quicker in action, shorter in duration and must be given every 8-12 hours, but it causes less diarrhoea.
Debrisoquine Sulphate B.P. ('Declinax') *presentation* Tablets 10 and 20mg; *dose* 10-400mg daily subdivided 8-12 hourly. On withdrawal nightmares and disturbed sleep can occur. Debrisoquine unlike guanethidine does not deplete the neurones of noradrenaline but only blocks nerve transmission. This may make side effects less likely. **Guanoclor Sulphate** ('Vatensol') and **Guanoxan Sulphate** ('Envacar') are less used and available in 10 and 40mg tablets and the daily dose is 10-160mg. **Guancydine,** Guanadrel ('Hylorel'), Guanabenz and Guanfacine are new guanidines.
Methyldopa ('Aldomet', 'Dopamet', 'Medomet') is very widely prescribed and reduces both standing and lying blood pressure by a central and a peripheral action, though postural hypotension can occur. *Presentation* Tablets B.P.125, 250 and 500mg and capsules ('Co-Caps'), Methyldopate Hydrochloride Injection B.P. and U.S.P. available as a solution in ampoules 5ml 50mg/ml. *Dose* orally 125mg 8 hourly increasing if needed to 2g or more daily. The i.v injection is given for hypertensive crises 250-500mg in 100ml of 5% Dextrose given over a period of 30-60min. Tolerance can occur. *Adverse effects* on the whole it is well accepted but tiredness and sedation are prominent. Less common are fever, dizziness, dry mouth, abdominal distension, diarrhoea, weight gain, oedema, depression, haemolytic anaemia, hepatitis both acute and chronic, galactorrhoea, tremor, nightmares and leg fatigue. Methyldopa is valuable for treating hypertension in pregnancy.

Vasodilators
These include hydrallazine, minoxidil and the alpha blocker prazosin. **Hydralazine Hydrochloride** ('Apresoline') is used with beta blockers to combat the tachycardia and raised cardiac output it causes. It is also used in hypertension in pregnancy. *Presentation* Tablets B.P. (1963) 25 and 50mg, ampoules containing 20mg. The *oral dose* is kept below 200mg daily to reduce the risk of systemic lupus erythematosus, parenterally it is given 20-40mg i.v. (1mg/min) or i.m. for the emergency control of blood pressure. **Prazosin Hydrochloride** ('Hypovase', 'Minipress') is claimed to cause no impotence, lethargy or depression. Chemically it is a quinazoline derivative. *Presentation* tablets 0.5, 1, 2 and 5mg; *dose* 3-20mg daily. *Adverse effects* include tachycardia, dizziness, weakness and light-headedness from hypotension. Some patients unpredictably get severe syncope or even loss of consciousness, usually within twenty-four hours of taking the first dose. The risk is reduced by giving all patients initially a test dose of 250µg (0.25mg), in the evening in the safety of the home or hospital, and by warning the patients of the symptoms of postural hypotension. **Minoxidil** is a 'last ditch' potent drug causing hirsuties, fluid retention and reflex cardiac stimulation. *Dose* for hospital use 2.5-10mg up to 80mg daily, for severe hypertension.

Clonidine Hydrochloride ('Catapres') an imidazoline works by reducing sensitivity to catecholamines by central and peripheral actions. *Presentation* tablets 100 and 300µg; *dose* 50 or 100µg orally thrice daily with increments no less than every 2-3 days of 50 or 100µg up to 2mg daily. *Adverse effects* drowsiness, dry mouth, constipation, weight gain, impotence, depression hypomania, dizziness, headache, rash and pruritus. Sudden stopping o clonidine can cause a dangerous rise in blood pressure with insomnia, palpitation, agitation and increased catecholamine production (countered by labetalol). This is important since patients often stop therapy by themselves The drug must be withdrawn slowly, over at least 4 days.

Ganglion Blockers
These are rarely used except perhaps for those refractory to simpler measures. **Mecamylamine Hydrochloride** ('Inversine') is fully absorbed and works in an hour or so and lasts 6-12 hours. *Presentation* Tablets B.P. 2.5 and 10mg; *dose* 2.5mg b.d. increasing by 2.5mg every 2-3 days up to 60mg daily. *Adverse effects* those of ganglion blockers plus tremor, weakness, mental upsets, diarrhoea or constipation.
Pempidine Tartrate is well absorbed and rapidly excreted. *Presentation* Tablets B.P. 1 and 5mg; *dose* 2.5mg 6 hourly up to 80mg daily.

Refractory Hypertension
Single (monotherapy) is rarely sufficient and a combination of drugs is needed For some patients control even with all the existing medications is very difficult. At times oral **Diazoxide** 50-800mg daily may work, but hyperglycaemia and frank diabetes may result. Tablets B.P. 50 and 100mg are available. Beta-blockers, diuretics and **Pargyline** ('Eutonyl') can be given to the depressed hypertensive.

MANAGEMENT OF HEART FAILURE
Treatment is based on mental and physical rest, improvement of heart action with digitalis, and a reduction of blood volume and extracellular fluid by diuresis and occasionally curtailing sodium intake. Peripheral resistance (impedance) is reduced by *vasodilators* (oral or i.v. trinitrin, hydralazine, prazosin, nitroprusside). Vasodilators are contra-indicated in aortic stenosis mitral stenosis, pulmonary hypertension, constrictive pericarditis and hypertrophic obstructive cardiomyopathy since with obstruction the peripheral resistance is needed to maintain the circulation. *Acute left heart failure* causes pulmonary oedema and the breathless patient has to sit upright. He can be nursed in bed, or in a chair with arm rests. Morphine or heroin has a calming effect, but the most useful measure is i.v. frusemide 20-40mg. Digoxin is given orally and i.v. aminophylline 250mg may be helpful given slowly over 15 min. *Congestive heart failure* is nursed the same way. Bed rest improves renal function Digitalization and diuretics are given and salt restriction is not usually needed The response is judged by urine output, weight loss and clinical symptoms. The staff should know which foods and medicines contain sodium and which drugs can worsen heart failure. *Fluids:* it is customary to allow several pints daily and more in feverish states and hot weather. *Mechanical removal of fluid* from the pleural cavity can be lifesaving and helpful for leg oedema when diuretics fail Oxygen in pharmacological amounts is valuable in cyanosis and heart failure with few exceptions (Chapter 20). *Antibiotics* infections provoke arrhythmias

and heart failure and can supervene in waterlogged lungs. *Sedation* is treated by a benzodiazepine, but underlying ventilatory lung disease should be excluded. Confused patients can settle with a phenothiazine, or chlormethiazole. Venesection is worth a trial in patients with polycythaemia, but this may provoke vessel clotting so anticoagulants should be given. Pulmonary emboli may cause, or complicate, heart failure and are treated by anticoagulants. *Bowels and bladder* avoidance of constipation and abdominal distension helps breathing and lowers the diaphragms. Faecal impaction should be excluded. Modern powerful diuretics may induce acute retention of urine. *Reversible heart failure* includes anaemia, hypertension, arrhythmia, thyrotoxicosis, avitaminosis, alcoholism, drugs (e.g. beta blockade), thromboembolic disease, valvular stenosis and constrictive pericarditis.

Infective Endocarditis

Early and precise diagnosis is important. In district hospitals about 75% of organisms are penicillin sensitive and of low virulence and *Streptococcus viridans* is likely. In cardiothoracic units with prosthetic valve surgery diphtheroids, staphylococci, Gram-negative organisms and fungi are met. In addicts and those on renal dialysis staphylococci are common. In non-surgical patients penicillin G i.m. 2 mega units 4-6 hourly gives a concentration of $1-5\mu g/ml$; i.v. therapy (say 20-40 mega units daily) is reserved for organisms

TABLE 12
INFECTIVE ENDOCARDITIS

Type	*Organism*	*Therapy*
Naturally Occurring	Non-haemolytic Streptococci (*Str. viridans*)	Penicillin G i.m. or i.v., or oral Ampicillin, Amoxycillin or Phenoxymethylpenicillin
	Str. faecalis	Penicillin G and Streptomycin; Ampicillin and Streptomycin or Amoxycillin and Streptomycin or Gentamicin with a Penicillin
	S. aureus	Penicillin
	Rickettsiae	Tetracycline
Surgical Prostheses	*S. albus* *S. aureus*	Fusidic acid and Cloxacillin
	Gram-negative Fungi	Gentamicin Amphotericin
Addicts (Narcotic)	*S. aureus*	Fusidic acid and Cloxacillin

that need high concentrations. The serum can be tested for bactericidal amounts of penicillin. Oral therapy has been given—ampicillin is less bound to plasma proteins than penicillin V and is given with probenecid 500mg 6 hourly at a dose of 500mg 6 hourly; blood levels are taken to exclude poor absorption. For staphylococci, cloxacillin and fusidic acid, and for *Streptococcus faecalis,* ampicillin and streptomycin or gentamicin are given. Rickettsial infections are difficult to treat; they are prescribed tetracycline or erythromycin. For resistant cases (intractable heart failure or infection) surgery is performed. When large amounts of penicillin are given it is wise to consider the sodium or potassium content to avoid excessive levels. When teeth need to be extracted during penicillin therapy cephaloridine, co-trimoxazole or tetracycline can be administered and for prophylaxis in surgery on those at risk 1 mega unit of penicillin G 4 hours before, and oral or injectable penicillin for 48 hours after, is advised (but not always effective). Before delivery ampicillin 1g and gentamicin 80mg i.m. or i.v. offers good prophylaxis. Injections as a method of prevention outside hospital are unpopular. 2g of phenoxymethyl penicillin 1-2 hours before dental extraction then 500mg 6 hourly for 3 days is an alternative.

New and Investigational Drugs
The treatment of arrhythmias is still unsatisfactory and certain additional therapies are available for specialist use.
Amiodarone is a benzfuran derivative and an analogue of thyroxine. Its main use is for supra- and ventricular arrhythmias especially the Wolff-Parkinson-White syndrome since it prolongs the refractory period of the accessory pathways. *Dose* is 5-10mg/kg B.W. i.v. and orally 200-300mg daily. *Adverse effects* skin pigmentation, thyroid dysfunction, and corneal deposits which do not interfere with sight and reverse on stopping therapy.
Aprindine is used for both supra- and ventricular arrhythmias. *Dose* 200mg i.v. at 2mg/min; 30min later 100mg at 2mg/min; 6h later 100mg at 2mg/min; orally loading dose 100mg 6-hourly day 1, 75mg 6-hourly day 2, 50mg 6-hourly day 3 thereafter 100-200mg daily in 6 or 12-hourly doses. *Adverse effects* tremor, ataxia, convulsions, hallucinations with toxic levels, agranulocytosis, cholestatic jaundice.
Tocainide is related to lignocaine but can be taken orally. It is used for ventricular ectopic arrhythmias in a dose of 800-2100mg daily. *Adverse effects* gastro-intestinal, tremor, twitching, headache, paraesthesiae, dizziness.
Disopyramide Phosphate ('Norpace') is now available as an injection 20mg/ml in 5 and 7.5ml ampoules which is not to be confused with 'Rythmodan' injections as the base (p. 149).

20 DRUGS AND RESPIRATORY DISEASES

INFECTIONS

Pneumonias. Antibiotics are the main treatment for pneumonia due to pneumococci, staphylococci, rickettsiae, mycoplasma, the capsulated strain of *H. influenzae,* and the rarer *Ps. aeruginosa, Proteus spp, Esch. coli,* and *Klebsiella pneumoniae.* In practice a high percentage cannot be proved by microbiology to have an infection and treatment then has to be empirical. Antibiotics are given and the results assessed clinically. Therapy is for 7 days at least. In the very ill parenteral administration is safer. Several choices are possible: **Amoxycillin** 250-500mg 8 hourly, or the cheaper and usually equally effective **Ampicillin. Penicillin G** 600mg 8 hourly, or **Penicillin G** 600mg with **Streptomycin** 500mg 12 hourly, unless the patient is elderly, or has poor renal function. With chronic underlying lung disease **Tetracycline,** Minocycline or Amoxycillin have the advantage of wider activity. With tetracycline and **Erythromycin** there is also cover against mycoplasma pneumonia and psittacosis. For those allergic to penicillin **Co-trimoxazole,** tetracycline, erythromycin, novobiocin or **Clindamycin** can be tried or a **Cephalosporin** which, like **Flucloxacillin** or **Fusidic acid,** and be used for penicillinase-producing staphylococci. Chloramphenicol with its risks is little used, except in severe infections in the elderly, when it can be highly effective. The Gram-negative infections usually respond to **Gentamicin.** *Pneumocystis carinii* pneumonia occurs in subjects with immunodeficiency disease, or who are being treated with corticosteroids or cytotoxics. It may respond to pentamidine 4mg/kg B.W. daily i.m. for up to 14 days (see p. 45) or even better to co-trimoxazole. *Other measures* include attention to fluid and food intake, oral hygiene, adequate rest and sleep, relief of pain, cough and abdominal distension and the use of oxygen. Pneumonia, bronchopneumonia and purulent bronchitis are still major killers.

Acute bronchitis often responds to tetracycline, ampicillin, co-trimoxazole or a cephalosporin. Milder forms may recover without needing antibiotics. Acute laryngotracheitis and epiglottitis caused by *H. influenzae* can be rapidly fatal in infants and is treated by i.v. chloramphenicol.

Pleural space infection or empyema is treated by general and local antibiotics combined with surgical drainage.

Lung-abscess. Treatment depends on the organism. If sensitive penicillin G 1-2g 6 hourly may be necessary for several weeks.

BRONCHODILATORS OR ANTISPASMODICS

Bronchial muscle tone is a balance of sympathetic and parasympathetic nerve action plus the action of local hormones or chemicals such as prostaglandins and histamine. Antispasmodics act by reducing airway resistance in the bronchial tubes. Their name suggests that they reduce muscle spasm, but improved air flow can also result from lessening the swelling of the bronchial mucosa and by loosening and removing the secretions in the lumen.

Adrenergic or Sympathomimetic Drugs

Sympathomimetics produce bronchodilation by stimulation of the beta 2 receptors in the bronchial muscle. To a varying degree they cause unwanted side effects on the heart by stimulating the beta 1 receptors in the myocardium. Newer preparations are more selective, acting almost totally on the bronchial muscle. Chemically all the sympathomimetics have a similar structure. Some are catecholamines resembling adrenaline, others have slight but important alterations in structure slowing their breakdown by natural enzymes. They vary in speed of onset, duration of effect, selectivity, method of administration (oral, injection or inhalation) and cost. They may be given prophylactically e.g. before exercise or at night or for actual symptoms.

Adrenaline (Epinephrine U.S.P.) is a rapid antispasmodic which can be inhaled, or injected s.c., or i.m. (not i.v. in asthma). *Presentation* Adrenaline Acid Tartrate Injection B.P. is a 1:1000 solution (as adrenaline) in ampoules 0.5 and 1ml. It is kept away from the light. *Dose* 200-1000μg (0.2-1mg). It is most effective given early in asthma and it is used for the severe form. It must not be given concurrently with sympathomimetic inhalations and is best avoided in patients with hypertension or coronary artery disease. *Adverse effects* if adrenaline is given beta 1 receptor stimulation gives rise to palpitations and tachycardia commonly, and in overdosage, heart muscle injury with chest pain, breathlessness, headache, rising pulse and blood pressure, pulmonary oedema, ECG abnormalities and increase in serum transaminases.

Ephedrine Hydrochloride Ph. Eur. an ancient Chinese drug of plant origin, is slow to act taken orally, but its duration is more prolonged than either adrenaline or isoprenaline. *Uses* mild asthma. Like adrenaline it has both beta 1 and beta 2 receptor stimulating activity. *Presentation* Tablets B.P. 15, 30 and 60mg; *dose* 15-60mg. The hydrochloride or sulphate salt of ephedrine can be injected. It takes an hour to work and lasts 4 hours. The U.S.P. Injection is Ephedrine Sulphate 25 or 50mg/ml. Ephedrine is contained in many official and proprietary mixtures e.g. Ephedrine Elixir B.P.C. 15mg/5ml, 'Amesec', 'Asmapax', 'Franol' and 'Tedral'. Another use is topical as a nasal decongestant 0.5 and 1% in normal saline. *Adverse effects* mental stimulation, palpitation, insomnia so it should not be taken late in the day; it also interferes with function in the compromised, elderly bladder leading to difficulty in micturition, dribbling and acute retention.

Isoprenaline Sulphate Ph. Eur. (Isoproterenol U.S.P. 'Aleudrin') acts quickly like adrenaline and is absorbed systemically when dissolved sublingually. It is the prototype of the synthetic adrenaline-like drug and has been very popular, but has been superseded by oral derivatives with less cardiac (beta 1) stimulation. *Presentation* Tablets B.P. 10 and 20mg; *dose* 5-20mg sublingually (not swallowed). (Inhaler see below; for other uses see Chapter 19). *Contraindications* to its use are hypertension, coronary artery disease, thyrotoxicosis and left ventricular failure. *Adverse effects* ulceration of tongue, tremor, angina, arrhythmias, tachycardia, ventricular fibrillation. Isoprenaline can paradoxically cause lowering of the oxygen tension in the blood by alteration in blood flow and ventilation, and by bronchoconstriction.

Predominantly Beta 2 Stimulators or Agonists

Orciprenaline Sulphate (Metaproterenol Sulphate, 'Alupent') by mouth works in 30 min and the duration of bronchodilatation lasts 4 hours, by injection acts in 10 min and lasts 30-90 min. *Presentation* Tablets B.P. 20mg, Elixir B.P.C. 10mg/5ml, Injection B.P. contained in ampoules 1ml 500μg/ml (Inhaler see below). *Dose* orally 20-80mg in divided doses and 500μg i.m.

Adverse effects palpitations, headache, abdominal discomfort and nausea.
Terbutaline Sulphate ('Bricanyl') is a long-acting bronchodilator stated to be
selective with little cardiac stimulation. *Presentation* tablets 5mg, syrup
300μg/ml for children in 300ml bottles, injections 500μg contained in 1ml
ampoule (inhalation see below). *Dose* 5mg t.d.s. in adults, or 250-500μg s.c.
Salbutamol Sulphate (Albuterol, 'Ventolin') *presentation* Tablets 2 and 4mg,
sustained release ('Sandets') 8mg, syrup 2mg/5ml, ampoules 5ml 50μg/ml for
slow i.v. injection undiluted, 1ml 0.5mg (500μg)/ml which can be diluted with
Water for Injections and 5ml 1mg/ml (inhaler see below). *Dose* 2-4mg 6
hourly or 8mg delayed release tablet one or two 12 hourly. Orally it works in 5
min and lasts 4 hours. The injection of 500μg (0.5mg) is given s.c., i.m. or i.v.
and the 5mg injection is for i.v. infusion starting at a rate of 5μg/min but varying from 3-20μg/min in Dextrose or Sodium Chloride Injections. It is excreted
renally. *Contra-indications* for the beta 2 stimulators are as for isoprenaline.
Isoetharine Hydrochloride ('Numotac') is an old drug recently re-introduced.
Presentation tablets 10mg; *dose* 10-20mg 3 or 4 times daily. *Actions, uses* as for
isoprenaline.
Methoxyphenamine Hydrochloride ('Orthoxine') is a sympathomimetic
related to methylamphetamine. *Presentation* tablets 100mg; *dose* 50-100mg
3-4 hourly to a maximum of 500mg daily. It is used like ephedrine. *Adverse
effects* dry mouth, nausea, dizziness.
Methylxanthines
These may be given orally, parenterally and rectally by suppository or solution. They are phosphodiesterase inhibitors preventing the breakdown of
cyclic AMP. They cross the blood-brain barrier causing headache, insomnia
and excitement. In action they enhance B_2 agonists (sympathomimetics)
therapeutically and in toxicity. Their value is sustained and efficacy remains
with chronic therapy and not just initially.
Aminophylline Ph. Eur. is theophylline with ethylenediamine. *Presentation*
Injection B.P. in ampoules 250mg/10ml for i.v. use and 500mg/2ml for i.m.
injection, Tablets B.P. 100mg ('Cardophylin'), suppositories 5, 25, 50, 100,
150 and 360mg. *Dose* orally 100-300mg daily, i.v. 250-500mg given over
10-15 minutes when it is valuable for bronchial or cardiac asthma; by suppository for adults usually at night 360mg. Rectal aqueous solutions work fast
in children with a peak level at 6 hours with the absence of nausea seen with
oral administration and a more predictable absorption than the suppository.
Slow release forms are available to reduce nausea which is usually related to
serum levels:— 'Phyllocontin' (tablets 100 and 225mg), 'Theograd' (tablets
350mg) and 'Slophyllin' (capsules 60, 125 and 250mg; tablets 100 and 200mg
and syrup 80mg/15ml. *Adverse effects* mental stimulation, excitement, insomnia, tachycardia (like coffee), ectopic beats, nausea, vomiting and convulsions.
With too fast injection i.v. cardiac arrest occurs. To avoid toxicity attention to
initial i.v. and infusion doses, and oral doses, is important and blood levels if
possible should be measured (normally 5-15mg per litre).
  Theophylline derivatives are used to avoid some of the gastric symptoms of
aminophylline. Examples are **Choline Theophyllinate** ('Choledyl') *presentation*
Tablets B.P. 100 and 200mg, Elixir B.N.F. 62.5mg/5ml; *dose* 400-1600mg for
adults. Others are theophylline piperazine derivatives acepifylline, ('Etophy-
late') proxyphylline ('Thean'), theophylline sodium glycinate, etamiphylline
camsylate ('Millophyline') and diprophylline ('Neutraphylline', 'Silbephyl-
line') which is well tolerated including by i.m. injection; *dose* 200-400mg

orally, 400mg by suppository, or 500mg i.v., or i.m.

Mixtures of ephedrine, barbiturates and theophylline reduce adverse effects, but continued administration of barbiturates causes liver enzyme induction and may reduce the effectiveness of corticosteroids.

Deptropine Citrate is an antihistamine with anticholinergic action taken as 1mg tablets ('Brontina'); *dose* 2-3mg daily. It is also available in a metered aerosol ('Brontisol'). Precautions as for the antihistamines.

Measures for Bronchial Asthma

Mild or early attacks of asthma respond to oral or inhaled antispasmodics, but if severe require i.v. or i.m. salbutamol, s.c. terbutaline, i.v. aminophylline and corticosteroids or ACTH. Patients with status asthmaticus must be in hospital. They need a calm environment with help at hand through the 24 hours. *Sedation is dangerous* if restlessness is due to anoxaemia or carbon dioxide retention. Hypnotics should not be prescribed. Hyperventilation and the distress of the illness often prevent adequate fluid and food being taken. Adequate hydration is essential. Water is a medication and will lessen viscid secretions; i.v. dextrose is given to the ill bed-fast patient. *Oxygen is usually needed* in the highest concentration possible with masks or spectacles to ease the dyspnoea and cyanosis (CO_2 narcosis is not usually a problem, but blood gases should be monitored). In many cases antibiotics are needed when asthma has been provoked by bacterial infection. It is dangerous to give isoprenaline to those who have already had adrenaline injections but injected terbutaline is helpful. Attacks may be *curtailed by corticosteroids,* in urgency i.v., as hydrocortisone 100-200mg 3-6 hourly often infused with aminophylline, or if feasible as oral prednisone 10-20mg 6 hourly for 24 hours then reducing as clinical improvement occurs. A week's course can be stopped without danger. In severe cases (coma, hypertension, heart strain, CO_2 narcosis) bronchial suction, lavage and assisted intermittent positive pressure respiration are life-saving. Drugs may induce asthma by stimulating histamine release, beta receptor blockade, by parasympathetic stimulation or by unknown means (see p. 256). Others produce an allergic IgE medicated response.

In recurrent asthma important problems are whether patients need steroids or ACTH, who gives it (hospital or G.P.) and who controls it, and if given whether treatment is continuous or intermittent. The treatment of asthma is unsatisfactory and many people die including children and young adults.

INHALANTS

Inhalers give symptomatic relief at a fraction of the dose required to get the same effect by mouth with less chance of cardiac side effects. Inhalers are more rapid and effective, but abuse easily occurs and patients may become resistant to their use. The technique of inhaling is often faulty and much is swallowed! For those who cannot hand-synchronize their spray in time with inhalation an auto breath-actuated inhaler can be prescribed.

(1) **Humidification.** A steam kettle is of value in croup and oxygen should be passed through water to prevent drying of the respiratory tract. Humidification of the airway is important after tracheostomy. Hot moist air eases tracheitis.

(2) **Corticosteroids.** Asthma may be brought under control without the need for oral steroids, or with a much smaller oral dose by using inhaled water insoluble steroids which are topically effective. **Beclomethasone Dipropionate B.P.** ('Becotide') contains $50\mu g$ per puff and the container gives 200 inhalations. The daily dose is usually $400\mu g$, in severe cases up to $800\mu g$. **Betamethasone**

Valerate B.P. ('Bextasol') delivering in metered dose 100µg has similar uses. Although systemic effects are unusual, local fungal infection with yeasts has frequently occurred in the pharynx and bronchi, but the incidence although not small is considerably reduced if the daily dose is kept under 400µg. These preparations are taken prophylactically daily, irrespective of wheeze. If acute illness supervenes oral corticosteroids are usually needed especially if corticosteroids have been given before.

(3) **Disodium Cromoglycate** (Cromolyn Sodium U.S.P.) is not a bronchodilator, but prevents some allergic or inflammatory responses e.g. to pollens or house dusts. In the form of 'Rynacrom' it is used for allergic rhinitis at a dose of 10mg (1 capsule) to each nostril 4 times daily or as a 2% aqueous solution as a spray or nasal drops. Sodium cromoglycate 20mg with isoprenaline 100µg is available as powder in capsules as 'Intal Co', or as Sodium Cromoglycate Cartridges B.P. ('Intal') without isoprenaline to prevent asthma. It is taken from 3-4 times daily by inhaling the contents of the 'Spincaps' irrespective of whether the patient has wheeze. It is moderately effective, but expensive. It may also help exercise-induced asthma.

(4) **Bronchodilators.** Official sprays are adrenaline and atropine compound and isoprenaline and isoprenaline compound. These liquids are used with hand sprays. 'Brovon' and 'Rybarvin' contain adrenaline and atropine. 'Medihaler Epi' contains adrenaline. **Isoprenaline** aerosol inhalations are *Ordinary* (80µg per puff, 'Medihaler Iso') or *Strong* (400µg per puff, 'Medihaler Iso-forte'). In view of the *reports of death* while taking isoprenaline patients should be educated to take no more than 10-12 puffs daily and not to increase this if ineffective. Isoprenaline has a quick peak of action in 5 minutes. It has been rendered obsolete by safer sympathomimetics.

Orciprenaline ('Alupent') is available as a 5% inhalant solution and metered aerosol, but is also liable to cardiac effects. **Salbutamol** ('Ventolin') aerosol inhaler delivers 100µg each time and the dose is 1-2 puffs every 4 hours. The canister contains 200 deliveries. **Terbutaline Sulphate** ('Bricanyl') delivers 250µg per inhalation; 1 or 2 doses are taken with an interval of several minutes between each and the dose is 8 per 24 hours. A respirator solution 10mg/ml is also available. **Rimiterol** ('Pulmadil') per puff provides 200µg and the container gives 300 inhalations. It is available as an auto-inhaler (breath-activated) as well as a hand-triggered pressurized aerosol. It is claimed to have little heart action, a quick onset, but is deliberately (half-life of 5 minutes) not as prolonged as salbutamol in effect. **Fenoterol** ('Berotec') is a sympathetic B_2 agonist and **Ipratropium Bromide** ('Atrovent') is an anticholinergic inhalant.

(5) **Antibiotics** can be inhaled e.g. penicillin, natamycin, and colistin.

(6) **Mucolytics** reduce sputum viscosity. They are mainly used for mucoid sputum. Inhaled water mist is probably as effective as detergents, or proteolytic substances which may cause allergy. **Sodium Acetylcysteine** ('Airbron') is an aminoacid derivative *presentation* 20% solution in 10ml vials; *dose* by nebulizer 2-5ml 3 or 4 times daily. Other measures include adequate hydration during chest infections and after operations. Muco-ciliary transport is also improved by stopping smoking. **Oral Mucolytics** include iodinated glycerol ('Organidin') and iodides in mixtures. **Bromhexine Hydrochloride** ('Bisolvon') acts within mucus-secreting cells and reduces viscosity by breaking the bonds which cross-link the components of mucins. When prescribed it is used during infection or after operations. *Presentation* tablets 8mg, elixir 4mg/5ml, ampoules 4mg/2ml for injection. *Dose* orally 8-16mg 3 or 4 times daily for

adults. 8-24mg daily deep i.m. or by slow i.v. infusion in dextrose. **Carbo-cisteine** ('Mucodyne') as a 5% syrup 250mg/5ml or capsules 375mg; *dose* 10-15ml t.d.s. or 2 capsules t.d.s. is said to act quicker than bromhexine. Both need to be avoided in those with peptic ulcers.

Cough Suppressants
Many remedies are used and their popularity rests on their colour, presentation and attractive flavour as much as anything. It is important to know why a patient has a persistent cough before treating it. Tubercle, cancer and heart disease should be excluded. Stopping smoking helps bronchitics and so may warming the bedroom. Reduction of allergenic dust of animal, vegetable, chemical or human origin is worth trying in asthmatics. Post-nasal drip and bronchial infection can also be treated. After operations a cough may be protective and should not be suppressed. The useless, painful or unproductive cough of inoperable cancer should be controlled.
Simple cough remedies. Soothing fluids include honey, treacle with hot water or Simple Linctus B.P.C.
Cough suppressants are usually opium derivatives or synthetic narcotics which depress the medullary cough centre. **Codeine** is popular in official and branded forms e.g. Codeine Phosphate Syrup B.P.C. 2.5-10ml, Codeine Linctus B.P.C. 5ml and Codeine Phosphate Tablets B.P. 15, 30 and 60mg. Codeine constipates. Related are **Hydrocodone (Bi)Tartrate U.S.N.F.** ('Dicodid') which is unsuitable for long-term use as it is addictive and a Controlled Drug. **Dihydrocodeine Tartrate** ('DF 118') is effective and in tablet form is not a Controlled Drug. Squill Opiate or Gee's Linctus B.P.C. is popular; 5ml contains 800μg of morphine. **Diamorphine** (Heroin) Linctus B.P.C. is a Controlled Drug of powerful action finding a special place in the U.K. for terminal bronchial cancer; *dose* 2.5-10ml. **Pholcodine Ph. Eur.** is stronger than codeine and less addictive than heroin. Pholcodine Linctus Strong B.P.C. contains 10mg/5ml and Pholcodine Linctus 5mg/5ml. Pholcodine is contained in many proprietary formulations. **Methadone** ('Physeptone') is a synthetic addictive narcotic, a Controlled Drug, and is avoided in children; *dose* 2-5mg taken as Methadone Linctus B.P.C. 5ml contains 2mg, or as the 5mg tablet. **Dextromethorphan Hydrobromide** ('Cosylan', 'Syrtussar') is available as 15mg tablets and syrup in varying strengths. It has a low risk of abuse.
Other non-narcotic cough suppressants include pipazethate hydrochloride and isoaminile citrate ('Dimyril').

Cough Expectorants
Increase in bronchial secretion may be helped by hot fluids like tea and salt and water, e.g. Sodium Chloride Compound Mixture B.P.C. Bronchial secretion is said, but not proven, to be increased by ammonium chloride, ammonium bicarbonate, potassium iodide, ipecacuanha, squill and senega in sub-emetic amounts. These form the basis of the B.P.C. Mixtures whose dose is 10ml e.g. Ammonia and Ipecacuanha, Ammonium Chloride and Morphine, Potassium Iodide and Ammonia. Sodium-containing expectorants are avoided in heart failure. Some expectorants contain antihistamines e.g. 'Benylin Expectorant'.

Respiratory Stimulants ('Analeptics')
Their aim is to increase the rate or depth of ventilation by stimulating the respiratory centre. They are of limited value. **Nikethamide Ph. Eur.** *presentation* Injection B.P. in ampoules 2 and 5ml 250mg/ml; *dose* 500mg-2g which

can be repeated every 30-120 minutes. Amiphenazole, Dichlorphenamide and Ethamivan are now out of favour.

Aminophylline given i.v. 250-500mg is effective and a concentration of 10µg/ml is aimed for and an i.v. dose of 5.6m'g/kg B.W. over 15-30 minutes followed by a maintenance dose of 900µg/kg B.W. should achieve this level. Rapid injection will cause agitation, convulsions, tachycardia, hypotension and cardiac arrest. **Prethcamide** ('Micoren') is a mixture of equal parts of crotethamide and cropropamide in capsules 400mg. *Dose* 400mg orally thrice daily. **Doxapram Hydrochloride** ('Dopram') has been shown to be moderately effective and without harmful repercussions. *Presentation* infusion 2mg/ml in Dextrose Injection 5% and ampoules 5ml 20mg/ml; *dose* 1-1.5mg/kg B.W. hourly if needs be. *Adverse effects* tachycardia, tremor, agitation, hypertension.

RESPIRATORY FAILURE
This exists when oxygen or carbon dioxide levels are abnormal because of nerve, muscle or chest disease. Treatment is based on first localizing the disorder to the airways, lung tissue or blood supply. *Obstructive airway disease* when under-ventilation is caused by infection and sputum retention, antibiotics, coughing, postural drainage, bronchial suction, tracheostomy or bronchoscopy are more effective than respiratory stimulants, though they occasionally avoid the need for artificial ventilation. In severe ventilatory failure ventilation, with intubation and intensive care nursing are the only effective remedies. For bronchial spasm, oedema and cell thickening steroids may be required. Patients with *restrictive airway* disease with decreased vital capacity need controlled amounts of oxygen. In *diffusion defects* or *uneven perfusion-ventilation* high concentrations of oxygen are needed as with stiff fibrotic lungs. In *defective perfusion* anticoagulants and improving right heart function with digoxin may be helpful. *Parenchymal* infective lesions are dealt with by antibiotics and non-infective produced oedema, fibrin, proteinaceous fluids, or fibroblastic tissue may clear with steroids, or in pulmonary oedema with diuretics.

Oxygen Ph. Eur.
Pure or air-enriched oxygen is used pharmacologically with known concentration, flow and continuous administration. In hypoventilatory disorders hypoxia is the stimulus for breathing and its correction can lead to dangerous carbon dioxide narcosis. It is usual to start with 23 or 25% oxygen by a 'Venturi' apparatus with a flow rate of 1-4 litres/min and gradually increase the concentration. In perfusion and diffusion defects the higher concentrations required are given by masks, nasal tube or tent. However, stated concentrations are not necessarily accurate. Pulmonary oedema, cardiac infarction, and arrest, near-drowning, electrocution, poisoning and shock require 40-80% oxygen at a flow rate of 4-10 litres/min with an oronasal mask ('Polymask', 'Pneumask'). In premature babies both low and high concentrations are dangerous and very great specialist skill is needed to adjust ventilatory pressures, inspiration and expiration times and duration of treatment.

Hyperbaric oxygen at 2 or 3 times normal atmospheric pressure has been used for carbon monoxide poisoning and gas gangrene.

Cor-Pulmonale is right ventricular failure due to chest disease. Treatment aims to reverse lung disease with antibiotics, antispasmodics, corticosteroids, oxygen, anticoagulants plus the treatment for heart failure.

21 DRUGS AND THE ALIMENTARY SYSTEM

Control of gastric secretion is by vagal nerve stimulation leading to a pepsin-rich juice and hormonal stimulation by gastrin formed in the pyloric antrum causing an acid-rich juice. The brain and vagal nerves are responsible for hunger and appetite secretion. Gastric secretion can be reduced by bland foods, sedatives, antivagal drugs and vagotomy. Histamine is a potent stimulator of gastric secretion and drugs which block acid production at H2 receptor sites will reduce acidity e.g. cimetidine. In those too frail for surgery gastric secretion has been reduced by radiotherapy.

Oesophagitis may be controlled by weight reduction and avoidance of corsets so reducing intra-abdominal pressure and reflux, avoidance of gastric stimulants such as caffeine, tea and coffee and local irritants like hot fluids and citrus fruits. Antacids reduce pH which leads to gastrin secretion and this 'tightens up' the gastro-oesophageal junction by direct hormonal action (i.e. sphincter pressure rises as the pH of the stomach is made less acid). 'Mucaine' is a suspension of aluminium and magnesium hydroxide with oxethezaine a local anaesthetic used for symptomatic relief. Anticholinergics should be avoided since they lower sphincter tone, but metoclopramide and bethanechol chloride ('Myotonine') may increase it with symptomatic improvement.

Hiatus Hernia may be helped by weight reduction, antacids and the avoidance of fats which delay pyloric opening as well as postural measures in bed.

Peptic Ulcer in the acute stage is helped by physical and mental rest. Rest in bed if economically possible relieves pain. It is usual to prohibit smoking, to give small, frequent, bland meals, sedatives and antacids. In severe pain a continuously flowing intragastric drip of fluid food helps. Food is an excellent buffer and the frequency of giving it is as important as the content. Ulcerogenic drugs (e.g. aspirin, phenylbutazone, indomethacin and corticosteroids) should be avoided. **Cimetidine** ('Tagamet') is often effective in reducing basal and nocturnal acid secretions in treating gastric and duodenal ulcers, oesophagitis, Zollinger-Ellison syndrome, and acute gastro-intestinal bleeding from stress ulcers. *Presentation* Tablets 200mg, syrup 200mg/5ml and ampoules 2ml 100mg/ml. *Dose* 200-400mg t.d.s. plus 400mg nightly for at least 4 weeks. Cimetidine is no panacea and it is uncertain how long to continue therapy, but a nightly maintenance dose of 400mg can be given. *Adverse effects* nausea, vomiting, drowsiness, rashes, dizziness, vertigo, myalgia, gynaecomastia, upset glucose homeostasis confusion, impotence.

ANTACIDS

Antacid therapy is less agressive in the U.K. than in the U.S.A. partly from tradition and now because of H2 blockers. Peptic ulcer pain is relieved and ulcers heal with intensive therapy as shown by endoscopy. Frequency of administration is important. They are ideally taken 2 hourly and 1 hour after meals and also last thing at night. With antacids a pH of 4-5 can be reached and this means most of the acid is neutralized. All forms have their advantages and disadvantages but aluminum and magnesium salts are the most popular. By altering urinary pH the renal excretion of some drugs taken concurrently may be delayed or enhanced. **Aluminum Hydroxide** is formulated as a 4% w/w Mix-

ture or Gel B.P., the *dose* of which is 5-15ml 2-4 hourly and as Tablets B.P. 500mg of dried gel which are convenient to carry. *Adverse effects* chelation of iron, calcium and tetracyclines with reduction in their absorption. It may prevent phosphorus absorption (it may deliberately be used for this in hyperphosphataemia) and excessive dosage causes depletion with hypophosphataemia, weakness, anorexia, bone pain and osteomalacia. Aluminium salts constipate, and occasionally predispose to intestinal obstruction. Aluminium hydroxide is a mild antacid. Many official and brand forms contain aluminium e.g. **Aluminium Glycinate B.P.** ('Glycinal', 'Prodexin') and Aluminium Hydroxide ('Aludrox', 'Gaviscon', 'Gelusil', 'Maalox'). **Calcium Carbonate Ph. Eur.** is effective, quick and often combined with magnesium carbonate to overcome its constipating effect. *Presentation* Tablets (U.S.P.) and various mixtures; *dose* as tablets is 1-4g 2 hourly. 'Titralac' which dissolves readily in the mouth contains calcium carbonate. *Adverse effects* large doses cause hypercalcaemia and contribute to the milk-alkali syndrome with renal failure. Belching occurs. **Magnesium Carbonate Ph. Eur.** exists in 2 forms — the light usually made-up in mixtures and the heavy employed in powders and tablets. It is a mildly acting antacid, laxative, poorly absorbed and changed to the chloride with liberation of carbon dioxide in the stomach. On its own the *dose* is 250-500mg. It is combined with sodium bicarbonate in **Magnesium Carbonate Mixture B.P.C.** and **Aromatic Magnesium Carbonate Mixture B.P.C.** the *dose* of which is 10-30ml. **Magnesium Hydroxide Mixture B.P.** ('Cream of Magnesia') contains 550mg of magnesium oxide in 10ml; the *dose* is 5-10ml. It is also converted into magnesium chloride in the stomach, but without carbon dioxide production. **Magnesium Trisilicate Ph. Eur., B.P.** is an insoluble powder, long-acting and causing no alkalosis, but it is slower to act than the above. *Presentation* Powder; *dose* 500mg-2g, or half a teaspoonful in water. Tablets 500mg U.S.P.; *dose* 500mg-2g. **Magnesium Trisilicate Mixture B.P.C.** contains 500mg/10ml of magnesium trisilicate plus equal amounts of light magnesium carbonate and sodium bicarbonate; *dose* 10-20ml. **Magnesium Trisilicate Compound Powder B.P.C.** contains equal parts of magnesium trisilicate, heavy magnesium carbonate, chalk and sodium bicarbonate; *dose* 1-5g. **Magnesium Trisilicate Compound Tablets B.P.C.** contain 250mg of magnesium trisilicate and 120mg of aluminium hydroxide gel; *dose* 1-2 tablets. Magnesium mixtures are cheap and in wide use. In renal failure some may be absorbed and magnesium silicate renal stones are a possibility. **Magnesium Aluminate** (Magaldrate, 'Riopan' in U.S.A.) as tablets or suspension has good neutralization effect with low sodium content.
Sodium Bicarbonate Ph. Eur. is soluble, rapidly absorbed, effective, but prolonged use and large doses of the powder cause alkalosis and renal impairment. The dose is 1-4g. A major drawback to its use alone, or as part of other mixtures, is sodium overload and the induction of heart failure.
Bismuth Salts are weak antacids and expensive and are contained in 'Bislumina Suspension', 'De-Nol' and 'Roter Tablets', but in few official formulations. Antacids with milk and proteins are pleasant to take, but contain calories (many patients gain unwanted weight on the frequent meal regime); examples are 'Gelusil Lac', 'Nulacin' and 'Neutrolactis'.

ANTICHOLINERGIC DRUGS
These stop vagal action at post-ganglionic nerve endings. Most are synthetic and reduce acid production and spasm in the stomach. They act like atropine

and in therapeutically effective doses side effects such as dry mouth, blurred vision and disturbances of micturition are almost inevitable (but may later wane). Their use is better for acute episodes of pain and when given at night. There is no proof that they heal ulcers. They should be avoided in those with acute angle closure glaucoma (but are safe in those with open angle glaucoma), prostatic enlargement, gastro-oesophageal reflux and in incipient pyloric stenosis as anticholinergics further delay gastric emptying. **Atropine** (Chapter 14) and belladonna are contained in many formulations e.g. **Phenobarbitone and Belladonna Tablets B.P.C.**, 'Bellergal' and 'Fenobelladine'.

Synthetic parasympatholytics include **Propantheline Bromide** ('Pro-Banthine') *presentation* Tablets B.P. 15mg, vials 1ml containing 30mg for injection in biliary and renal colic. *Dose* orally 15mg before meals. **Dicyclomine Hydrochloride** (included in 'Debendox', 'Merbentyl') *presentation* Tablets B.P. 10mg, Elixir B.P.C. 10mg/5ml; *dose* 30-60mg orally daily in 3 divided doses. **Hyoscine Butylbromide** ('Buscopan')*presentation* tablets 10mg, ampoules 1ml containing 20mg; *dose* 30-100mg orally daily in 3 or 4 divided doses. **Pipenzolate Bromide** ('Piptal') tablets 5mg; *dose* 5-10mg. **Poldine Methylsulphate** ('Nacton', 'Nacton Forte') Tablets B.P. 2 and 4mg; *dose* 8-32mg orally daily in divided doses and **Mebeverine Hydrochloride** ('Colofac') tablets 135mg; *dose* 135-270mg q.d.s. is used for colic and colon-spasm and irritability.

Mucosal Protectives
These are liquorice derivatives.
Carbenoxolone Sodium ('Biogastrone') is the semisynthetic derivative of glycyrrhizic acid, a glycoside (sugar compound) extracted from liquorice. It accelerates the mucosal healing of gastric ulcers even in out-patients, but does not prevent relapse or the long-term outlook. *Presentation* tablets 50mg; *dose* 300mg daily in 3 divided doses for one week then 50mg b.d. or t.d.s. orally daily. *Adverse effects* it has mineralocorticoid activity causing fluid retention, oedema and hypokalaemia which are dose dependent. Hypertension, muscle weakness and heart failure can result in the elderly so caution is needed especially if there is previous cardiac or renal disease. 'Duogastrone' is a 50mg capsule designed for release in the duodenum in duodenal ulcer.
Deglycyrrhizinated Liquorice is the residue of liquorice root after glycyrrhizic acid has been removed. It is contained in 'Caved S' (plus bismuth, magnesium, aluminium and sodium salts) to avoid the mineralocorticoid activity of carbenoxolone for gastric ulcer. It may not be so effective in healing, but it would appear to be suitable for the unfit and the elderly. The dose is 6 tablets daily in divided doses.
Gefarnate ('Gefarnil') a terpene-like substance has been used without clear proof of efficacy. *Presentation* capsules 50mg; *dose* 50mg 3 or 4 times daily.

Flatulence and Anorexia
Symptomatic treatment is unsatisfactory for the cause should be sought and treated specifically. Carminatives induce belching and relieve distension. Usually they contain peppermint, ginger or cardamom mixtures. **Polymethylsiloxane** (Dimethicone, 'Asilone') is also used for flatulence. *Presentation* tablets 250mg with 500mg aluminium hydroxide, suspension and a gel 125mg/5ml with antacids and for paediatric use a suspension containing 25mg/5ml; *dose* 1-2 tablets (or equivalent) before meals. Stimulation of appetite is attempted with Gentian Mixtures with Nux Vomica B.P.C. (almost a harmless old-

fashioned placebo) and with alcoholic beverages. **Cyproheptadine Hydro-chloride** ('Periactin') is an antihistamine used to promote appetite. *Presentation* Tablets B.P. 4mg, Syrup U.S.N.F. 2mg/5ml; *dose* 2-4mg 3 or 4 times daily orally. In anorexia nervosa chlorpromazine and sometimes insulin are used to restore appetite as well as psychotherapy. Care must be taken to forestall dangerous hypoglycaemia. Some drugs undesirably suppress appetite e.g. sulphonamides and morphine while corticosteroids (useful in malignancy) and isoniazid improve appetite. Weight increase also may occur with the tricyclic antidepressive drugs and the benzodiazepines.

Vomiting
Emetics may be needed when children swallow poisons. Homely measures are pharyngeal stimulation, mustard powder 1-3 teaspoonfuls in a glass of tepid water, a teaspoonful of salt (no more) in 100ml of warm water and if available 10-15ml of Ipecacuanha Emetic Draught, Paediatric B.P.C. or Syrup of Ipecacuanha U.S.P. Apomorphine is little used. Children have been given 50µg/kg B.W. followed by a narcotic antagonist.

Anti-Emetics suppress vomiting in Ménière's syndrome, after irradiation, in malignancy, terminal cancer, pregnancy, alcoholism, and liver disease. Examples are chlorpromazine ('Largactil'), cyclizine ('Marzine', 'Valoid'), dimenhydrinate ('Dramamine'), meclozine ('Ancoloxin'), promethazine theoclate ('Avomine'), prochlorperazine ('Stemetil')', thiethylperazine ('Torecan') and trifluoperazine ('Stelazine'). **Metoclopramide Hydrochloride B.P.** ('Maxolon', 'Primperan') structurally related to procainamide, is an anti-emetic with central and peripheral actions. It is also used for gastro-oesophageal reflux. Given i.v. for diagnostic radiology it accelerates gastric emptying by increasing peristalsis, relaxes the pylorus, dilates the duodenum and increases the transit time through the small intestine. It may also be used for emptying the stomach before anaesthesia. *Presentation* Tablets B.P. 10mg, syrup 5mg/5ml, ampoules 10mg/2ml; *dose* orally 10mg t.d.s., i.m. 10-30mg daily, i.v. 10mg for adults. Its use in children is not advised. *Adverse effects* dystonic reactions like the phenothiazines e.g. opisthotonos and hallucinations. A dose should not exceed 500µg (0.5mg)/kg B.W. so as to avoid these extrapyramidal symptoms.

Adsorbents are believed to absorb 'toxins'. Examples are kaolin; *dose* 12-15g or more, or charcoal 4-8g. Their value is dubious.

TREATMENT OF DIARRHOEA
For logical treatment the cause must be identified. Small bowel malabsorption has many causes. Patients suffer from under-nutrition and need a diet high in energy and rich in protein. In steatorrhoea fat can worsen the condition and lead to further fluid and electrolyte loss. Median chain triglycerides are often better absorbed. *Coeliac disease* or gluten enteropathy usually improves when a gluten free diet is given. In non-responsive cases steroids may help. Gluten is a protein of wheat and rye flour and is contained in bread, biscuits, cakes, custards, ice-cream and soups. *Dermatitis herpetiformis* may also improve on a gluten-free diet and so reduce the need for dapsone. In children small bowel diarrhoea may be due to congenital or acquired enzymatic inability to deal with sugars such as lactose or sucrose. *Bacterial overgrowth* and activity in the small intestine (as met in patients with tropical sprue, blind loops, diverticula or strictures) splits bile salts into irritant bile acids causing steatorrhoea and

vitamin B_{12} deficiency. The bacteria can be suppressed by tetracycline, or clindamycin. The same antibiotics will treat Whipple's disease, and bacterial stagnation in scleroderma. In severe diarrhoea replacement of fluid and electrolytes orally, or i.v. may be necessary and in malabsorption calcium, iron, vitamins (A, D, K and B_{12}) and folic acid supplements have to be given.

After ileal resection watery diarrhoea from colonic irritation from unabsorbed bile salts (cholerrhoeic diarrhoea) occurs. This may be helped by the binding resin **cholestyramine** 4g t.d.s., plus oral water-soluble vitamins, injected fat soluble vitamins D, K and A and perhaps median chain triglycerides which can be absorbed irrespective of bile salts. *Ulcerative colitis* requires a high energy, protein and vitamin intake, ACTH i.m. or corticosteroids orally, parenterally or by enema in the acute phase, plus in severe forms i.v. fluid, nutrients, electrolytes and blood. Oral sulphasalazine on a long-term basis prevents relapses of colitis. Antibiotics are little help and oral broad spectrum forms may upset the bowel, as may oral iron. Surgery is often needed eventually.

Infective causes viruses have no specific therapy, some fungi respond to oral nystatin. With *bacillary dysentery* widespread transferable resistance occurs to many antibiotics and the modern view is that their administration is not indicated in the common variety *Shigella sonnei,* but in the toxic forms of *Shigella flexneri* therapy is often needed and i.v. co-trimoxazole is valuable. *Shigella dysenteriae* and *Shigella boydii* also need appropriate antibiotics. *Cholera* kills many thousands in the East and now El Tor is spreading into Europe. Special oral glucose- Na, Cl, K electrolyte solutions (e.g. Dacca solution) help, plus i.v. fluids. Tetracycline, chloramphenicol or co-trimoxazole reduce stool volume, bacterial count and duration of diarrhoea. Prevention is by public health measures, rather than vaccines and co-trimoxazole has been given to contacts. *Typhoid* is treated by chloramphenicol, unless resistance is present when ampicillin or co-trimoxazole is used. Other forms of salmonellosis from food poisoning are treated symptomatically (except in the young, elderly or those with bacteraemia) since antibiotics delay natural cure or prolong the carrier state.

Giardia lamblia is a common cause of sea-goer, tourist or traveller's diarrhoea and may complicate immunological disorders (see p. 46). There is suggestive evidence that certain enteropathic strains of *Esch. coli* causing diarrhoea in travellers can be prevented with 'Streptotriad'.

Antidiarrhoeal agents used for symptomatic treatment are astringents (tannin), adsorbents (bismuth, chalk, charcoal, kaolin, kaolin and pectin compounds 'Kaopectate' and magnesium aluminium silicate), antiperistaltics (opium, morphine, codeine, chlorodyne) and antispasmodics (atropine). Official B.P.C. Mixtures are Aromatic Chalk with Opium, Kaolin, and Kaolin and Morphine. **Diphenoxylate and Atropine** Tablets U.S.P. and 'Lomotil' contain Diphenoxylate Hydrochloride B.P. 2.5mg and Atropine Sulphate B.P. 25µg; *dose* 4 tablets initially then two 6 hourly. A syrup is available 5ml is equivalent to the tablet and is supplied in 60ml and 500ml bottles. 'Lomotil' poisoning in children, by accidental or therapeutic error, can be fatal. Diphenoxylate is structurally related to pethidine and prolongs the passage of contents in the gut by its action on the muscle. It is slower to act, but more prolonged in duration than codeine or pethidine and is contra-indicated in the first year of life, in patients taking barbiturates and those with liver disease. Atropinism with high fever, flushing and tachypnoea occurs early but up to a day later drowsiness, coma, small pupils, hypotonia, loss of tendon reflexes, nystagmus, convulsions, respiratory depression and apnoea can still be noted. The atropine slows the absorption of the opioid diphenoxylate. Treatment is by emptying the stomach, gastric lavage, resuscitation and naloxone. **Loperamide Hydrochloride** ('Imodium') is said to act locally on gut muscle and not to have the opioid-like side effects of diphenoxylate. *Presentation* capsules 2mg, syrup 1 mg/ml; *dose* 6-8mg daily in divided doses. **Difenoxin** ('Motofen' in U.S.A.) was introduced in 1978.

Partial gastrectomy leads commonly to energy, protein and iron deficiency from malabsorption and less frequently to folic acid, vitamin B_{12} and D depletion. All need to be anticipated and corrected. In Crohn's disease suppression of the process often requires corticosteroids, or azathioprine, in addition folic acid and vitamin B_{12} are often prescribed. Trials also indicate the benefits of long-term sulphasalazine.

APERIENTS (Evacuants, Cathartics, Laxatives, Purgatives)
Constipation has various causes—faulty habits, diets lacking in fluid and fibre roughage, decreased colonic activity with age, lack of exercise, dehydration, confinement to bed, disease, and drugs. Drugs cause constipation by:
(1) *reducing peristalsis* by an anticholinergic action, e.g. ganglion blockers, tranquillizers and antidepressives. Narcotics like opium and morphine reduce peristalsis,
(2) *absorbing moisture* and hardening stools e.g. antacids, iron, aluminium salts,
(3) *abuse of purgatives;* constipation following diarrhoea.

Aperients work by adding fluid to the motion, increasing bulk, or by stimulating peristalsis. They are used clinically to: (1) aid poor colonic function especially in the elderly, (2) produce a soft stool in painful anal fissure, haemorrhoids, or when strain would be undesirable as after cardiac infarction, subarachnoid haemorrhage, lumbago and haematemesis, (3) counteract drugs which constipate, (4) evacuate blood in the gut as in cirrhosis with coma and (5) expel worms, ingested poisons and faeces before surgery or radiology.

Abuse and purgative addiction may lead to loss of fluid, hypokalaemia with muscle paralysis, renal failure, metabolic acidosis, hypocalcaemia and hypomagnesaemia, as well as protein loss from malabsorption. Damage to the colonic nerve plexuses with megacolon can result from habitual use. Aperients should be avoided in unexplained pain since they can worsen appendicitis. Water attracting colloids occasionally cause bowel obstruction. Oxyphenisatin was withdrawn because it caused hepatitis. Purgatives should not be used before instituting regular habits, trying adequate fluids, and fibre roughage (e.g. 'All-Bran' or Ispaghula husk contained in 'Fybogel' which also contains 6mmol of sodium per sachet). A great deal of research is now going on into the chemistry and biological actions of natural dietary fibre. The dietician will supply information about fibre containing foods and preparations.

Saline Laxatives or Hypertonic Solutions
Magnesium Sulphate B.P. (Epsom salts) and **Sodium Sulphate B.P.** (Glauber's salt) are unabsorbed and retain excess water, which mechanically stimulates peristalsis. *Dose* 2-16g of the crystals dissolved in water. Taken before breakfast it acts in a few hours. Repeated use causes loss of body sodium and potassium. Mist Alba is **Magnesium Sulphate Mixture B.P.C.,** 10ml contains 4g of

180   THERAPEUTICS

magnesium sulphate and 500mg of magnesium carbonate. Similarly acting are magnesium hydroxide mixture, Magnesium Citrate Solution U.S.N.F.; *dose* 60-200ml and Seidlitz powders.

Bulk Laxatives or Physical Peristaltic Stimulants
These are safe, non-irritant, water-attracting solids. By absorbing fluid they increase and soften the bowel contents, e.g. **Methylcellulose Granules B.P.C.**; *dose* 1.5-6g and 'Celevac', 'Cellucon' (tablets) and 'Cologel' (suspension). Agar-Agar is obtained from sea-weed; *dose* 4-16g. 'Isogel' comes from tropical seeds and like the plant preparations 'Metamucil', and 'Normacol' is usually given in a dose of 1-2 teaspoonfuls once or twice daily. Granules are swallowed in water without chewing. *Adverse effects* bolus colic, faecal impaction.

Vegetable Laxatives
Chemically of the anthraquinone glycoside group, these comprise aloes, cascara, senna and rhubarb. They mildly irritate the colon and work in 8-12 hours so they are taken at night. *Aloes* is the strongest; the active˙principle is aloin. Because it gripes it is not given alone, or in pregnancy. Aloin is included in 'Alophen', 'Taxol' and Phenolphthalein Compound Pills B.P.C. (30mg phenolphthalein, aloin 15mg, belladonna dry extract 5mg). The belladonna combats griping. *Dose* 1-3 pills at night. **Cascara Sagrada Ph. Eur.** is gentler than aloes. *Presentation* Cascara Tablets B.P. a dry bark extract containing between 17 and 23mg of total hydroxyanthracene derivatives and Cascara Liquid Extract B.P. containing 1g of cascara powder in each ml. *Dose* 1 or 2 tablets, or 2-5ml of extract or as 'Cascara Evacuant' containing 2g of the bark extract/5ml and is flavoured; *dose* 2.5ml morning and night, or 2.5-5ml at night. 'Veracolate' contains bile salts and phenolphthalein as well. **Rhubarb** is contained in Gregory's Powder (Compound Rhubarb Powder B.P.C.) and Compound Rhubarb Pill B.P.C., as well as the B.P.C. Mixtures — Gentian and Rhubarb, Rhubarb Compound, Rhubarb, Ammonia and Soda the dose of which is 10ml. **Senna** is the best of this group, and is either the powdered leaf or the pods of the plant. *Dose* 500mg-2g. Senna Tablets B.P. contain 7.5mg of sennosides and the dose is up to 30mg as sennoside B. 'Senokot' is available as tablets containing sennosides A and B, equivalent to 7.5mg of sennoside B, granules equivalent to 6.5mg/g of sennoside B (a teaspoonful 2.8g contains 15mg), and syrup equivalent to 1.8mg/ml sennoside B. *Dose* 2-4 tablets, 1-2 teaspoonfuls of granules, or 2-4 teaspoonfuls of syrup. Children over 6 have half doses. Senna is widely used for long-term use in the aged.
Castor oil derived from castor seeds on digestion in the small gut liberates ricinoleic acid a strong irritant. It is rarely used; *dose* 4-16ml. **Cathartics** are very irritant. Colocynth and jalop are contained in vegetable laxative tablets; *dose* 1-3 tablets.

Non-Vegetable Laxatives
Phenolphthalein is used in various chocolate flavoured laxatives. It acts on the colon, part is absorbed and then excreted in the bile so prolonging the effect. *Dose* 60-300mg. *Adverse effects* red rash, often a fixed eruption. Liquid Paraffin and Phenolphthalein Emulsion B.P.C. contains 30mg phenolphthalein/10ml; *dose* 5-20ml. It is also in Pill Phenaloin and 'Agarol Emulsion. Like Bisacodyl it is a diphenolic derivative.

Bisacodyl ('Dulcolax') *presentation* enteric-coated Tablets B.P. 5mg; *dose* 5-10mg taken morning or night. 'Dulcodos' contains 5mg bisacodyl and 100mg dioctyl sodium sulphosuccinate.

Dioctyl Sodium Sulphosuccinate B.P.C. ('Dioctyl') is a detergent stool softener. *Presentation* as dioctyl sodium sulfosuccinate capsules and tablets (U.S.P.), liquid and syrup (U.S.N.F.); *dose* 100-500mg. In Britain tablets 20 and 100mg, and syrup 12.5mg/5ml are available.

Liquid Paraffin (Liquid Petrolatum U.S.A.) is an unabsorbed, lubricant mineral oil which softens stools. *Presentation* the B.P.C. Emulsion is 50% strength; *dose* 10-30ml. Other B.P.C. Emulsions are with magnesium hydroxide, phenolphthalein, or cascara. A disadvantage is that liquid paraffin seeps through the anus soiling underclothes. It may prevent absorption of vitamins and other drugs and in dysphagic patients, or habitual consumers, accidentally enter the lungs causing a paraffinoma. Long-term use is not advised.

Lactulose is a synthetic disaccharide composed of fructose and galactose which is unabsorbed since the enzymes of the small intestine cannot hydrolyze it. In the colon it is fermented into simple organic acids such as acetic and lactic acids which stimulate the colon and also make the contents more acid. The latter action may help in portal-systemic encephalopathy (liver coma) by reducing the absorption of nitrogenous substances. *Presentation* 'Duphalac' and 'Gatinar' syrup 670mg/ml (plus 5% w/w lactose and 8% w/w galactose) in bottles 300ml and 1 litre; *dose* initially 30ml for constipation and 30-50ml for portal-systemic encephalopathy and smaller amounts for maintenance.

INTRARECTAL THERAPY

Suppositories are solid firm conical-shaped bodies designed for rectal insertion. The base is non-irritant and melts at body heat. Their advantage is they can be administered by the patient, relative or nurse. For 'aesthetic' reasons they have not been popular in Britain, in contrast to the Continent. They have several uses:

(1) To stimulate bowel actions by softening stools e.g. **Glycerin Suppositories B.P.** 1,2,4 and 8g mould sizes which are 70% glycerin. **Bisacodyl** ('Dulcolax') which contains 5 or 10mg of active substance in 1.7g base chemically stimulates the rectal mucosa. 'Beogex' acts by physical distension liberating CO_2 from its components, anhydrous sodium phosphate and sodium bicarbonate. A successful suppository avoids the side effects of oral laxatives and the bother of an enema.

(2) To treat haemorrhoids and fissures by astringents (protein precipitants), hamamelis, zinc oxide, bismuth subgallate; local anaesthetics, corticosteroids and anti-infective agents e.g. Bismuth Subgallate Compound Suppositories B.P.C. which contain 200mg bismuth subgallate, plus castor oil, resorcinol and zinc oxide and 'Anusol', 'Anusol H.C.', 'Anugesic H.C.', 'Nestosyl' and 'Proctosedyl'.

(3) Anti-inflammatory to treat ulcerative colitis e.g. hydrocortisone and sulphasalazine.

(4) For systemic action by absorption from the rectum. Here suppositories help to avoid gastric side effects of the same drug taken orally, or the need to inject it. Dyspnoea of cardiac or respiratory origin may be helped by aminophylline, diprophylline or proxyphylline. Ergotamine tartrate and caffeine ('Cafergot') is given for migraine and prochlorperazine ('Stemetil') for vertigo and vomiting, including after operations. Chlorpromazine ('Largactil')

helps quieten the elderly. In rheumatic diseases morning stiffness may be helped by phenylbutazone, or indomethacin, inserted at night. Pain may be relieved by pentazocine ('Fortral') not a Controlled Drug, or oxycodone, dextromoramide ('Palfium') and morphine which are Controlled Drugs.

Enemas are fluid preparations given via the rectum. They are used to stimulate the colon in constipation, soften faeces, or to relieve partial obstruction and faecal impaction. **Soap Enema B.P.** contains 30g in 600ml of water. Fletcher's disposable enema contains phosphate. Another use has been to dehydrate patients with cerebral tumours with magnesium sulphate, but this has been superseded by systemic dexamethasone or i.v. mannitol. Enemas can be a vehicle for soluble corticosteroids used topically in ulcerative colitis. **Prednisolone Enema B.P.C.** ('Predsol') is prednisolone sodium phosphate equivalent to 20mg prednisolone in 100ml buffered solution. Hydrocortisone acetate is now available in a foamy base ('Colifoam') 10g in one application inserted rectally. **Hydrocortisone Sodium Succinate B.P.** 100mg can be infused as a rectal drip, or hydrocortisone can be given as a retention enema ('Cortenema') 100mg in 60ml of fluid. Sulphasalazine in enema form is now available.

LIVER COMA

Coma results from accumulation of toxic nitrogenous waste products derived from bacterial action in the gut absorbed into the blood. It occurs late in cirrhosis, or early in acute hepatitis or liver necrosis from drugs. *Precipitating factors* in cirrhosis are the unwise use of *constipating drugs* which increase bacterial decomposition of proteins; the *use of sedatives* normally metabolized by the liver such as morphine and quick-acting barbiturates; the giving of ammonia compounds, *large quantities of protein,* or *haemorrhage* into the gut; *fluid and electrolyte* disturbance caused by excessive diuretics or removal of ascites.

Treatment depends on early diagnosis (apathy, shakes, drowsiness). All protein is stopped and calories are given as 400g of carbohydrate daily, preferably orally, but if coma or vomiting exist i.v. dextrose is given. Fluid intake, output, and blood electrolytes are monitored. Blood lost is replaced and balloon compression of oesophageal varices are attempted. Purgatives: since stale blood in the gut is poisonous to cirrhotics evacuation by purging, or enema is desirable. **Neomycin** reduces bacterial action causing coma, at a dose of 1-1.5g 6 hourly given by gastric tube. It may be combined with lactulose initially 30-50ml t.d.s. Lactulose is expensive and excessive diarrhoea and hypokalaemia may result. Sedation: all drugs are dangerous. Restlessness may be controlled by benzodiazepines. For irreversible fulminant hepatic coma charcoal haemoperfusion has proved successful in nearly 50%, as compared with 10-20% survival not so treated.

PANCREATIC DISEASE

The pancreas if diseased may from enzyme lack cause malabsorption. Enzyme replacement may help. **Pancreatin B.P.** is available as Granules or Tablets. The dose is 2-8g daily. 'Nutrizym' contains bromelains (protein digesting enzymes), pancreatin (obtained from animal pancreas) and ox bile containing bile acids. The tablets are so made that the bromelains are liberated in the stomach and the other components in the duodenum. *Dose* 1 or 2 tablets, during or after, meals swallowed whole with liquid. Pancreatic preparations include 'Combizym', 'Cotazym', 'Enzypan', 'Panar', 'Pancreatin' and 'Pancrex' in varying strengths and formulations. Children are best given Pancreatin as the contents of 'Pancrex V' capsules, or as the (Pancrex V) strong powder sprinkled on food or milk at a dose of 1-2g. *Fibrocystic disease* of the pancreas is treated in addition with prophylactic antibodies and curtailment of fat intake. **Cimetidine** ('Tagamet') (see p. 174) is used in chronic pancreatitis and in patients taking pancreatin to reduce destruction of gastric acid.

Gall Bladder

For **cholecystitis** ampicillin or **cephamandole** which is excreted in the bile in high concentrations would be the first choice.

    Chenodeoxycholic Acid ('Chendol') reduces the cholesterol content of bile. Gallstones are increasing in frequency and related to obesity, diabetes mellitus and hyperlipidaemia. Gallstones occur if bile is supersaturated with cholesterol. Chenodeoxycholic acid if taken by mouth dissolves cholesterol gallstones and may also prevent their recurrence and formation. It does not cure the underlying metabolic defect. The requirements for successful dissolution of stones are:

(1) The gall bladder should be functioning.
(2) The stones should be of cholesterol and radiotranslucent.
(3) It is not advised in women of childbearing age.
(4) It is to be considered in those in whom surgery is contraindicated or refused. It is not advised in patients with liver disease or chronic bowel disease.
Presentation capsules 125mg; *dose* 10-15mg/kg B.W. in divided amounts though giving the greater part at night is more effective. The duration of therapy is unknown but is either for years or permanent. This is important since the cost is high. *Adverse effects* diarrhoea, pruritus.

Ursodeoxycholic Acid an epimer of chenodeoxycholic acid reduces cholesterol content of bile, but also expands the bile acid pool. This Japanese introduced therapy is laxative and the dose is 150-600mg daily.

22 RENAL DISEASE

RENAL TRACT INFECTION

Incidence. In children and women who are virgins it is about 1-2%, otherwise in women it is 5-7% with a special risk in pregnancy. The incidence in geriatric practice is very high. Outside hospital infection is in 95% due to *Esch. coli*. In hospital this falls to about 50-60% with *Proteus spp, Str. faecalis, Ps. aeruginosa* also important. For **effective therapy** the infection must be *bacteriologically confirmed* since symptoms are a poor guide and the organism *must be identified* as well as the strain to distinguish re-infection (which is a defect in defence mechanisms) from relapse which is a failure of therapy. Renal antibodies indicate renal involvement. If the kidneys are involved infection is more difficult to cure and high tissue levels are needed. Neither nalidixic acid nor nitrofurantoin is suitable for upper renal tract infection because tissue concentrations are inadequate. The chance of cure is less in pregnancy and when there is anatomical or functional abnormality, or if there is a continued intake of *analgesic drugs*.

After treatment eradication must be ensured by adequate follow up and appropriate investigations. Acute infections particularly first attacks when treated usually do not recur and the urine remains sterile. After repeated or persistent infection complete eradication is unusual. Renal infection (pyelonephritis) is a special problem in women and children and predisposes to renal failure and hypertension though not as much as was thought. Drug treatment needs ideally to be prompt, effective, bactericidal to bacteria, to be taken orally and reach high urinary and kidney concentrations. Therapy is for at least 7-14 days to prevent relapse. A good fluid intake, frequent voiding of urine, especially after sex and perineal hygiene may be added measures, and also a vaginal lubricant to prevent recurrences of cystitis.

Acute Infections

Sulphonamides are suitable for most infections. Quick-acting preparations are sulphadimidine or sulphafurazole 2-3g initially then 1g 6 hourly. They are best for *Esch. coli*. Modern varieties are safe and act in acid or alkaline urine. Although more expensive **co-trimoxazole** which contains a sulphonamide is even more effective and is also valuable for *Proteus spp*. The dose is 2 tablets twice daily. **Nitrofurantoin** is useful in *Esch. coli* and *Str. faecalis* infections and gives high urinary, but low renal levels, so it is less good for pyelonephritis. The adult dose is 100mg q.d.s. For precautions and adverse effects see p. 26. Streptomycin kills bacteria such as *Proteus spp*, but is dangerous in conventional doses if renal failure exists. If prescribed the urine is kept alkaline since this enhances its action. Gentamicin, tobramycin or carbenicillin are used for Gram-negative infections particularly *Ps. aeruginosa*. The levels of gentamicin are measured to ensure therapeutic as well as toxic values; the dose is 80-120mg which may be 8, 12 or every 24 hours or more, depending on the levels. Such infections may be accompanied by Gram-negative bacteraemia, other causes include abdominal surgery, biliary disease, and any disease causing reduced cellular or humoral immunity. Drugs used are shown in Table 13.

TABLE 13

ANTIBIOTICS USED IN GRAM-NEGATIVE BACTERAEMIA

Name	Dose		Route	Comments	Uses
	Adult	Paediatric (daily)			
Ampicillin	500mg-3.0g 6 hourly	400mg/kg B.W.	i.v., i.m.	Avoid in penicillin allergy	Escherichia coli, Proteus mirabilis, Salmonella typhi, Haemophilus influenzae
Carbenicillin	5.0g 4 to 6 hourly	400mg/kg B.W.	i.v.		Pseudomonas aeruginosa
Cefuroxime	750mg 8 hourly	30-100mg/kg B.W.	i.v., i.m.	Avoid in penicillin allergy	Escherichia coli, Klebsiella aerogenes, Haemophilus influenzae
Cephaloridine	1.0g 6 to 8 hourly	30-60mg/kg B.W.	i.v., i.m.	Avoid with frusemide and aminoglycosides. Check renal function	Escherichia coli, Klebsiella aerogenes
Cephalothin	1.0-2.0g 4 to 6 hourly up to 12g daily	40-80mg/kg B.W.	i.v.	i.m. painful. i.v. preferred: better than cephaloridine in renal failure	"
Cephradine	500mg-1.0g 6 hourly	50-100mg/kg B.W.	i.v., i.m.		"
Chloramphenicol	1.0g 6 to 8 hourly	neonates: 25mg/kg B.W. others: 50mg/kg B.W.	i.v., i.m.		Salmonella typhi (Typhoid), Haemophilus influenzae
Gentamicin	40-80mg 8 hourly (5mg/kg B.W. daily)	6mg/kg B.W.	i.v., i.m.	Dose depends on renal function; monitor blood levels	Pseudomonas aeruginosa, Proteus species, First choice in undiagnosed bacteraemia
Lincomycin	600mg 8 or 12 hourly	12-20mg/kg B.W.	i.v., i.m.	Systemic clindamycin may be better	Bacteroides
Penicillin G	600mg-1.2g or more 6 hourly	15-40mg/kg B.W.	i.v., i.m.	In sensitive subjects sulphonamides or chloramphenicol	Meningococcus
Streptomycin	0.5-1.0g 12 hourly	20-40mg/kg B.W.	i.v., i.m.	ototoxicity limits course	Brucellosis
Ticarcillin	5g 8 hourly up to 20g daily	200-300mg/kg B.W.	i.v.		Pseudomonas aeruginosa and many others
Tobramycin	3-5mg/kg B.W.	3-5mg/kg B.W.	i.v., i.m.	as for gentamicin	Pseudomonas aeruginosa
Co-Trimoxazole	800-1200mg Sulphamethoxazole and 160-240mg Trimethoprim 12 hourly	30-40mg Sulphamethoxazole and 6-8mg Trimethoprim kg B.W. divided into two equal doses	i.v.	Must be diluted in infusion fluid	Most Gram negative, except Pseudomonas aeruginosa

Carbenicillin is given 1g 6 hourly for Proteus infections. The **Cephalosporins** are also effective against *Esch. coli*. **Kanamycin** is restricted because of toxicity but like gentamicin can be highly effective when *Esch. coli* renal infection has caused bacteraemia. **Ampicillin** or amoxycillin is also a popular remedy and is effective for *Str. faecalis* and for *Esch.coli* but resistance to it is increasing. The dose is 250-500mg 6 hourly usually orally. Parenteral injection is necessary when the patient is ill, vomiting or unable to swallow. Tetracyclines 500mg 6 hourly have a wide range, but the risk of worsening renal function curtails their use. Other antibiotics find occasional use such as **Penicillin G, Colistin** and **Carfecillin**. Sometimes *Esch. coli* responds to cycloserine 250mg orally every 8 hours. In pregnancy beta-lactam antibiotics, erythromycin, nitrofurantoin and sulphonamides are best. Tetracycline, nalidixic acid and co-trimoxazole are not advised.

Chronic or recurrent infections are usually due to resistant bacteria and guidance is needed from the laboratory. In some patients all antibiotics fail often because there is an underlying defect which impedes natural drainage such as stones, or prostatic enlargement. Rotation of antibiotics may be tried and if eradication is achieved twice weekly co-trimoxazole may keep the urine sterile.

Certain antibiotics (basic lipid soluble and active when ionized in the acid prostatic fluid) are able to diffuse into the prostate and prostatic fluid, namely erythromycin, clindamycin and co-trimoxazole. The latter is useful for chronic prostatitis.

Urinary Antiseptics
These are tried when antibiotics or chemotherapy fail or as alternatives.
Nalidixic Acid ('Negram') is well absorbed and excreted into the urine in high concentrations. It is bactericidal to Gram-negative organisms especially *Esch. coli* and some *Proteus spp.* but not *Ps. aeruginosa*. *Presentation* Tablets B.P.C. 500mg, Mixture B.P.C. 60mg/ml; *dose* 500mg-1g q.d.s., children 60mg/kg B.W. in 4 divided doses daily. *Adverse effects* nausea, vomiting, rashes, photosensitivity, paraesthesiae, haemolytic anaemia (if red-cell enzyme deficiency), headache and raised intracranial pressure in those with poor renal function.
Oxolinic Acid chemically related to nalidixic acid is no longer available in the U.K.
Hexamine when excreted into an acid urine breaks down to yield formaldehyde and was the first pro-drug. *Dose* 600mg-2g before meals. The urine is made acid with ammonium chloride.
Mandelic Acid is taken as the calcium or ammonium salt. It works in an acid urine. The patient is taught to adjust the urine acidity to a pH of 5 or less with an indicator paper. *Dose* 2-4g.
Hexamine Mandelate (Methenamine Mandelate U.S.P. 'Mandelamine') *presentation* tablets 250 and 500mg; *dose* 1g q.d.s. The urine is made acid with ammonium chloride 450mg tablets up to 12 daily, or methionine 4-12g daily.
Hexamine Hippurate ('Hiprex', 'Hiprex 250') is used prophylactically and to treat urinary infections. *Presentation* tablets 250mg and 1g; *dose* for adults 1g 2 to 4 times daily. Children take 250-500mg twice daily. The urine is acidified with 2g daily of ascorbic acid. *Adverse effects* rashes, gastric irritation, bladder discomfort. It should not be given with sulphonamides or alkalies.

RENAL FAILURE

Prevention is possible by the avoidance of excessive analgesics, and the treatment of renal infection, hypertension, gout and hypercalcaemia.

In **acute renal failure** there is inability to excrete urea, water, sodium, chloride, potassium and organic acids. Anaemia, bleeding and hypertension ensue. It arises in medical, surgical, accident or obstetric practice from severe renal parenchymal, glomerular or tubular infections or damage, blockage to urinary outflow, poisons, mismatched blood transfusions, circulatory failure, shock, blood, plasma and salt and water loss, and injury. *Treatment.* The underlying cause when possible is corrected. In **acute glomerular nephritis** the patient is kept in bed, fluids are restricted according to the urinary output—the intake is usually 500-700ml, salt intake is drastically curtailed and diet rich in carbohydrates, but low (e.g. 40g) in protein is given. Food is given orally but culinary skill is required to give about 400g of carbohydrate in only a small amount of fluid and to make it palatable. If persistent vomiting occurs i.v. feeding is undertaken. Associated infection requires antibiotics. Curtailment of fluid and salt reduces the risk of hypertension, heart failure and convulsions. Most patients recover on medical measures. *Progressive renal failure* of glomerular origin is sometimes treated with heparin, (intravascular coagulation), immunosuppressives and steroids with poor results.

Temporary measures to reduce hyperkalaemia which can cause cardiac arrest are **Oral Sodium Polystyrene Sulphonate** ('Resonium A') an ion-exchange resin; *dose* 15g t.d.s. suitably flavoured, or more rapidly intravenous dextrose 50g, soluble insulin 50 units, sodium bicarbonate 50-100mmol or 40-50ml of 10% calcium gluconate. Should medical measures fail *haemodialysis* or *peritoneal dialysis* is tried particularly when renal failure follows accidents or septic abortion.

Patients should be isolated and *barrier nursed* so as to reduce infection which is a frequent killer. One source is the indwelling catheter. Weighing of the patient is important to achieve the correct fluid intake.

Chronic Renal Failure

In some patients renal failure may be reversed by relieving renal obstruction, and in others by stopping damage by analgesics, gout or hypercalcaemia. Renal transplantation and home or hospital dialysis schemes do not suffice for all those who need it so medical treatment is still required. Chronic peritoneal dialysis is safe for long-term use in children who can continue to grow and diabetics who are at less risk for retinal haemorrhage.

(1) **Increase in metabolism** of the body proteins is prevented by giving adequate calories and avoiding starvation, infection, injury or operations.

(2) **Derangement** of water, sodium, potassium, calcium, magnesium, and hydrogen ion balance is corrected if feasible, as is anaemia, heart failure and hypertension.

Sodium Chloride: many patients with chronic renal disease lose salt excessively. These patients do not have oedema or marked hypertension. Diarrhoea and vomiting also cause sodium and fluid loss with further deterioration in renal function. Renal function improves with oral supplements of sodium chloride 3-20g or more daily which may be given as Slow Sodium 600mg tablets (10 mmol of sodium) more palatably, or i.v. as Sodium Chloride Injection B.P. if the patient is vomiting or unconscious.

Hydrogen ion: metabolic acidosis is often best. ignored. Correction with sodium bicarbonate (orally 3-12g daily) carries the risk of tetany and the serum bicarbonate should not be raised above 15mmol/litre.

Protein is restricted if the blood urea is raised above 100mg/dl(16mmol/l) or more informative when the glomerular flow rate as measured by the creatinine clearance drops to a critical level. A diet based on egg and 200ml of milk, low protein bread, pasta (Carlo Erba), or biscuits (Salza-Pisa); calories as liquid glucose ('Hycal'), or as 'Caloreen', alcohol or double cream is prescribed. Some diets are in a form largely of essential aminoacids so there is little waste. Egg albumin and potato are suitable but such diets are boring and tend to elevate the blood potassium. Protein portions or units (exchanges) may make the diet more interesting.

Anaemia is difficult to correct. Transfusion of blood carries a risk of depressing renal function. Every attempt should be made to avoid transfusion because of risks of hepatitis and iron overload and also it may make future transplantation (because of incompatibility) more difficult. In those in whom transplantation is not possible transfusion may be unavoidable if the haemoglobin is below 6g. Iron and folates if lacking should be supplied and vitamins B complex, vitamin B_{12} monthly and androgens may have some beneficial effect.

Hyperkalaemia can be treated by ion-exchange resins e.g. Calcium Polystyrene Sulphonate which for long-term use is better than the sodium cation exchange resin. Potassium containing medicines, potassium sparing diuretics, acidosis and anaesthesia should be avoided.

Hyperphosphataemia is treated by reducing phosphorus intake and using phosphate binders such as aluminium hydroxide 20ml 4-5 times daily, or as dried gel ('Alu-Cap' 8-10 capsules daily). The dietary intake of calcium is low in patients taking Giovenetti diets and they should have supplements of 1g daily especially if they are having dialysis.

Hypermagnesaemia can be temporarily counteracted by 1-2g of calcium gluconate. Medicines with magnesium e.g. antacids should be avoided.

Renal bone disease may respond to vitamin D or its metabolites (1α 25 dihydroxycholecalciferol, 1 α 25 dihydroxy D_3 known as **Calcitriol** officially, or the analogue **Alfacalcidol** or 1α hydroxy D_3 available as 'One Alpha').

Hypertension requires hypotensives (unless it causes deterioration in renal function) and in some restriction of sodium. Congestive failure is treated with digoxin and diuretics. Frusemide is valuable as it increases urine volume and glomerular flow.

Hyperlipidaemia and associated cardiac and cerebrovascular disease are common events in dialysis patients and predispose to mortality. If treated by clofibrate there is a risk of toxicity if there is hypoalbuminaemia. Free or unbound clofibrate in the plasma can cause fever and muscle pain.

Infection causes deterioration of function and must be treated. It affects the dose of drugs such as digoxin and also the choice and dose of antibiotics e.g. gentamicin (see p. 256). This applies to drugs in general. They should be avoided if possible and if given either the dose or the times of administration have to be modified.

Terminal care involves the relief of distressing symptoms such as hiccough, vomiting and pericarditis.

Nephrotic Syndrome

Nephrotic syndrome is a state of generalised oedema and marked protein loss from the kidneys. The underlying cause should be treated if relevant (nephritis, diabetes mellitus, lupus erythematosus, amyloidosis, malaria, renal vein thrombosis, and some drugs). Treatment is usually symptomatic—oedema is controlled by salt restriction to 500mg-1g daily, supplemented by diuretics. A low serum protein contributes to oedema formation and can be temporarily improved by infusions of salt-free albumin and giving a protein-rich diet. Bacterial infection by pneumococci or streptococci is a hazard. Steroid therapy with prednisone (or allied drugs) up to 80mg daily may be helpful. Children respond better than adults. The types that do well have no abnormality, or minimal changes only on microscopy. Should steroids fail, or if the child cannot be weaned off them, success may be obtained with cyclophosphamide 3mg/kg B.W. daily for 8 weeks or azathioprine 50-100mg daily. Cytotoxic agents have the advantage that unlike corticosteroids, stunting of growth does not occur. With low-dose schemes alopecia, leucopenia and infection are also avoided. Testicular damage and sterility are drawbacks. The use of diuretics in steroid sensitive nephrotic syndrome in young children is not advised since fatal hypovolaemia can occur. If hypovolaemia is induced then i.v. plasma can be given.

Enuresis

Imipramine or amitriptyline 25-75mg for adults and 10-20mg for children may help (beware accidental overdose).

Nocturia

Emepronium Bromide ('Cetiprin') *presentation* tablets 100 and 200mg; *dose* 200mg thrice daily. *Uses* relief of nocturia in the elderly. If retained in the mouth or oesophagus they can cause ulceration. **Flavoxate Hydrochloride** ('Urispas') is used for dysuria and nocturia. It has anticholinergic actions and side effects. *Presentation* tablets 100mg; *dose* 200mg thrice daily. Mistakes occur in the use of these anticholinergic preparations since the elderly male with nocturia often has prostatic enlargement with urinary retention. Such drugs then precipitate acute urinary retention.

Renal Stones

If uric acid crystals form without reason long-term alkalinization of the urine to pH 8 helps solubility. Primary hyperoxaluria can be cured by giving magnesium hydroxide orally. This alters the urinary ionic concentration.

23 DRUGS AND BLOOD CONDITIONS

Anaemia results from decreased formation, excess destruction or loss of blood. Impaired formation results from lack of essential protein, iron, vitamin B_{12}, vitamin C and folates.

IRON DEFICIENCY

Iron containing foods are meat, eggs, peas, beans and cereals as haem iron or ferric iron complexes. A poor diet, blood loss (menstrual, gastro-intestinal from peptic ulcer, cancer, worms, haemorrhoids, drugs, hiatus hernia), poor absorption (intestinal disease, gastrectomy) and increased demands (infancy, pregnancy) cause iron deficiency anaemia. This anaemia is common in women, infants and the aged and a reason should be sought so the case may be treated. Only 10% of ferrous iron is absorbed from the diet and a woman needs to absorb 1-2mg, and a man 500μg-1mg daily. The body stores are 4g of iron. 2.5g in haemoglobin and a small amount in myoglobin, tissue enzymes and circulating in the plasma and 1g in liver, spleen and marrow. The iron stores of an adult male normally last 6-8 years.

TABLE 14
PREPARATIONS OF ORAL IRON

Ferrous Salt	Tablet (mg)	Iron (mg)	Brand
Sulphate Ph. Eur., B.P.	300	90	
Sulphate Compound B.P.C.	170	51	
Gluconate Ph. Eur., B.P.	300	36	Fergon; Sidros
Succinate B.P.	100	35	Ferromyn
Fumarate B.P.	200	65	Fersamal
	290	100	Fersaday; capsule Galfer
Glycine Sulphate	225	40	Kelferon

Choice of route

The oral route is safest and cheaper. Many preparations exist. The ferrous forms are best. In iron deficiency at least 100mg of elemental iron is needed daily and is readily absorbed when body stores are depleted. The dose of ferrous salts is usually 1 tablet t.d.s. before food. Many preparations exist (Table 14) the cheapest is **Ferrous Sulphate Compound Tablets B.P.C.** Adults preferring fluid forms can take Ferric Ammonium Citrate Mixture B.P.C. 10ml containing 2g of ferric ammonium citrate, or mixtures or syrups e.g. Ferrous Fumarate Mixture B.P.C. ('Fersamal') 45mg Fe/5ml. Sodium Ironedetate ('Sytron') 27.5mg Fe/5ml, Ferrous aminoacetosulphate ('Plesmet') 25mg Fe/5ml and Ferrous Sulphate Mixture B.P.C. 10ml. Babies and children can have Ferric Ammonium Citrate Paediatric B.P.C. 5ml containing 400mg/5ml, or Ferrous Sulphate Mixture B.P.C. 5ml containing 60mg ferrous sulphate equivalent to 18mg of iron (Fe). They are given thrice daily in milk. **Slow release iron** is convenient as it can be taken once daily, but preparations are expensive and its absorption (which normally takes place in the duodenum and upper jejunum) may not be adequate. One or 2 tablets provide 90-130mg of iron e.g. 'Feospan', 'Ferro-Gradumet', 'Fersaday', 'Ferrocap', 'Fersamal' and 'Slow Fe'.

A course of iron treatment lasts at least 2 months. The aim is to treat the anaemia and to replenish body stores. Therefore iron is continued for a month or so after the haemoglobin is normal. In women several courses may be necessary each year. In addition to iron deficiency anaemia some resistant mucocutaneous forms of candidiasis may only clear up after a course of iron, irrespective of anaemia. Dermatologists have also noted that idiopathic pruritus may at times also respond to iron therapy and some patients with the restless leg syndrome may also respond.

If suboptimal, or no response occurs in anaemia it may mean (1) failure to take the iron, (2) failure to absorb iron because of slow-release, poor disintegration, or intestinal malabsorption states, (3) blood loss is taking place perhaps from cancer, or (4) the diagnosis is wrong e.g. thalassaemia minor, anaemia of infection, or sideroblastic anaemia. A response to iron starts in 4-6 days. The haemoglobin rises optimally 1.5g per week. A response to iron does not exclude a serious underlying cause and iron wrongly given, by mouth or injection, can eventually cause haemosiderosis and liver disease.

Disadvantages of Oral Iron
Gastric and intestinal discomfort, sickness, constipation and diarrhoea occur in about 25%. These complaints depend on how much iron is taken and absorbed and may be lessened by starting or limiting the daily dose to 1 or 2 tablets taken with food. Iron pills may be mistaken for sweets with fatal or serious consequences in children, causing haematemesis, shock and liver damage. The antidote is desferrioxamine (p. 241). The patient is told the stools will go black.

Injectable Iron
Only a few patients need parenteral iron (it should not be given to children). Such patients are those who fail to absorb iron, have persistent intolerance as in ulcerative colitis, or are uncooperative or unreliable. Total dose infusions are sometimes given for convenience and in late pregnancy. Iron injections have their risks. Given i.m. they cause pain, redness, and tissue staining. Total dose infusions and intravenous bolus injections can cause anaphylaxis with sweating, nausea, flushing, chest pain, circulatory failure, shock and rarely death. Some arm or shoulder pain is common as is phlebitis. Injected iron is quickly excreted and can cause bladder irritation. Oral and injected iron should not be given concurrently. If the plasma carrier protein is saturated by oral therapy, iron injections may be followed in a few hours by toxic (due to free plasma iron) symptoms such as headache, nausea, vomiting, dizziness, loss of taste, myalgia, abdominal pain, lacrimation, chest pain, shock and death. If a patient has taken oral iron continuously and iron injections need to be given an interval of several days should occur after stopping oral iron. Iron injections are harmful in aplastic and haemolytic anaemias as iron overload of the liver and splenic stores results. In paroxysmal nocturnal haemoglobinuria iron can precipitate an haemolytic crisis.

Preparations
Iron Sorbitol Injection B.P. ('Jectofer') *presentation* ampoules 2ml containing

50mg Fe/ml; *dose* 1.5mg Fe/kg B.W. which is 100mg, or 1 ampoule daily for an average adult. For a complete course 20-30 injections may be necessary. They are given deeply i.m. **Iron Dextran Injection B.P.** ('Imferon', 'Ironorm') *presentation* ampoules 2, 5 and 20ml (for total dose infusion) 50mg Fe/ml; *dose* 1-5ml daily by deep i.m. injection as it stains the skin, or by a series of i.v. injections, or infusions including total dose. Disposable syringes containing 2ml are available ('Imferon D'). An infusion should be given at 10 drops/min for the first 30 min.

MEGALOBLASTIC ANAEMIAS

These arise from vitamin B_{12}, folic acid and perhaps vitamin C lack and from the adverse effects of cytotoxic and other drugs. Vitamin B_{12} compounds are present in meat, milk and eggs. To be absorbed they combine with the intrinsic factor made by the stomach. Absorption occurs in the terminal ileum, storage in the liver and they act on the bone marrow. Body stores are maintained by 2-5μg daily and if not replaced last 3-4 years. Dietary deficiency occurs in strict vegans (common in certain Indian sects). The cobalamins are destroyed by heat and alkalies. A pint of milk 580ml contains 1-2μg, 1 egg 0.3μg and an average mixed diet 2-5μg. Vegetable sources include yeast extract vegetable savoury 10μg/30g 'Barmene', a vegetable milk 'Plamil' 10μg/28ml, and 'Velactin' 2.8μg/28ml. Deficiency also occurs where there is lack of intrinsic factor (pernicious anaemia post gastrectomy, or when cancer destroys the gastric mucosa), failure to absorb (coeliac disease, tropical sprue, ileal disease e.g. Crohn's disease) or competition for it as a nutrient by bacteria (blind loops, intestinal strictures, diverticula post-gastrectomy) or by fish tapeworm. The megaloblastic anaemia caused by bacteria utilizing vitamin B_{12} can be reversed by tetracycline therapy.

Hydroxocobalamin ('Cobalin H', 'Neo-Cytamen') is preferable to cyanocobalamin because being highly bound to plasma proteins less is excreted and it is retained longer. Most people require supplements every 2-3 months. A few are 'short responders' and need more frequent doses. *Presentation* Injection B.P. a solution in ampoules 1ml containing 250 and 1000μg; *dose* 250-1000μg every other day initially then 1000μg i.m. every few months. Hydroxocobalamin is used for tobacco amblyopia and for continued nitroprusside therapy. **Cyanocobalamin** ('Cytamen', 'Hepacon-B_{12}') is a semi-synthetic pharmaceutically stable derivative used orally and parenterally. Parenteral use should be confined to the Schilling test and the rare patient allergic to hydroxocobalamin. *Presentation* Injections Ph. Eur., B.P. a solution containing 250 and 1000μg; *dose* 1000μg (1mg) daily for several days then 250μg i.m. weekly until the anaemia is cured thereafter 250μg every 3-4 weeks. **Oral Vitamin B_{12}** ('Cytacon') as tablets or syrup can be absorbed in Addisonian anaemia if massive pharmacological amounts are given. Normally this is unnecessary as it is expensive and injections are better. However, rarely allergy can result from injected B_{12}. Oral B_{12} in physiological amounts can be given to strict vegans, or alternatively they can be given injections. There is also a case for giving oral B_{12} to all pregnant vegan women. It is of interest that B_{12} lack can cause infertility. A dietary history must be taken in all Asians.

A poor or suboptimal response to B_{12} therapy in megaloblastic anaemia usually means associated infection, hypothyroidism, co-existing iron lack, a wrong diagnosis, or cancer of the stomach. *Adverse effects* allergy, rarely hypokalaemia, fluid retention.

Folic Acid Deficiency
Folic Acid (Folates) occurs in all foods containing yeast, liver, green vegetables, cereals, nuts and fruit. Cooking however destroys folic acid. Folates are absorbed in the jejunum. Folate lack is the commonest vitamin deficiency in the world. Its function is to aid DNA synthesis and aminoacid metabolism. The normal requirements are about 50-70µg daily. Stores only last a few months. Deficiency arises from:
(1) a poor diet in the elderly, in alcoholics and in the chronically physically and mentally ill, and after prolonged i.v. feeding in intensive care units.
(2) small gut malabsorption in partial gastrectomy, coeliac disease, tropical sprue, and dermatogenic enteropathy.
(3) increased needs in pregnancy, lactation, malignancy, haemolytic, sickle cell and myeloproliferative anaemias, rheumatoid arthritis, Crohn's disease, and psoriasis.
(4) loss in renal dialysis, and interference with folate metabolism by anticonvulsants, methotrexate, oral contraceptives, co-trimoxazole, alcohol, and pyrimethamine.
Folic Acid ('Folvite') *presentation* Tablets B.P. 5mg (Tablets U.S.P. 100 and 250µg, 1mg and 5mg, and an injection 5mg/ml); *dose* orally 5-15mg daily. A major indication is pregnancy and many preparations exist combining iron with physiological amounts of folic acid e.g. 'Folex 350', 'Pregaday'.
Cytotoxic drugs cause megaloblastic anaemia by interference with DNA synthesis.

HAEMOLYTIC ANAEMIA
Often red cells are destroyed by infections e.g. malaria or mycoplasma, chemical poisons or drugs. Here the treatment is of the cause. Auto-immune haemolysis may be secondary to a variety of diseases (e.g. reticuloses, connective tissue diseases, some leukaemias), or have no obvious cause. In this group corticosteroids, immunosuppressives and splenectomy are of help. Red cells deficient in glucose 6-phosphate dehydrogenase (an enzyme) are haemolysed by many oxidant drugs (see p. 249) and this particularly afflicts Negroes and Mediterranean peoples. Repeated blood transfusions in the haemoglobinopathies e.g. thalassaemia cause iron overload which needs correction.

LEUKAEMIA
The treatment of acute leukaemia is best carried out in special units which may use varying schedules. Details of the drugs used, the cytotoxics and corticosteroids, are discussed in Chapters 9 and 11. Problems arise from long-term toxicity of the drugs and from infection.

Acute Leukaemia
Cytotoxic drugs are usually employed with corticosteroids, blood and platelet transfusion and antibiotics. Combined therapy causes remissions in 90% of children with *acute lymphoblastic leukaemia,* by using prednisone 60mg daily or 40mg/m^2 daily with vincristine. Possibly, even better results may occur if doxorubicin, daunorubicin, or colospase are added. Remissions are maintained with intermittent methotrexate i.v., or i.m. 30mg/m^2 twice weekly, cyclophosphamide, or mercaptopurine. Cranial-spinal x-ray therapy, and intrathecal methotrexate 10mg/m^2, 5 or more injections in spaced courses, prevent relapse from meningeal leukaemia since not all cytotoxics cross the

blood-brain barrier to eradicate malignant cells there. In *acute myeloblastic leukaemia* perhaps 50-60% improve with cytotoxic drug combinations e.g. cytarabine with doxorubicin, daunorubicin or thioguanine. The results are poor in adults over 60. One schedule is thioguanine 120mg daily orally for 5 days, daunorubicin 40mg i.v. on the first day, cytarabine 50mg i.v. daily for 5 days and prednisolone 50mg orally daily. There is an interval of 9 days between courses and there may be 6 courses. Stimulation of the immunological system nonspecifically with B.C.G. or whooping cough vaccine or specifically with irradiated tumour cells from donors (allogenic) may prolong survival in acute myeloblastic leukaemia. This may be given weekly with monthly 7 day consolidation courses of drugs (Day 1 doxorubicin 60mg i.v., vincristine 2mg i.v., days 1-5 prednisolone 100mg daily and days 5, 6, 7 cytarabine 160mg i.v.).

Chronic Leukaemia
Lymphatic. Often treatment is not necessary in the early stages, otherwise **Chlorambucil** 100-200μg/kg B.W. (e.g. 5-12mg) is given daily initially with a maintenance dose of 1-4mg daily. For associated haemolysis corticosteroids help and for local lymphadenopathy if marked radiotherapy. If there is hypogammaglobulinaemia injections of human immunoglobulins can be tried.
Myeloid. Here the most suitable drug is **Busulphan;** the dose is initially 2-6mg reduced later to 500μg-2mg daily. The aim is to achieve a white cell count of about 20 000/mm^3 and a rise in haemoglobin. If busulphan loses its effect alternatives are available (Chapter 9). Death occurs in about 3-4 years as a result of transformation to an acute myeloblastic anaemia. In chronic leukaemias radiotherapy although useful is not as affective as drug therapy. Anaemia is controlled by transfusions and bleeding by platelet transfusions and local measures. Splenectomy in selected cases may help.

HAEMORRHAGIC DISORDERS
Bleeding is due to coagulation or clotting defects, platelet deficiency or capillary damage.
(1) *Lack of clotting factors* is seen in haemophilia (Factor VIII deficiency) and Christmas disease (Factor IX deficiency). Haemophilia is treated with human antihaemophilic globulin (AHG) either cryoprecipitate, lyophilized freeze-dried AHG or occasionally fresh blood or plasma, but the latter contain a low concentration of AHG (see Chapter 28 on blood-products). Human AHG is the treatment of choice, but animal AHG derived from beef or pig is also available. AHG is used to control spontaneous haemorrhage, or for planned surgical procedures. Christmas disease is treated by Factor IX concentrates available from special centres or as 'Proplex' (Hyland-Travenol) or 'Prothromblex' (Immuno Ltd).
(2) *Low Platelet Disorders.* Platelets stop bleeding largely by sticking to and mechanically plugging defects in small vessels. In addition they liberate a platelet factor which initiates clotting. Thrombocytopenia may be due to blood disorders, infection, drug sensitivity and cirrhosis. The idiopathic form is treated with corticosteroids, cytotoxics, or splenectomy. Platelet concentrates are available from the National Tranfusion Centres for use in selected cases.
(3) *Capillary Diseases.* Scurvy is treated by vitamin C.

MARROW DAMAGE
Agranulocytosis is often due to drugs such as chloramphenicol, phenylbutazone, or amidopyrine. Death may occur from infection.

Marrow Failure (aplastic and hypoplastic anaemias). The marrow fails to produce red cells, white cells or platelets either singly or collectively. The reason may be unknown, or due to drugs, industrial poisons, or radiation. Treatment is withdrawal of cause if known and if due to arsenic or gold dimercaprol can be given. Treatment otherwise is by: (1) blood transfusions (2) patient isolation to prevent infection and antibiotics for infection which because of a low white cell count is common (3) platelet transfusions for bleeding episodes (4) corticosteroids are occasionally helpful (5) anabolic steroids. **Oxymetholone** ('Anapolon 50') is the one of choice although testosterone derivatives may also be tried. *Presentation* Tablets B.P. 50mg; *dose* 2-5mg/kg B.W., or 250-350mg daily for an average adult. The steroid has to be given for months before improvement may occur and success is more likely in children. *Adverse effects* commonly fluid retention, occasionally jaundice and the possibility of the development of hepatoma a liver cell cancer. (6) marrow transplants have been performed with success in some patients.
Myeloproliferative Disorders. Polycythaemia rubra vera is treated initially and rapidly by venesection and maintenance of lower levels is achieved by radioactive phosphorus in a dose of 2-5millicuries. Thrombosis is common and is treated by anticoagulants. Other complications which require therapy are acute leukaemia, marrow failure and gout. Busulphan is useful in the treatment of myelofibrosis. Primary thrombocythaemia is treated by radioactive phosphorus. This takes time to work and pyrimethamine can be used to lower platelet levels until the phosphorus works.

SIDEROBLASTIC ANAEMIAS
These are disorders of iron incorporation into haem. Drug-induced causes are pyridoxine antagonists (isoniazid, cycloserine, pyrazinamide, alcohol, chloramphenicol, phenacetin). In primary cases oral pyridoxine 100mg thrice daily is worth trying. Folic acid and vitamin B_{12} status should be assessed as megaloblastosis can co-exist. In some patients blood transfusions are needed and parenteral desferrioxamine may prevent overload of iron.

24 VITAMINS

These are essential for growth and nutrition. Vitamins are either fat soluble A,D,E, and K or water soluble B complex and C. Deficiency results from dietary neglect from poverty or apathy in the elderly, in poorly-fed children, the insane, those with gut disease, alcoholism, inborn errors of metabolism or drug addiction. Vitamin deficiency is common among Asian immigrants who may suffer from rickets or osteomalacia. In India millions are suffering from vitamin lack which can cause blindness. Adequate vitamins are necessary in those growing fast, in pregnancy, lactation and those on special diets lacking essential vitamins.

Fat Soluble Vitamins
Vitamin A, or retinol. Natural sources including its precursor carotene are the dairy products milk, butter, marine foods, fish and liver oils and carrots. Deficiency leads to a dry skin, corneal damage and night blindness. *Therapeutic* daily dosage is 10 000-25 000u, *prophylactic dose* 2500-5000u. *Presentation* Halibut Liver Oil Capsules B.P. 3500-4700u each; other sources are Cod-liver Oil B.P. and 'Ro-a-vit' tablets 50 000u. Roche supply an injection 'Arovit' 300 000u/ml on a named patient basis for use i.m. in malabsorption. *Hypervitaminosis* with doses of 100 000u daily for months, anorexia, itching, weight loss, liver and spleen enlargement, skin desquamation, painful bones and joints may result and if acute raised intracranial pressure.
Vitamin D. Natural sources of vitamin D_3 or cholecalciferol are dairy products and fish oils. It can be produced by the action of ultra violet light on the skin. *Function* it is really a hormone and is converted into the active metabolite by first the liver and then the kidneys (into 1,25-dihydroxycholecalciferol) and it aids the calcification and maturation of bone. Other actions are on the gut and kidney. *Uses;* to treat rickets, osteomalacia and hypocalcaemia when they are caused by vitamin deficiency, or resistance to its action and for its parathyroid hormone-like action. *Doses* For therapy vitamin D_2 or **ergocalciferol** is used. This is produced from irradiated yeast. The potency varies between batches and brands which is a disadvantage in stabilizing a patient. *Therapeutic amounts* daily for ordinary rickets or osteomalacia are 5000-50 000u and for renal rickets up to 400 000u. *Prophylactic amounts* are 400u daily. *Preparations* Calciferol Tablets Strong (High Dose) B.P. 50 000u (1.25mg) and the weaker Calcium with Vitamin D Tablets B.P.C. containing 500u (12.5µg).
Dihydrotachysterol is chemically similar, acts quickly and is used postoperatively after parathyroidectomy. It is available as a solution 250µg/ml ('AT 10'); *dose* 1-10ml or 200µg tablets ('Tachyrol'). Because supplies of calciferol are decreasing **cholecalciferol B.P.** (Vitamin D_3) will be increasingly used. It is equipotent with Vitamin D_2 and less likely to be oxidized.
   Vitamins A and D Capsules B.P.C. contain 4000u of vitamin A and 400u (11µg) of vitamin D. Calciferol Solution B.P. contains 75µg/ml in vegetable oil for oral use, Calciferol Injection B.P.C. is supplied in ampoules 2ml 300 000u/ml, 'Sterogyl 15' contains 600 000u/ml in 1.5ml ampoules. *Hypervitaminosis* children receiving 1800u daily, may have poor appetite; toxicity occurs with over 20 000u daily and leads to sickness, headache, polyuria, renal

calcification, and renal damage. Barbiturates and other anticonvulsants change vitamin D to inactive metabolites and hypocalcaemia and osteomalacia can result.

Vitamin K. *Source* there are two natural vitamins: K_1 present in green foods and vegetables, and K_2 produced intestinally by bacteria. *Function* essential for prothrombin synthesis in the liver. The natural vitamins are fat soluble and require bile salts for absorption. *Deficiency* leads to hypoprothrombinaemia, bleeding and delayed clotting and is caused by malabsorption, obstructive jaundice and drug therapy.

Synthetic Vitamin K_3. These are naphthaquinones with vitamin K activity. **Menaphthone Sodium Bisulphite** (Menadione Sodium Bisulfite) and the **Menadiol derivative** ('Synkavit') are water soluble and injected, the latter can be taken orally as well.

Natural Vitamin K_1 Phytomenadione (Phytonadione U.S.A.) is the preferred preparation and is indicated when speed is required to neutralize anticoagulants, and in hypoprothrombinaemia in the newborn. *Presentation* Tablets B.P. 10mg ('Konakion'), Injection B.P. in ampoules 1mg/0.5ml and 10mg/1ml ('Aquamephyton', 'Konakion') as an aqueous colloidal solution, and a water miscible solution 1mg/0.5ml ('Konakion'). *Dose* orally 5-20mg, s.c., or i.m. 5-20mg; i.v. in emergencies 5-50mg for adults slowly at a rate of 5mg/min, and for infants $500\mu g$-1mg. For liver disease with biliary obstruction especially if laparotomy is to be performed, and intestinal malabsorption 10mg is injected i.m. For the prophylaxis of hypoprothrombinaemia of the newborn $500\mu g$-1mg is given i.m. and for actual haemorrhage 1mg. Babies born of mothers taking anticonvulsants should be given prophylactic vitamin K_1 as they are liable to spontaneous haemorrhage. In pregnancy should the mother who is being treated with oral anticoagulants go into early labour (before being changed to heparin) she is given vitamin K_1. If not the baby is liable to bleed from trauma into the brain, body cavities and from the umbilicus. The baby with hypoprothrombinaemia is given vitamin K_1, fresh frozen plasma or fresh blood (e.g. 40ml) or even an exchange transfusion. In anticoagulant overdosage, if mild, oral doses 10-20mg suffice, or if severe, up to 50mg i.v. Rapid administration causes facial flushing, sweating, chest constriction, circulatory shock. Large doses of vitamin K_1 should be avoided if it is intended to continue with anticoagulants. For severe haemorrhage fresh blood is advised. Neonates may not respond to vitamin K_1 because of hepatic immaturity.

Vitamin E or **Alpha Tocopheryl Acetate Ph. Eur., B.P.** has been used for acanthocytosis in children (an anaemia with lipoprotein deficiency and brain disease). Brand product 'Ephynal' tablets 3,10, 50 and 200mg.

Water Soluble Vitamins

Vitamin B complex includes vitamins B_1 (thiamine), B_2 (riboflavine), nicotinic acid and nicotinamide, B_6 (pyridoxine) and pantothenic acid. They are concerned with carbohydrate, fat and protein metabolism.

Vitamin B_1 Ph. Eur. (Aneurine, Thiamine) natural sources are egg, liver, wheat germ, peas, beans, and fresh vegetables. *Function* the oxidation of carbohydrates and the metabolism of brain and nervous tissue. Adult requirements are 1-2mg daily. *Deficiency* occurs with high carbohydrate diets such as polished rice, with starvation, diarrhoea, alcoholism, liver disease, and thyrotoxicosis. Symptoms are painful neuritis, cardiac enlargement and failure, oedema, nausea, vomiting in beri-beri; Wernicke's encephalopathy (mid-brain haemorrhages and ocular palsy) and Korsakow's syndrome of mental confusion and confabulation. *Presentation* Thiamine Hydrochloride, Tablets, B.P. 3, 10, 25, 50, 100 and 300mg, Injection B.P. solution in ampoules 25 and 100mg/ml; *dose* 50-100mg daily orally, i.m. or in cardiac failure i.v. Brand products include 'Benerva'.

Riboflavine Ph. Eur. (Vitamin B₂) means the yellow substance. Natural sources are liver, milk, yeast and green vegetables. *Requirements* are 1-3mg daily. *Deficiency* causes angular stomatitis, sore magenta coloured tongue, and seborrhoeic dermatitis. *Presentation* Tablets B.P.C. 3mg, Injection U.S.P. for i.m. or i.v. use. *Dose* therapeutic 6-60mg.

Nicotinic Acid (Niacin) is changed in the body to the active form nicotinamide. Natural sources; meat e.g. liver, yeast, unpolished rice, milk, vegetables. *Requirements* 15-30mg daily. *Deficiency* causes pellagra (dermatitis, dementia, diarrhoea, stomatitis, raw tongue, anorexia, tiredness). Secondary deficiency occurs in carcinoid syndrome and Hartnup's disease. *Presentation* Tablets B.P. 50mg; *dose* 100-500mg. Other uses are for peripheral vascular disease, Ménière's syndrome and hypercholesterolaemia. *Adverse effects* flushing, burning skin, hyperglycaemia. **Nicotinamide Ph. Eur.** (Niacinamide) is used in pellagra and is less likely to cause side effects. *Presentation* Tablets B.P.C. 50mg, Injection B.P. (1963) solution 50mg/ml.

Pyridoxine Ph. Eur. Vitamin B₆: natural sources include liver, yeast and cereals. Requirements are 1-2mg daily. *Deficiency* is rare but can occur with drugs like isoniazid and in rare childhood and adult sideroblastic anaemias, and pyridoxine responsive convulsions. *Presentation* Pyridoxine Hydrochloride Tablets B.P.C. 20 and 50mg; *dose* 20-150mg daily. Pyridoxine ('Benadon') is also prescribed as an anti-emetic in pregnancy, alcoholism, and irradiation sickness.

Vitamin B deficiency is usually multiple so compound preparations are available e.g. Vitamin B Compound Tablets B.P.C. (ordinary) and Vitamin B Compound Strong B.P.C. as well as 'Becosym', 'Benerva Compound', and Vitamins B and C Injection B.P.C. ('Parentrovite') containing aneurine (thiamine) hydrochloride 100 or 250mg, nicotinamide 160mg, riboflavine 4mg, pyridoxine hydrochloride 50mg and ascorbic acid is given i.m. or i.v. The contents of the paired ampoules are mixed just before use.

Ascorbic Acid Vitamin C ('Redoxon'): natural sources are citrus fruits, oranges, lemons, blackcurrants, rose hips, green vegetables. Cooking lowers the content. *Function* formation and maintenance of bone, cartilage and blood. *Requirements* in health vary from 20-75mg or more daily. *Deficiency* causes scurvy, anaemia, bone pain, and bleeding gums and can occur in bottle-fed babies, those inadequately fed, in the elderly and the mentally ill. *Presentation* Tablets B.P. 25, 50, 100, 200, 500 and 1000mg, Injection Sodium Ascorbate B.P.C. ampoules 5ml containing 500 and 1000mg.

Multivitamin preparations have few indications clinically. Vitamin Capsules B.P.C. (contain A 2500u, Thiamine 1mg, Riboflavine 500μg, Nicotinamide 7.5mg, C 15mg and D 300u) taken 2 or 3 daily. Vitamins A and D are present in 'Adexolin'. Multivitamin preparations include 'Abidec', 'Juvel', 'Multivite', 'Orovite'; vitamins and minerals are present in 'Minadex'. 'Multibionta' is a multivitamin supplement to accompany parenteral nutrition. (Vitamin A 10 000u, thiamine 50mg, riboflavin 10mg, nicotinamide 100mg, pantothenyl alcohol 25mg, ascorbic acid 500mg. αtocopheryl acetate 5mg. pyridoxine hydrochloride 15mg per 10ml ampoule).

25   OBESITY AND DIABETES MELLITUS

Obesity, the commonest nutritional disorder in developed countries, brings a decreased life expectancy and an increased risk of cardiac disease, diabetes mellitus, osteoarthritis, gallstones and psychological disorders. Treatment is based on a low energy diet with ample protein, iron and vitamins, but small amounts of fat (for palatability) and carbohydrates. The diet may have to be modified if type II or IV hyperlipidaemia is present. It is usual to start with 1000 Calories (4.2 mega Joules) composed of 100g of carbohydrate, 40g of fat and 60g of protein. With diets of 400 Calories or below the patient should be in hospital. Total or severe partial starvation is dangerous unsupervised and if prolonged is associated with sudden death from cardiac muscle disease and hypokalaemia. Dieting must take into account the patient's dietary habits, customs, religion, intelligence, finance and emotional state. Both the patient and relatives must be involved. Bulk diets of filling green foods and water may help, or artificial bulk such as methylcellulose which swells in the stomach so reducing hunger e.g. 'Celevac' and 'Cellucon'. Special powdered foods enriched with vitamins, proteins and vegetable oils are available but expensive e.g. 'Limmits' and 'Metercal'. When dieting genuinely fails drugs are tried. Diuretics cause temporary weight loss which encourages the patient, but otherwise have no merit unless obesity-heart failure or water retention is present. Psychotherapy may by relief of anxiety or depression help curb appetite. Exercise is encouraged.

Appetite Suppressants
Because of addiction and cardiac and C.N.S. stimulation non-amphetamines are preferred. In fact, however, three of the most popular anorexigenic drugs are amphetamine derivatives chemically, but they are not Controlled Drugs.
Fenfluramine Hydrochloride ('Ponderax') is widely prescribed. *Presentation* tablets 20 and 40mg and sustained action tablets 60mg; *dose* 40mg in divided amounts increasing to 120mg or 2mg/kg B.W. or slow-release tablet once or twice daily. Both increase and decrease of dosage should be in a stepwise manner.
Diethylpropion Hydrochloride ('Tenuate') *presentation* Tablets U.S.N.F. 25mg and slow release tablet 75mg; *dose* 25mg thrice daily, or once as 75mg delayed form. 'Apisate' contains diethylpropion. Insomnia, habituation and addiction occur. Diethylpropion is much cheaper than fenfluramine.
Phentermine ('Duromine', 'Ionamin') *presentation* capsules 15mg, or 30mg in slow release form. *Dose* one capsule at breakfast. Because of their sympathomimetic potential they are not prescribed with monoamine oxidase inhibitors, nor to people likely to be addicts because of personality defects. Fenfluramine can make patients drowsy, or depressed and can be given to anxious patients since it rarely makes them high, though aggression has been noted. Fenfluramine should be avoided in depression. It also causes diarrhoea. Another use for fenfluramine is to treat obese diabetics and it may be given to hypertensives and with hypotensive agents though it may potentiate their effects. Alcohol should not be taken while on fenfluramine. Phentermine and diethylpropion have mild stimulant actions, and can cause insomnia, agitation, tremor, convulsions, palpitation and dry mouth.

Mazindol ('Teronac') is an indole compound neither related to, nor metabolized to amphetamine but is a central nervous sytem stimulant. *Presentation* tablets 2mg; *dose* 2mg before the midday meal. *Adverse effects* are mild insomnia, dizziness, nervousness, chills, headaches. This is an expensive drug.

DIABETES MELLITUS

In diabetes mellitus there is either an actual lack or a relative insufficiency of insulin. Insulin made in the pancreatic islets of Langerhans is derived commercially from cattle or pigs. Insulin lack causes failure to utilize efficiently carbohydrates, fats, or proteins. Hyperglycaemia, glycosuria, hyperketonaemia and fluid and electrolyte loss may occur. Insulin lowers the blood glucose, increases stores of liver glycogen, abolishes glycosuria and promotes the use of ketones, fats, glucose and aminoacids.

Types of diabetes acute insulin deficiency is typical of those under 40 years of age. The mature onset type with relative insufficiency is milder and usually occurs in overweight middle-aged women, who are treated by weight reduction.

Aims of treatment are to ensure the patient feels well and can work. The urine before meals should be relatively sugar free and the blood glucose between meals below 200mg/dl (11 mmol/l).

Carbohydrate if insulin is used the dietary carbohydrate is usually limited and apportioned through the day to suit the time relationships of the insulin. For adults 100-200g is enough since larger amounts need more frequent injections unless the patient is a heavy manual worker or is pregnant. *Portions* the carbohydrate foods for breakfast, mid-morning, lunch, tea, supper (dinner) and at night are prescribed in portions or amounts containing a fixed quantity of carbohydrate which may be 5, 10 or 15g. This ensures variety. The Diabetic Association recommend 10g portions be adopted in the U.K. so that diet sheets are interchangeable (Table 15).

Foods with little or no carbohydrates are *vegetables:* artichokes, asparagus, french beans, broccoli, brussel-sprouts, cabbage, cauliflower, celery, leeks, marrow, mushrooms, onions, spinach, turnips and swedes; *salads:* cress, cucumber, lettuce, radishes, tomatoes; *fruits:* gooseberries, grapefruit, melon, rhubarb; clear soups, tea, coffee, soda water, 'Oxo', 'Bovril', 'Marmite', diabetic fruit drinks, salt, pepper, vinegar, mustard and lemon.

Protein is not limited except in renal failure and 2g/kg B.W. is allowed for children. Fat is curtailed in the obese and those with hyperlipidaemia.

INSULIN

Insulin is given when control is impossible by other means. It is usually injected s.c. into either upper arm, thigh, buttock or abdomen.

TABLE 15

WEIGHTS OF COMMON FOODS
CONTAINING 10g OF CARBOHYDRATE*

Food	Weight (oz)	How weighed
Apples	4	with skin
	3	peeled
	5	stewed without sugar
Bananas	2	without skin
Beetroot	4	boiled
Biscuits	½	average plain
Bread	⅔	white or brown
Carrots	8	boiled
Cereals		
(breakfast)	½	as bought
Cherries	4	raw with stones
	4	stewed without sugar
Damsons	5	stewed without sugar
Grapefruit	12	with skin
Grapes	2	fresh
Horlicks	½	
Milk	7	fresh
Milk evaporated	3	
Onions	14	boiled
Onions, spring	4	raw
Oranges	5½	with skin
	4	peeled
Ovaltine	½	
Parsnips	3	boiled
Peaches	4	fresh whole
Pears	4	fresh with skin
	5	stewed unsugared
Peas (green)	4½	young boiled
	3	average boiled
	2	tinned
Pineapple	3	fresh eatable portion
Plums	4	ripe Victoria
	6½	ripe smaller varieties
	8	stewing plums
Potatoes	2	boiled
	1	fried
Ryvita	½	
Strawberries	6	fresh ripe
Swedes	9½	boiled
Toast	½	
Tomatoes	12	raw, cooked, tinned

*Based on recommendations of the British Diabetic Association.
1 oz=30g

Rapid Action (Under 8 Hours)
Insulin Injection Ph. Eur., B.P. an acid solution pH 3 of beef origin ('soluble', 'clear', 'regular' or crystalline insulin) is effective, simple, safe and widely used. It is the insulin of choice in diabetic coma and during the stress of infection, operation, labour or injury. It is a popular twice or more daily regime because of its flexibility for use in children and active adults. It may be combined with long-acting insulins e.g. protamine zinc or isophane. *Administration* it is rapidly absorbed given s.c., acts in 20-30min with maximum effect in 3-4 hours and has little action after 6 hours. It may also be given i.m., or i.v. but the duration of action is brief. *Presentation* strength 20, 40, 80 and 320u/ml. *Dose* usually 20-60u 30min before breakfast and the main evening meal. The diet is arranged so that most carbohydrate is taken in the 4-6 hours after each injection.
Neutral Insulin Injection B.P. is a clear neutral solution (pH 7) of pork ('Actrapid MC', 'Leo Neutral'), or beef ('Nuso') origin. It begins to work in 30 min, with a peak effect at 2-4 hours and total duration of 6-8 hours. The strengths are 40 and 80u/ml and its uses and administration are as for soluble insulin, but it can be given in the same syringe as delayed acting insulins. Being a neutral solution it may cause less local reactions than the acidic Insulin Injection B.P. Ordinary, monocomponent and rarely immunogenic forms are available.

Delayed Action (Intermediate) Insulins
Globin Zinc Insulin Injection B.P. acts in 2 hours with peak effect at 6-12 hours and a duration of 16 hours. It is a clear solution with a pH of 3-3.5 used for mild diabetes and now largely superseded. Strength 80u/ml; administration s.c.
Isophane Insulin Injection Ph. Eur., B.P. (NPH) is a neutral cloudy suspension of beef insulin crystals in protamine and zinc with a pH of just over 7 which acts after 2 hours, has a peak effect in 10-12 hours and total duration of approximately 24 hours. It is poorly soluble in body fluids. Isophane insulin may be given once or twice daily, either alone, or with soluble or neutral insulins in the same syringe. It acts like globin insulin and its advantages over protamine zinc insulin are that it contains less protamine, and it has a shorter action thus being less likely to cause nocturnal hypoglycaemia. When mixed with soluble insulin it interferes less with its rapid action than PZI. 'Leo Retard' is a rarely immunogenic highly purified form.
Insulin Zinc Suspensions have no added protein which lessens the chances of allergic reactions. By altering the size of the suspended particles the speed of absorption and duration of action can be altered.
Insulin Zinc Suspension (Amorphous) Ph. Eur., B.P. with a pH of 7-7.5 (Semi-Lente Insulin) is composed of small rapidly absorbed particles of beef origin and behaves like soluble insulin acting in 30 minutes, with peak action at 2-4 hours but a duration of 12 hours and is given twice daily. It is now available as 'Semitard MC' a highly purified monocomponent porcine insulin. I.Z.S. Crystalline has larger crystals and hence a more delayed action and longer duration (see below).
Insulin Zinc Suspension Ph. Eur., B.P. (Lente Insulin) is a cloudy neutral suspension of water insoluble beef insulin crystals in zinc chloride which is made up of 3 parts of the quick I.Z.S. Amorphous and 7 parts of I.Z.S. Crystalline, the combination acts in 30-60 min with a peak effect at 4-8 hours and lasts up

TABLE 16
STRENGTHS AND TYPES OF INSULIN IN THE UK

Rapid Action Insulins

Insulin Injection (Soluble)
- 20u/ml
- 40u/ml
- 80u/ml
- 320u/ml

Neutral ('Nuso', 'Actrapid M.C.'
  'Leo Neutral')
- 40u/ml
- 80u/ml

Delayed Action Insulins

Globin Zinc   80u/ml

Isophane (Standard and 'Leo Retard')
- 40u/ml
- 80u/ml

I.Z.S. Amorphous ('Semi-Lente', 'Semitard M.C.')
- 40u/ml
- 80u/ml

I.Z.S. Crystalline ('Ultra-Lente', 'Ultratard M.C.')
- 40u/ml
- 80u/ml

I.Z.S. ('Lente', 'Lentard M.C.', 'Monotard M.C.')
- 40u/ml
- 80u/ml

Biphasic ('Rapitard M.C.', 'Leo Mixtard', 'Leo Initard')
- 40u/ml
- 80u/ml

Protamine Zinc
- 40u/ml
- 80u/ml

to 24-36 hours. It is used both for the initial control and for the maintenance of stabilized diabetics, of mild to moderate severity. Dose initially 20u increasing by 4-8u every few days up to 80-100u daily. Many patients are suited to this mixture, but the 3:7 ratio is not suitable for every person's eating habits and escape from control readily occurs with infection, trauma, operation and pregnancy and after a time, inexplicably. Novo Lente has been replaced by monocomponent 'Lentard M.C.' of beef and pork origin and by 'Monotard M.C.' which is 100% porcine of similar duration.

Biphasic Insulin Injection B.P. ('Rapitard M.C.') is composed of 1 part of a neutral (pH 7) solution of pork insulin mixed with 3 parts of crystalline undissolved insulin of beef origin together making a cloudy mixture. It works in 30 min with a peak action at 4-12 hours, and total duration of 18-22 hours. It has similar uses to I.Z.S. and is now monocomponent.

Prolonged Action Insulins

Protamine Zinc Insulin Injection Ph. Eur., B.P. (P.Z.I.) is a cloudy suspension pH 6.9-7.4 of insulin in protamine a fish sperm protein and zinc chloride. Given before breakfast it starts to work 4-6 hours later with a peak effect at 8-20 hours and total duration of 24-36 hours. Mild diabetes can be controlled on this alone in a dose up to 40u daily. Its main use is with soluble insulin and it is given once daily. The soluble form is drawn up first and then the P.Z.I. so as to prevent it entering the soluble insulin bottle. Alternatively, separate syringes are used. Allergy to it may arise. The carbohydrate portions are spread evenly throughout the day as they are with the other delayed action insulins though some transfer of portions may be necessary according to the blood sugars and symptoms.

Insulin Zinc Suspension (Crystalline) or Ultra-Lente Insulin is a cloudy neutral solution which acts in 2-3 hours with peak effect at 7-10 hours and total duration of 24-36 hours. It is usually mixed with I.Z.S., I.Z.S. Amorphous or Insulin Injection in varying proportions. It is now available in the highly purified 'Ultratard M.C.' of bovine origin.

All insulins are labelled according to their animal source, pork or beef insulin. All British insulins in practice are bovine. Imported insulins are porcine (Nordisk) or porcine, bovine or mixed (Novo). In the U.S.A. ordinary insulins are porcine, bovine or mixed. In some patients a change from bovine to a non-British porcine insulin may help and at times a change in brand. Biologically, porcine insulin is closer to human insulin. Bovine and partially bovine insulins being more antigenic are liable to cause insulin resistance and on transferring to a pork insulin the dose *may have to be reduced significantly.* Crystalline insulin is impure containing pro-insulin, a larger molecule which by cleavage forms insulin, intermediates and dimers (two insulin molecules bound together) as well as insulin. Purification is achieved by chemical and physical means. Highly purified insulins are finding increasing use (e.g. new patients) extraction yields having increased to satisfactory levels. They greatly reduce antibody formation, and reactions and fat atrophy at injection sites are less. Highly purified insulins available in the U.K. are from **Nordisk** (via Leo Laboratories)—Neutral ('Leo Neutral'), Isophane ('Leo-Retard') and Biphasic ('Leo-Mixtard 30/70' and 'Initard 50/50') all porcine; and from **Novo** the monocomponent 'M.C.' insulins 'Actrapid', 'Semitard', and 'Monotard' all porcine; 'Lentard' and 'Rapitard' bovine and porcine, and 'Ultratard' bovine, Single component insulins are produced by Lilly (for U.S.A.) and are U-100 strength only, and supplied as porcine, or bovine insulin by special order, (Lente, Regular, Isophane, P.Z.I.).

Shaking the bottle the clear insulins (Soluble, Neutral or Globin) need no shaking before use, P.Z.I. and Isophane are cloudy and settle in a deposit and require gentle shaking. The cloudy I.Z.S. preparations need vigorous shaking.

Strengths of insulin are shown in Table 16. They are supplied in 5 and 10ml multidose vials. Identification of type of insulin and strength is by the writing on the vial label rather than colour codes. In the U.S.A. the usual strength is U-100 (orange cap) with a U-100 syringe; but U-40 (red cap) and U-80 (green cap) are available. Lilly also make a U-500 strength for use in insulin resistance. Identifying letters on American labels are R (insulin injection), G (Globin zinc insulin), N (Isophane insulin suspension), L (Lente insulin), S (Semilente), U (Ultralente) and P (Protamine zinc insulin).

Storage insulin is kept cool, but not frozen. An expiratory date is on the label.

Measurement of dosage British clinics use the B.S. 1619 syringe with 1 and 1.5ml capacity with Luer fittings and needles. The barrel has 20 equal divisions/ml. The number of units of insulin contained in each division varies with the strength of the insulin. The patient frequently gets the dose wrong; the syringe, insulin strength and amount drawn up should be checked frequently in the clinic. Nurses and, at times doctors, confuse between marks on the syringe and the dose in units. If a doctor, or a nurse, injects a patient not known previously to them they should ask the patient to show his insulin dose card, or to write down the dose he is taking. *Care of syringes and needles* Disposable syringes and needles are best and cheaper in the long run and are more convenient for carrying around. The injection sites should be varied systematically so that no one site is used more than once per month.

Where treated if a patient needs insulin it is advantageous to start therapy in hospital where he can be instructed how and where to inject, the care of syringes and needles, diet, hygiene and given information about his illness. It is possible to teach these matters as an out-patient or by the district nurse. Close follow-up with careful control of diet and insulin dosage should be emphasized.

Complications of Insulin Therapy

Hypoglycaemia. Insulin overdosage causes apprehension, blurred vision, shakiness, hunger, sweating, weakness, difficulty in thought and speech, aggressive behaviour, convulsions, dementia and coma. It is the commonest cause of coma in a diabetic. Other features are angina, cerebrovascular insufficiency, fatigue and hunger pain. A reactive hyperglycaemia may follow (a Somogyi effect with see-saw control). Hypoglycaemia results from delayed or omitted meals, extra exertion, uneven absorption of insulin, insufficient carbohydrate content of diet, varying sensitivity to insulin action of a hormonal nature e.g. adrenal or pituitary disease and accidental or deliberate overdosage of insulin. Quick acting insulins cause rapid symptoms which respond to treatment. Long-acting insulins often produce headaches, and, relapsing hypoglycaemia after treatment is not uncommon. *Treatment* **Dextrose Injection Strong B.P.C.** a 50% solution is supplied in 50ml ampoules and at least 20ml (10g) is given i.v. If no i.v. dextrose is available **Adrenaline** 0.5-1ml of a 1:1000 solution is injected s.c. which promotes glucose formation from liver glycogen providing some is present. An alternative is **Glucagon** a pancreatic hormone which raises the blood sugar by mobilizing hepatic glycogen and will also correct hypoglycaemia. *Presentation* Glucagon Injection B.P. is a solution made from vials of powder containing 1 and 10u (previously mg) of Glucagon Hydrochloride with ampoules of suitable solvent 1ml and 10ml. *Dose* 0.5-1u s.c., i.m., or i.v. The dose may be repeated, if necessary every 20 min. Larger doses of 2u or more have been used to terminate insulin coma in psychiatry. If the patient is rousable he may be able to swallow sugar lumps, or take other food.

Acquired insulin resistance occurs when patients need more than 200u daily. The cause is formation of insulin antibodies (especially to bovine insulin), or the development of endocrinal disease. Improvement may follow corticosteroid therapy, or a change of insulin from bovine to porcine.

Local insulin allergy is common a few hours after injection and resembles inflammation. Typically seen in new diabetics it may settle spontaneously, or after changing the type or brand of insulin.

Generalized sensitivity to insulin is uncommon and rare with the protein free insulin zinc suspensions or the specially purified monocomponent insulins. It is manifested by rash and pruritus.

Local fat atrophy occurs at injection sites and consists of an ugly hollow. Fat hypertrophy and fibrotic areas occur which interfere with insulin absorption. Injections should not be repeated at the same site but rotated over a wide area.

DIABETIC COMA

The best results are obtained when one specially interested physician and his team undertake the care of all patients with diabetic coma in a hospital and the care is of 'intensive therapy unit' standard (care of coma, metabolic observations, accurate monitoring and charting of vital functions, results and treatment; nursing of precipitating illnesses and complications) and when there is a fully comprehensive round-the-clock laboratory back-up. Regimes vary, but common denominators are enthusiasm, expertise, flexibility and excitement over the management of this serious, but interesting condition.

(1) Therapy starts when seen at home, or if not, immediately on arrival at hospital.

(2) Fluid and electrolytes are replaced. Typical losses are fluids (3-12 litres), sodium (500mmol), chloride (400mmol), potassium (350mmol), magnesium (40mmol) and phosphorus (150mEq). An i.v. infusion is set up and **Sodium Chloride Injection B.P.** 0.9% is given rapidly at a rate of 120 drops/min for 1 or 2 litres. This helps to restore the blood pressure. In hyperosmolar coma 0.45% Sodium Chloride is usually given. Partial correction of the acidosis with **Sodium Bicarbonate Injection** 1.4% is a debatable procedure. When given the amount should be moderate (e.g. 1 bottle for every 3 of sodium chloride) since alkaline fluids can induce hypokalaemia and possibly cerebral oedema. **Potassium Chloride** may be needed from the onset if serum levels are low or indicate depletion (e.g. normal levels with a low blood pH). The accepted rate conventionally is up to 20mmol/h providing there is an adequate renal flow, but in expert hands this amount is often exceeded. In the recovery phase there is a diuresis and potassium and other electrolytes may be needed.

(3) Soluble insulin is always given, but the dose and mode of administration vary. Some regimes base the dose, which may be 40-200u, on the height of the initial blood sugar and it is given partially i.v. or i.m. Thereafter, insulin is injected 2-4 hourly until control occurs. Insulin counteracts acidosis by stopping the formation of ketoacids. Another technique is deliberately to give small but regular doses e.g. 6-10u i.m. hourly. This seems simple, safe and suitable for district hospitals as nurses can give it and there is less need for stringent biochemical control. A modification is to give 6-10u i.v. hourly in albumin solution, which stops the insulin sticking to the infusion apparatus. This needs a constant infusion pump.

(4) The stomach is decompressed by stomach tube as acute dilatation may occur, and most therapists would also have the bladder catheterized.

(5) When the blood sugar has fallen to 300mg/dl, (15mmol/l) or lower, Dextrose Injection B.P. 5% is commenced. The i.v. line is maintained until the ability to eat without feeling, or being, sick is demonstrated and ketosis has disappeared.

(6) The precipitating cause (infection, cardiac infarction, gastro-intestinal upset) is also treated.

(7) When measured hypoxia is often present and may require treatment.

(8) On recovery treatment is as for pre-coma.

Pre-coma is diabetic ketosis without impaired consciousness. Soluble insulin is given 4-6 hourly on a varying scale according to the amount of sugar in the urine and blood. If the patient is not vomiting 20g of carbohydrate is taken in a fluid or easily digested form 2 hourly. Salt supplements are needed.

Prevention of coma or ketosis. Fit diabetics will develop ketones in the urine if insulin is stopped, and unwell diabetics are more likely to do so. In infections insulin will need increasing under medical control. The patients must not stop insulin though the dose may have to be adjusted. If the appetite is poor insulin is given and the usual portions taken in fluid form. Two large lumps of sugar, 2 teaspoonfuls of glucose or sugar dissolved in water, or a cup of milk (7 oz) equal 10g of carbohydrate.

ORAL HYPOGLYCAEMIC AGENTS

Indications. *Control of mild diabetes* The patient who responds best is middle aged, has never had ketonuria and is not markedly overweight. If previously on insulin, control occurs with 40u or less. These drugs are relatively weak and provide poor control during stress. Liver and renal disease and probably pregnancy are contra-indications. However, sulphonylurea compounds are being used in pregnancy in some countries, for those who do not require insulin, do not show ketoacidosis and who maintain when treated a blood sugar below 150mg/dl (7mmol/l). Dieting is still necessary for those controlled by oral therapy. About a quarter of all diabetics can be treated with oral agents and diet. Reports from the U.S.A. have indicated the strong suspicion that there is an excess of vascular disease associated with the intake of tolbutamide and phenformin so that a re-interest is taking place in control by strict dieting alone. A response to oral therapy is usually evident within days of starting (unless there is primary failure). Loss of control through secondary failure may occur months or years after satisfactory control, and at times of intercurrent illness insulin may be needed. Chemically there are two main groups — sulphonylureas and biguanides.

Sulphonylureas

These lower the blood sugar by stimulating the pancreas to make and release insulin. **Tolbutamide Ph. Eur.** ('Orinase', 'Pramidex', 'Rastinon') was the first satisfactory compound. *Presentation* Tablets B.P. 500mg; *dose* 500mg q.d.s. with, or after meals at first, reduced to 500mg 2 or 3 times daily. The effect only lasts 8 hours and therefore it has been considered suitable for the elderly since prolonged hypoglycaemia is avoided. *Adverse effects* nausea, sickness, rash, alcohol intolerance and possibly vascular complications. **Chlorpropamide** ('Diabinese', 'Melitase') is widely used and has a prolonged action of 24-36 hours. *Presentation* Tablets B.P. 100 and 250mg; *dose* 100-350mg daily taken at breakfast. *Adverse effects* since it is slowly excreted it can cause dangerous hypoglycaemia especially in the aged and when intercurrent illness causes anorexia. By inappropriately potentiating ADH (anti diuretic hormone) it causes hyponatraemia and fluid retention which may induce or worsen heart failure and nocturnal angina. This water retaining effect is said not to occur with tolazamide, acetohexamide and glibenclamide. *Adverse effects* occur in about 5-10% and include gastro-intestinal disturbances (nausea, sickness, occasional cholestatic hepatitis), rashes (erythema multiforme, exfoliative dermatitis, phototoxic reactions), progressive rise in serum alkaline phosphatase and less frequently aplastic anaemia, leukopenia, alcohol intolerance (shown by vasomotor reactions with flushing, giddiness, tachycardia, headache, muscle weakness, and ataxia). **Tolazamide** ('Tolanase') *presentation* Tablets U.S.P. 100 and 250mg; *dose* 100-250mg up to 1g in divided doses daily. *Adverse effects* are mainly gastro-intestinal (nausea, vomiting and diarrhoea in about 2%). Hypoglycaemia and alcohol intolerance are claimed less than with chlorpropamide. **Acetohexamide** ('Dimelor') is rarely used as the first choice and few patients benefit from it when other sulphonylureas have failed. *Presentation* tablets 500mg; *dose* 1000-1500mg initially then 500mg once daily for maintenance, taken before breakfast. *Adverse effects* are as for the sulphonylureas (toxicity on the liver and marrow), allergy (skin, liver), gastro-intestinal, hypoglycaemia and headache.

Glibenclamide ('Daonil', 'Euglucon') introduced in 1967 is a second generation sulphonylurea. *Presentation* Tablets B.P. 2.5 and 5 mg; *dose* 2.5mg increasing by 2.5mg once daily up to 15mg and rarely beyond 20mg. *Adverse reactions* as for the other sulphonylureas including severe hypoglycaemia (it may stimulate fasting plasma insulin levels). **Glipizide** ('Glibenese', 'Minodiab') is rapidly absorbed, metabolized and excreted and claimed like glibenclamide to have little antabuse reaction, or to be accumulative and hence not to cause problems with hypoglycaemia. This makes it suitable for the elderly as does the small tablet size. *Presentation* tablets 5mg; *dose* 2.5-5mg once daily with food increasing if necessary to 20mg daily in divided doses. **Glibornuride** ('Glutril') *presentation* tablets 25mg; *dose* 12.5mg initially once daily increasing to 75mg in divided amounts morning and night is the latest in this series. **Glybutamide** is in wide use in France and **Gliclazide** ('Diamicron') is a French preparation with anti-platelet action and prolonged hypoglycaemic action.

Drug interactions may occur with salicylates, sulphonamides and phenylbutazone which displace the sulphonylureas from their binding by serum proteins and so by releasing extra unbound (free drug) enhances their action. The hypoglycaemic effect is also potentiated by beta-blockers, monoamine oxidase inhibitors, chloramphenicol and ethionamide, and opposed by the corticosteroids, adrenaline, thiazide diuretics and the oral contraceptives. The sulphonylureas may also predispose to hypothyroidism.

Biguanides
Biguanides are given when sulphonylureas fail, or are used with them, or with insulin in severe diabetes. Obese diabetics unable to diet may find their anorexic qualities useful. Historically these compounds were tried before insulin was introduced, but the original compounds were too toxic. They lower the blood sugar independently of pancreatic insulin stimulation, or release, and presumably work by a peripheral tissue action. Any response is usually apparent in a few days. The biguanides, particularly phenformin have lost popularity. While they are still prescribed in Europe they are no longer available in N. America. This is because of the risk of lactic acidaemia, but a total embargo is unwarranted. It appears that metformin which is eliminated only by renal mechanisms is less likely to cause lactic acidaemia. Phenformin is excreted by hepatic and renal means. Patients are being changed from phenformin to metformin (or sulphonylureas), but on the whole control of blood sugars is poorer and patient acceptability is less. The risks of lactic acidosis are less if precautions and contra-indications are observed and the dose of phenformin kept to 50-75mg daily. The liver fails to utilize lactate if the blood pH is below 7.1 so

treatment is to raise the pH with i.v. sodium bicarbonate. **Phenformin Hydrochloride** ('DBI', 'Dibotin'),*presentation* Tablets B.P. 25mg, capsules 25 and 50mg; *dose* initially 25mg b.d. up to 75mg b.d. taken after meals. **Metformin Hydrochloride** ('Glucophage') *presentation* Tablets B.P. 500 and 850mg; *dose* 1500-3000mg daily in 3 divided amounts after food. *Adverse effects* nausea, vomiting, diarrhoea, intestinal malabsorption of folates and vitamin B_{12}, metallic taste, lassitude, ketonuria and lactic acidaemia, often without marked hyperglycaemia or glycosuria. The biguanides should not be given if there is liver or renal disease, or any illness (e.g. circulatory failure) predisposing to lactic acidaemia.

Pyrimidine Derivatives
Glymidine ('Gondafon') although not a sulphonylurea it is like them a sulphonamide derivative and acts on functioning islet tissue. *Presentation* tablets 500mg; *dose* initially 1-1.5g then 500mg-1g given daily at breakfast. *Uses* and *reactions* resemble the sulphonylureas and it does not seem to possess any advantages.

Hypoglycaemia
Apart from overdosage of insulin and oral hypoglycaemic agents hypoglycaemia is seen with alcohol intoxication, leucine sensitivity and insulin producing tumours. Leucine can be reduced in the diet. Treatment of idiopathic, leucine and some inoperable cases of insulinoma is possible with **Diazoxide** ('Eudemine') which prevents the release of insulin. *Presentation* Tablets B.P. 50mg; *dose* 5-20mg/kg daily in 2 or 3 equal amounts every 8-12 hours. Adults with malignant tumours may require up to 1400mg daily. *Adverse effects* hypertrichosis, oedema, nausea, anorexia, vomiting, hyperuricaemia, tachycardia, hypotension, ketoacidosis, hyperglycaemia. **Streptozotocin** and **tubocidin** are cytotoxic antibiotics which have been used for insulinomas. Streptozotocin lowers gastrin, glucagon and insulin levels and will induce remissions (given i.v. 2-4g at intervals) in malignant insulinoma, malignant gastrinoma and pancreatic 'cholera'. Its use is limited by renal toxicity.

NEW DRUGS
Gliquidone ('Glurenorm') is a sulphonylurea introduced in late 1979. *Presentation* tablets 30mg; *dose* 45-60mg up to a maximum of 180mg daily by mouth in divided doses before meals. The indications, precautions, contra-indications and adverse effects are as for the sulphonylureas.

26 DRUGS IN ENDOCRINE DISORDERS

There has been great progress recently in the isolation of hormones from the hypothalamus and the pituitary. Some have diagnostic uses, others have therapeutic uses.

The **hypothalamus** makes both releasing and inhibitory hormones. **Protirelin** or **Thyrotrophic Releasing Hormone** (TRH) as 40mg tablets or 200µg injection is used diagnostically and has been made synthetically. Both **Growth Hormone Releasing Hormone** (GHRH) and **Growth Hormone Release-Inhibiting Hormone** (GH-RIH) or somatostatin are available and the latter has been tried in acromegaly and breast cancer. A **Gonadotrophin Releasing Hormone** (FSH/LH-RH) Gonadorelin is used for the diagnosis of pituitary-ovarian failure and has been tried for the correction of sterility. The usual dose is 100-500µg s.c., i.m., or i.v.

PITUITARY HORMONES
Anterior Lobe
The *large molecular weight polypeptides* may contain many aminoacids. **Growth Hormone** or **Somatotrophin** ('Crescormon', 'Ascellarcrin') contains 159 in a single chain and is obtained at autopsy from human pituitaries. The dry weight of the human pituitary is 100mg of which 10-15mg is growth hormone and 20-300µg prolactin. It is given i.m. two injections weekly 10 or 20u in divided doses for growth retardation due to GH lack. GH administration is supervised in special centres where measurements of height can be exact and the results charted on percentile graphs. **Prolactin** is believed to have a role greater than just milk production. Certain tumours are thought to be prolactin dependent. Anti-prolactin compounds such as levodopa and bromocriptine have been given for these tumours as well as for alleviation of galactorrhoea. **Bromocriptine Mesylate** ('Parlodel') is a long-acting dopamine agonist. *Presentation* Tablets 2.5mg and capsules 10mg. *Dose* as bromocriptine base of 2.5-10mg (maximum 60mg) taken initially at night, it suppresses abnormal growth hormone production in acromegaly. In hyperprolactinaemia in addition to stopping galactorrhoea it also restores sexual potency and gonadal function (overcomes amenorrhoea). It is also useful to suppress puerperal lactation, but is too expensive for routine use. *Adverse effects* include nausea, vomiting, postural hypotension, constipation, nasal congestion, leg cramps, cardiac dysrhythmias, psychosis. It should be taken with food at night time.

Small Molecular Weight Polypeptides
Adrenocorticotrophic hormone (ACTH) is a 39 aminoacid polypeptide. This stimulates the adrenal cortex to make hydrocortisone and other hormones and so therapeutically mimics the actions of hydrocortisone and has similar uses. It is preferred by some to corticosteroids in selected patients with asthma, rheumatoid arthritis, ulcerative colitis, retrobulbar neuritis and Bell's palsy. The advantage of ACTH in children e.g. in asthma or Crohn's disease is that it does not suppress growth rate, or interfere with growth hormone response to stress, or the production of the anabolic tissue building hormones androgens and oestrogens, whereas corticosteroids do. The hypothalamic-pituitary-

adrenal axis is less disturbed so that cortisol (hydrocortisone) secretion is relatively unimpaired.

Short-Acting Injections

Corticotrophin Ph. Eur. ('Acthar') is a preparation of pork origin used s.c., or i.m. Corticotrophin powder is freeze-dried and dissolved in sterile water to make **Corticotrophin Injection B.P.** For s.c. and i.m. use 25 and 40u are available; the dose is 10-100u daily. *Adverse effects* antibody formation, allergy and in excess, Cushing's syndrome.

Long-Acting Injections

Delayed or depot preparations include **Corticotrophin Gelatin Injection B.P.** ('Acthar Gel') a solution in Water for Injections of corticotrophin with suitably hydrolyzed gelatin. The low melting point of 25°C allows easy self-injection. *Presentation* vials 2ml 40u/ml and 5ml 20, 40 and 80u/ml for s.c. and i.m. use. The action lasts 8-24 hours. The preparation is kept cool at 2-10°C. *Dose* 10-100u an average is 40u 1 or 2 times daily. ACTH gel has a physiological advantage in that it allows the natural secretion of endogenous ACTH for part of the 24 hours (because the duration of its action is usually less than this period). For asthma the starting dose is 40u b.d., then with improvement 40u daily, 20u daily, alternate days, then thrice weekly, twice and then 20u weekly. The same regime can be used for the nephrotic syndrome.

Corticotrophin Zinc Injection Ph. Eur., B.P. is an aqueous solution of corticotrophin in zinc hydroxide. *Presentation* vials 5ml 40u/ml. Administration and dose as for Corticotrophin Gel. It is given i.m. once daily.

Synthetic ACTH-like Preparations

Tetracosactrin Acetate B.P. ('Synacthen') a short-acting injection contains the first 24 aminoacids of ACTH. It is used to test adrenal cortex function. *Presentation* ampoules 250μg; *dose* 250μg i.m., or i.v. **Tetracosactrin Zinc Injection B.P.** ('Synacthen-Depot') is a long-acting preparation (up to 2 days) meant to be a less allergic alternative to the depot preparations of ACTH. Reactions, occasionally fatal, have been reported and it is recommended that the patient remains under medical observation for at least an hour after injection and self injection is not allowed. *Presentation* vials 2ml 1mg/ml and ampoules 1ml 1mg/ml. *Dose* 1mg i.m.

Glycoproteins

These are large polypeptides in which about one third is carbohydrates and they include TSH and the gonadotrophins. **Thyrotrophic hormone,** (TSH, 'Thytropar') is mainly used as a diagnostic test, but it has also been given to increase the uptake of radioactive iodine in certain forms of thyroid cancer.

Gonadotrophic hormones are the follicular stimulating hormone FSH acting on ovarian follicles or testicular tubules and the luteinizing hormone LH which stimulates the corpus luteum or the interstitial cells of the testis. Sources of gonadotrophins—**Chorionic Gonadotrophin B.P.** (HCG or Human Chorionic Gonadotrophin) is obtained from the urine of pregnant women and acts like LH. It is used only after endocrinological assessment for the treatment of delayed puberty, undescended testicles, hypogonadism, infertility from hypopituitarism and other forms of pituitary caused infertility. *Presentation* ampoules 100, 500, 1000, 1500, 2000 and 5000u ('Pregnyl', 'Profasi', 'Gonadotraphon L.H.'); the dose is 500-3000u twice weekly i.m. for 3-6 weeks which can be repeated later. To achieve pregnancy in anovulatory infertility when pituitary drive is lacking, stimulation of the ovaries can be achieved (in centres with special facilities) by injecting FSH derived, either from human pituitaries (**Human Pituitary Gonadotrophin** or HPG), or more usually from **Menotrophin** (human post-menopausal urine, HMG). Injection B.P. a sterile solution in Water for Injections. 'Pergonal' contains 75u of FSH and 75u of LH per ampoule with accompanying solvent of 1ml sodium chloride. In one regime 3 ampoules or 225u are given on days 1, 4 and 8 the FSH ripening the Graafian follicle and this is followed on day 10 by an injection of 4500u of HCG which acts like LH to induce ovulation and progesterone secretion.

Clomiphene Citrate B.P. ('Clomid') an antioestrogen is structurally related to chlorotrianisene, an oestrogen. It is used to treat anovulatory infertility when the pituitary and ovaries are capable of stimulation (e.g. Stein-Levanthal syndrome). When prescribed it acts as a pituitary gonadotrophin activator. The dose is usually 50mg, or one tablet daily for 5-10 days. Improved results may occur if HCG is injected a week after the course. With clomiphene and HCG overstimulation can cause multiple pregnancies and the hyperstimulation syndrome of enlarged painful and, at times, bleeding ovaries. Clomiphene is probably safer than gonadotrophin injections, but can cause hot flushes, headache, visual symptoms, nausea, vomiting, constipation, allergies and reversible hair loss. It is contra-indicated near the menopause, and in those with primary ovarian or pituitary failure, liver disease or ovarian cysts. Clomiphene 25-200mg daily can also be used in oligospermia due to failure of gonadotrophin production. **Danazol** ('Danol') has been introduced to suppress gonadotrophin secretion in precocious puberty and endometriosis.

Posterior Pituitary
Unrefined extracts containing both vasopressin and oxytocin are obsolete.
Oxytocin Injection Ph. Eur., B.P. ('Pitocin', 'Syntocinon') which acts on the uterus at term (oxytocic) is synthesized and is largely free from vasopressin. *Presentation* ampoules 0.5, 1 and 5ml 10u/ml, 1ml 5u/ml, and 2ml 1u/ml. The dose for the active management of the first stage, or accelerated labour, whereby labour is induced varies between hospitals; 1-8u can be added to 500 or 1000ml of Dextrose Injection 5% and then given i.v. In the author's hospital 2u are added to 500ml and according to response an i.v. drip rate at 15, 30, and then 60 drops/min is given; the increases occurring every 30min. If there is no response then 4u/500ml strength is given at 30 drops/min then 60 drops/min and the final strength is 8u/500ml again starting at 30 drops and then 60 drops/min. In general rates under 5mu/min are preferred. For accuracy the infusion may be given by a pump with a controlled drip counter which may be controlled by feed-back information from uterine contractions. (1u/litre = 1mu/ml; 15-17 drops = 1ml). For post-partum haemorrhage 20u can be added to a litre of Dextrose Injection 5% and given i.v. at a rate 60 drops/min. *Overdosage* may lead to foetal distrss and alter the Apgar rating by interfering with placental blood flow; uterine rupture is a rare possibility, other adverse effects are cardiac arrhythmias, hypotension and because of an antidiuretic effect water intoxication from fluid retention. **Oxytocin Tablets B.P.** ('Pitocin Buccal') contain 200u of Oxytocin Citrate and they have been used to start or

aid labour. The dose is half a tablet dissolved under the tongue repeated at 30min intervals to a total of 22 tablets. Absorption is unreliable and i.v. oxytocin is safer.

A widely used drug in labour is **Ergometrine Maleate Ph. Eur.** (Ergonovine Maleate U.S.P.). It is not a pituitary hormone, but an ergot derivative. It is used to arrest bleeding after delivery of the baby and placenta. *Presentation* Injection ampoules 1ml containing 125 and 500µg; *dose* 125-1000µg i.m., 125-500µg i.v. (only up to 250µg if the patient is hypertensive) and 500-1000µg (1mg) orally using Tablets B.P. 125, 250 and 500µg. 'Syntometrine' is **Ergometrine and Oxytocin Injection B.P.** containing 5u of oxytocin and 500µg of ergometrine in 1ml and is given almost routinely i.m. when the anterior shoulder is free, before delivery of the baby and placenta to prevent postpartum haemorrhage. Methylergometrine has similar uses to ergometrine but is unavailable in the U.K.

Prostaglandins
These are also used in labour, but are not of pituitary origin. They are fatty acid derivatives with wide biological presence and pharmacological and physiological activity. All natural prostaglandins have the same 20 carbon structure prostanoic acid. Structurally they are divided into 4 main categories A,B,E and F and these are again subdivided on a chemical basis. Two forms are commercially available **Dinoprostone** ('Prostin E_2') and **Dinoprost** ('Prostin F_2 alpha'). They are used to induce abortion or labour. They may be given orally e.g. 'Prostin E_2' tablets 500µg (0.5mg), i.v., or extra-amniotically and they are powerful oxytocics. They are at least as safe as oxytocin though more expensive. They are also effective in hastening delivery of the dead, or of the anencephalic foetus. For i.v. infusion PG F_2 α can be given at a rate of 50µg/min and a total dose averaging 36 000µg; for the E_2 series 0.5-2µg/min for the induction of labour to a total dose of 150-600µg and for inducing abortion 2-5µg/min to a total dose of 2000-5000µg. *Adverse effects* thrombophlebitis frequently, diarrhoea, vomiting, facial flushing, fever and rigors.

Sympathomimetic drugs have been used to delay the onset of labour, but the results are not impressive. **Orciprenaline Sulphate** ('Alupent Obstetric') 5mg is given in 500ml of Dextrose Injection 5% at a rate of up to 60µg/ml. **Mesuprine Hydrochloride** a derivative of isoxsuprine has been given i.v. at a dose starting with 10µg/min rising to 40µg/min to a total of 1.5mg over 60min. Other preparations are **Isoxsuprine Hydrochloride** ('Duvadilan') and **Ritodrine Hydrochloride** ('Yutopar') and **Salbutamol.**

Antidiuretic Hormone
Vasopressin (ADH) is used to treat diabetes insipidus when it is due to lack of the natural hormone arginine vasopressin a peptide of 9 amino acids. ADH acts on the renal tubules causing most of the filtered fluid to be reabsorbed. *Preparations* **Vasopressin Injection** ('Pitressin') is an aqueous solution of mammalian (e.g. porcine or bovine) posterior pituitary lobe. Since it only lasts 6-8 hours it is given several times daily. *Presentation* ampoules 1ml 20u/ml; *dose* 0.25-0.75ml (5-15u) s.c., or i.m. It has also been used to control bleeding from oesophageal varices as it lowers portal vein pressure; 20u are given in 200ml of Dextrose Injection 5% over 20-30min. **Vasopressin Tannate Injection** ('Pitressin Tannate Injection') has a delayed action of 36-48 hours but its

use in the U.K. has been discontinued. **Lypressin Ph. Eur.** ('Syntopressin') a pure synthetic lysine vasopressin is available as an aqueous nasal spray but has a short action of 3-4 hours. *Presentation* 5ml quantities of solution 50u/ml, *dose* 1-2 applications 3-7 times a day. It is simple to use but can cause nasal irritation. **Desmopressin** ([1-deamino-8-D-arginine] vasopressin, 'DDAVP'); *presentation* nasal drops in 2.5ml dropper bottle 100μg/ml, ampoules 1ml 4μg/ml. *Dose* intranasally 10-20μg once or twice daily, or 1-4μg i.m. or i.v. once daily. It is as effective and longer lasting than vasopressin without its pressor effects, (because of deamination and the substitution of D-arginine for L-arginine). Desmopressin also raises blood factor VIII levels in haemophilia. *Adverse effects* of vasopressin are smooth muscle stimulation, vasoconstriction, intestinal cramps, diarrhoea, sickness and anaphylaxis. Overdosage causes water intoxication with headache, nausea, vomiting, oedema, cramps, ataxia, convulsions and coma. **Chlorpropamide** and **Carbamazepine** potentiate the renal response to ADH and have been used in adults with partial ADH lack and mild diabetes insipidus. **Clofibrate** stimulates vasopressin release from the hypothalamus. Chlorpropamide is dangerous in children because of the risk of hypoglycaemia particularly when there is associated anterior pituitary disease with ACTH deficiency. In nephrogenic diabetes insipidus the tubules are insensitive to ADH. Here, thiazide diuretics by reducing glomerular flow will reduce urine flow by about 50%.

THYROID DISORDERS
Functions; the thyroid stimulates the rate of metabolism. Overaction causes thyrotoxicosis, underaction cretinism and hypothyroidism. Iodine lack produces thyroid enlargement or goitre. The thyroid hormone contains iodine obtained from the diet (sea foods and water). Iodine is removed from the blood stream and concentrated in the thyroid. By a series of processes it is made into the hormones thyroxine and liothyronine (tri-iodothyronine) and stored as thyroglobulin and released as needed. The body converts a small fraction of thyroxine into liothyronine. **Thyroid hormones** are used (1) to treat all forms of *hypothyroidism,* (2) to *reduce the size of goitres* by suppressing the secretion of thyrotrophic stimulating hormone and (3) to *suppress the growth* of certain thyroid cancers. Thyroid hormones are enhanced in their cardiac actions by sympathomimetic drugs and tricyclic antidepressants. Thyroid hormone dosage can be controlled by measuring TSH levels.
Preparations **Thyroid Extract** (desiccated thyroid) is obtained from animals. Although cheap it is unreliable and keeps badly. *Presentation* Tablets B.P. 30mg; *dose* 30-240mg daily. **Thyroxine Sodium Ph. Eur.** ('Eltroxin') is pure, reliable, quickly absorbed and acts in 1-2 days. Tablets deteriorate if damp and they should be kept away from the light. *Presentation* Tablets B.P. 50 and 100μg; *dose* 25μg daily (50μg every other day) to start in the elderly and those with heart disease increasing by monthly increments of 50μg in later life to 100μg, and up to 300μg (0.3mg) daily in younger adults. Treatment is faster in hypothyroid infants and is controlled by x-ray bone age and clinical methods. **Liothyronine Sodium** ('Cynomel', 'Tertroxin', T3, Tri-iodothyronine Sodium) *presentation* Tablets B.P. 20μg, ampoules of powder containing 20μg for i.v. use. *Dose* 5-100μg orally daily. It works rapidly in a few hours and is used for (1) the rapid treatment of hypopituitary and hypothyroid coma 10-20μg i.v. 8 hourly and (2) to suppress thyroid function; 40μg is given 3 times daily orally for 7 days. The normal gland will absorb less iodine, in thyrotoxicosis iodine

uptake as measured by isotopes is unsuppressed. This test can be dangerous in the elderly and cause arrhythmias and angina; the TRH test is safer. (3) In patients who have angina liothyronine 2.5μg t.d.s. initially is given in some departments since it is both quick to work and to stop should it produce adverse symptoms. In cardiac patients thyroid hormones can be given with a beta-blocker. In practice, in the routine case, only thyroxine is given. *Equivalents,* approximately 60 mg thyroid extract equals 100μg thyroxine and 20μg of liothyronine. *Drug-interactions* thyroid hormones are potentiated by tricyclic antidepressives and the general anaesthetic ketamine which causes hypertension and tachycardia. Cholestyramine reduces the absorption of thyroxine.

Drugs Suppressing Thyroid Overactivity

These are used in hyperthyroidism to temporarily and reversibly interfere with the enzymes which make thyroid hormones either (1) to make patients *safe for surgery,* (2) as *an alternative to surgery* in children, adolescents, and young adult women and in pregnancy, (3) patients *too young for radio-iodine,* or who decline surgery and (4) as an adjunct to ^{131}I therapy until it works. Medical treatment must be for 18 months or more. Follow up is essential as some patients will relapse. *Action* these preparations either stop the incorporation of iodine into thyroid hormone, e.g. the thiourea derivatives carbimazole and methimazole, and the thiouracils, or block the iodine trapping ability of the thyroid e.g. potassium perchlorate.

Carbimazole ('Neo-Mercazole') is popular and reasonably safe. *Presentation* Tablets B.P. 5mg; *dose* 45-60mg daily initially divided 8 hourly according to the severity. After 4-6 weeks the dose is reduced to 2.5-20mg daily and can be given once or twice daily. Improvement occurs in 4-21 days and control in 1-3 months. The drug is stopped 10 days before surgery and replaced by Lugol's iodine or potassium iodide. **Methimazole** ('Tapazole') *presentation* and *dose* as for carbimazole. **Methyl-** and **Propyl Thiouracil** have similar uses; *presentation* Tablets B.P. 50 and 100mg, and 25 and 50mg respectively; *dose* 10 times that for carbimazole. *Adverse effects* of this group are drug fever, arthralgia, cholestatic jaundice, rashes, leucopenia, thyroid swelling and hypothyroidism. Patients who get a sore throat which can be a symptom of agranulocytosis, rash or fever should be advised to stop their drugs and report to their doctor. Patients who develop a rash while taking carbimazole may not do so on propylthiouracil.

Potassium Perchlorate ('Peroidin') is only given if there is intolerance to the above. It will not act if iodine is given simultaneously. *Presentation* tablets 50 and 200mg; *dose* 200mg q.d.s. reduced later to 200-400mg daily. *Adverse effects* rashes, itching, nausea, vomiting, neutropenia, marrow and renal damage. The risks are less with small doses.

Iodine

The only indication for iodine in pharmacological amounts is in iodine deficiency goitre and the pre-operative therapy of thyrotoxicosis. **Potassium Iodide Ph. Eur.** is an alternative to Lugol's iodine. *Presentation* tablets 60mg; *dose* for preparation for surgery in thyrotoxicosis is 30-60mg daily. It works because large doses temporarily suppress overactive glands. Lugol's iodine solution is 5 parts iodine and 10 parts potassium iodide made up to 100 parts. *Dose* 0.3ml t.d.s. Pharmacological doses of iodine given to euthyroid patients with Hashimoto's disease, or who have had thyrotoxicosis treated by surgery or radio-iodine may induce hypothyroidism.

Dietary iodine is added to table salt, 1 part potassium iodide to 100 000 parts salt in goitrous areas to prevent goitre. The normal dietary needs are 100-400µg daily. Increase in dietary iodine in iodine deficient areas may cause iodine induced thyrotoxicosis and pharmacological doses of iodine may do the same in certain patients in non-endemic areas. Iodine may be introduced into the body in large amounts in isotopic leg scanning and in radiographic media. **Radioactive Iodine** (^{131}I) is a colourless tasteless solution; the dose is 10-15 millicuries which may be repeated. Iodine concentrates in the thyroid and the effects of irradiation may take months to be apparent. *Uses* (1) thyrotoxicosis in men over 40 years and women after reproductive life, unless the gland is large and nodular when surgery is preferable, (2) thyroid cancer of the type which absorbs iodine. *Adverse effects* eventually a high percentage—at least 30%—will become hypothyroid.

Propranolol has been used effectively by some surgeons on its own to prepare patients with thyrotoxicosis for surgery and more conventionally to slow rapid pulse rates in severe disease and thyroid crisis. It is usual to choose a betablocker without I.S.A. such as propranolol or sotalol. Beta-blockers can be used alone in the last few weeks of pregnancy and in neonatal thyrotoxicosis. Some patients with marked exophthalmos may respond to large amounts of prednisone e.g. 60-100mg daily.

Thyrotoxic crisis is a rare but serious complication of untreated thyrotoxicosis, or may follow ill-judged surgery, or even radio-iodine therapy to a severe thyrotoxic. Treatment is by—(1) i.v. fluids and dextrose to replace fluid lost by sweating (2) sponging, fans and drugs such as chlorpromazine to reduce hyperpyrexia, (3) reduction of thyroid hormonal synthesis and release with i.v. sodium iodide 1-3g daily and carbimazole 100-150mg daily in divided doses, (4) support for circulatory failure with oxygen and digitalis, or reduction of tachycardia and sympathomimetic effects with propranolol, and hydrocortisone 300mg daily for 'adrenal exhaustion'.

Adrenal Disease

Cortical hormones are vital; deficiency leads to salt and water loss with weakness, tiredness, vomiting, circulatory failure and death. Acute adrenal failure results from adrenal or pituitary disease, or suppression of adrenal function by corticosteroids. Treatment is by i.v. hydrocortisone, supplemented by dextrose (glucose) and sodium chloride and the treatment of precipitating events such as infection. Chronic adrenal failure or Addison's disease is often treated with **Cortisone** orally 25-50mg daily in divided amounts. Although it is poorly and erratically absorbed, it works for many; in the failures **Hydrocortisone** 10-30mg daily is used since it is absorbed better and does not have to be converted by the body. To achieve the best results the larger dose should be given in the morning to emulate the normal diurnal rhythm and blood levels should be monitored. Its disadvantage is its short action. For patients with excess ACTH secretion and persistent pigmentation a small dose (0.25-0.5mg) of dexamethasone at midnight will stop nocturnal ACTH production and lighten skin colour. In the tropics a high salt intake is advised, but in temperate climes a salt-retaining mineralocorticoid is prescribed. e.g. **Fludrocortisone Acetate** ('Florinef',) *presentation* Tablets B.P. 100µg and 1mg; *dose* 1-2mg initially and then 100-300µg for maintenance. The dosage of hormones is regulated by the patient's feeling of vigour, well-being, weight, blood pressure, absence of oedema and blood chemistry findings. **Deoxycortone Acetate Ph. Eur.** has largely been superseded; it can be injected i.m., or taken as an implant. *Presentation* Injection B.P. ampoules 2, 5 and 10mg/ml in oily solution, implants B.P. 100mg; *dose* i.m. 2-5mg daily, implant s.c. 100-400mg monthly. A long-acting form is **Deoxycortone Pivalate** ('Percorten M'); it is a powder of microcrystals given as a suspension. *Presentation* Injection B.P. ampoules 1ml 25mg/ml; *dose* 25-75mg i.m. once or twice monthly. Congenital adrenal cortical over-activity or hypertrophy is due to an enzyme defect which by a decreased feed-back effect leads to excessive ACTH secretion and it responds to cortisone in sufficient amounts to reduce the urinary steroids to normal levels; some chil-dren are salt losers and require treatment for acute adrenal failure and long-term fludrocortisone.

Adrenal-overactivity in adult life can be blocked by inhibitors which reduce cortisol production. They include phenobarbitone, o,pDDD or Mitotane (used for adrenal cancer), metyrapone, amphenone and aminoglutethimide. They are tried when surgery is impossible. They may cause adrenal insuffi-ciency, nausea and vomiting. Plasma cortisol levels should be monitored.

In **hypopituitarism** cortisone or hydrocortisone is given as for Addison's dis-ease plus thyroxine and sex hormones.

Parathyroid Glands

These control calcium and phosphorus metabolism. Underactivity leads to hypocalcaemia which causes tetany, twitching, cataracts, convulsions and mental symptoms. Low levels of serum calcium also occur with vitamin D defi-ciency and malabsorption. The treatment for hypoparathyroidism is vitamin D_2 (calciferol) 50 000-200 000u (1.25-5mg) daily. Dosage is controlled by serum calcium estimation. Dihydrotachysterol B.P. ('AT10') is a quicker act-ing, 3-4 times more potent, but a more expensive alternative and is therefore suitable post-operatively after parathyroidectomy. *Presentation* bottles 15ml, 250µg/ml (0.25mg) in arachis oil; *dose* 0.25-2.5mg daily.

Calcium Salts

Calcium Gluconate Injection B.P. is used for the emergency relief of tetany from hypocalcaemia. *Presentation* ampoules 5 and 10ml of a 10% solution for i.v. or i.m. use; *dose* 10-20ml (1-2g).
Oral Preparations: **Calcium Gluconate** *presentation* Tablets B.P.C. 600mg; *dose* 1-6 tablets thrice daily or **Calcium Gluconate Effervescent Tablets B.P.C.** and the alternative 'Sandocal' an effervescent compound containing calcium lactate gluconate providing 400mg of calcium per tablet, *dose* 1-6 tablets daily. **Calcium Lactate Ph. Eur.** *presentation* Tablets B.P. 300 and 600mg; *dose* 3-15 thrice daily. They are used with vitamin D_2 in rickets and osteomalacia. The aim is to provide 1-3g of calcium daily.

Treatment of Hypercalcaemia

There is often vomiting, and renal fluid loss leading to dehydration which needs correction. **Frusemide** 100mg/h i.v. should be tried first as it quickly low-ers the serum calcium (quite unlike the thiazides). **Intravenous Phosphates** lower the serum calcium by exceeding the solubility product of calcium hyd-rogen phosphate. Renal clearance of calcium is decreased and calcium levels are lowered by inhibition of bone resorption and the complex of calcium and phosphate is deposited in bone and soft tissue. The effect occurs within 24 hours. **Sodium Phosphate** 0.75mmol/kg B.W. has been given i.v. over 8-12 hours. 'Inphos' solution is a commercial preparation used in the U.S.A. In 50ml there is 50mmol of phosphorus, 80mmol of sodium and 10mmol of potassium and this is diluted in 500-1000ml of 5% dextrose. 'Polyfusor Phosphate Injection' available in the U.K. contains sodium 162mmol, phosphorus 100mmol and potassium 19mmol per litre. *Adverse effects* include tetany from hypocalcaemia and hypomagnesaemia, hyperphosphataemia, hypotension, renal failure and pulmonary oedema. **Sodium Sulphate** or **Sodium Chloride** in isotonic solutions can be infused i.v. e.g. 3 litres over a period of 9 hours. This increases calcium excretion, but the effect is limited to the time of administration and the large amounts of fluid can be dangerous if there is poor renal or cardiac function because of the sodium load. Other measures are **Ethylene Diamine Tetra-acetate** (EDTA) 50mg/kg B.W. i.v., **corticosteroids** (either oral or parenteral which are slow to act, nor do they work in primary hyperparathyroidism), **Mithramycin** 25µg/kg B.W. i.v. and calcitonin. **Calcitonin** is a rapidly acting polypeptide hormone derived from human, porcine and salmon origin with a molecular weight of 3500 containing 32 aminoacids. Beside its use in hypercalcaemia it also relieves the bone pain of Paget's disease where it inhibits excessive resorption of bone. **Calcitonin (Pork) Injection B.P.** ('Calcitare') is a sterile solution in suitable solvent. *Presentation* 160u of lyophilized powder in vials with gelatin diluent. *Dose* s.c., i.m. for Paget's disease 40-160u daily initially and for hypercalcaemia 320-640u daily in divided doses according to the hypocalcaemic response. **Salcatonin** is a synthetic salmon calcitonin less expensive than the porcine form. *Presentation* multidose vials 2ml 200u/ml ('Calsynar'). *Dose* 50-100u. s.c., or i.m. daily or every other day for Paget's disease. For hypocalcaemia 400u 6 or 8 hourly ('Calsynar') or 5-10u/kg B.W. daily in 2 or 4 divided doses i.m. Because of expense calcitonin or salcatonin is reserved for Paget's disease unresponsive to analgesics and for nerve compression.

Oral Phosphate ('Phosphate-Sandoz') consists of sodium acid phosphate 68.1%, sodium bicarbonate 9.5% and potassium bicarbonate 8.5% and provides phosphorus 500mg, sodium 481mg (20.9mmol), and potassium 123mg (3.1mmol) in an effervescent tablet. The dose for hypercalcaemia is up to 6 tablets daily.

Diphosphonates

For selected patients with Paget's disease the choice includes one of the forms of calcitonin, mithramycin and **Etidronate Disodium** (Didronel in U.S.A.) or ethane hydroxy diphosphonic acid (EHDP). EHDP is a synthetic analogue of pyrophosphate. A P-C-P linkage replaces the P-O-P links or bonds in pyrophosphate. *Dose* orally 5mg/kg B.W. daily for a period not exceeding 6 months. Other uses for diphosphonates are to inhibit ectopic calcification and in excessive bone loss in some varieties of osteoporosis.

27 SEX HORMONES

Oestrogens secreted by the ovary are oestrone, oestradiol and oestriol. They promote the growth and development of the uterus and endometrium, vagina and its secretions, the breasts, muscles and subcutaneous fat. They help arrest bone growth and they influence temperament and sexual interest by an action on the brain. They are changed by the liver to water soluble forms excreted by the kidneys. The natural steroids were replaced in therapy by synthetic oestrogens because they were better absorbed orally, were cheaper, or could be injected but natural oestrogens are now back in vogue for menopausal flushes and oestrogen replacement since metabolic and vascular complications are less.

Indications
(1) natural or induced menopause.
(2) suppression of lactation except in older women and those with a history of venous thrombosis. Controlled trials do not uphold their wide use for this purpose and they may be superseded by bromocriptine (see p. 210).
(3) menstrual abnormalities usually with a progestogen. They suppress ovulation, abolish the pain of dysmenorrhoea and reduce the blood loss in metropathic uterine bleeding.
(4) oral contraception with progestogens.
(5) replacement therapy in primary ovarian failure to promote genital and secondary sexual growth.
(6) suppression of prostatic and breast cancers.
Oral preparations are listed in Table 17. Chemically some are steroids. Stilboestrol has been largely superseded. Ethinyloestradiol is cheap and widely used.
Stilboestrol Ph. Eur. (Diethylstilbestrol U.S.P.) *presentation* Tablets B.P. for range see Table 17; *dose* 50μg-1mg for menopausal symptoms and up to 15mg daily for milk suppression. The dose is up to 20mg daily for prostatic cancer, but recent evidence suggests that survival is better with 1mg daily than 5 or 10mg daily as there are less vascular complications.
The dose of **Ethinyloestradiol Ph. Eur.** for menopausal symptoms is the smallest possible e.g. 10-50μg daily with increments of 10μg (0.01mg); for ovarian replacement 50-250μg daily; for the suppression of uterine bleeding 0.5mg (500μg)-2mg, and for stopping lactation 100μg t.d.s. for 3 days reducing to 100μg daily for 6 days. The use of oestrogens to suppress lactation is under critical review. Oestrogens e.g. stilboestrol have been used for 'morning after' contraception, but except possibly for rape they should not be given if there is a possibility of pregnancy, or in known pregnancy, as there is a small risk of vaginal cancers in daughters in later life. Many gynaecologists prefer to give for the menopause natural oestrogens or compounds of them. **Piperazine Oestrone Sulphate** ('Harmogen') in each 1.5mg contains the equivalent of 0.93mg of oestrone. The dose is 1-3 tablets daily. **Oestradiol Valerate** ('Progynova') and **Oestriol** ('Ovestin') are 'natural' human hormones. 'Premarin' tablets are derived from an equine source and tablets are available 625μg, 1.25mg and 2.5mg.

Pessaries stilboestrol B.P.C. 500µg in 4g mould size are available for atrophic vaginitis.

Oestradiol implants e.g. 50mg are available for the treatment of oophorectomized patients and last for months.

TABLE 17
ORAL OESTROGENS

Name Approved	Proprietary	Presentation Tablets	Daily Dose* (mg)
Ethinyloestradiol B.P., Ph. Eur.	'Lynoral'	10, 50,100µg and 1mg	0.05-2
Quinestrol	'Estrovis'	4mg	4 for 2 days
Quinestradol	'Pentovis'	250µg (capsules) (0.25mg)	0.5
Mestranol B.P.		50µg	0.05-0.15
Oestradiol Valerate	'Progynova'	1 and 2mg	1-2
Oestriol	'Ovestin'	250µg (0.25mg)	0.25-0.5
Non-Steroidal Chlorotrianisene B.P.	'TACE'	24 12 (capsules)	12-48
Dienoestrol B.P., Ph. Eur.	'Synestrol' U.S.A.	10, 30µg 1 and 5mg	0.1-5
Methallenoestril		3mg	3-9
Stilboestrol B.P., Ph. Eur.		50, 100, 250 500µg; 1, 2, 5, 10, 25, 50 and 100mg	0.1-15

*for gynaecological use

Injectable Oestrogens
Oestradiol Benzoate Injection Ph. Eur., B.P. ('Benztrone') *presentation* ampoules of an oily solution 1ml containing 1,2 and 5mg/ml and 2ml 5mg/ml; *dose* 1-5mg i.m. several times weekly. **Oestradiol Valerate** (Estradiol Valerate U.S.P. 'Primogyn Depot') *presentation* ampoules 1ml of an oily solution 10mg/ml; *dose* 5-20mg i.m. every 2-4 weeks. Other esters are **Oestradiol Cypionate** and **Dipropionate**. These provide oestradiol in a long-acting form. For the large amounts used in prostatic cancer **Fosfestrol Sodium** ('Honvan') is prescribed which is stilboestrol diphosphate and is water soluble so can be given i.v. for rapid effect. *Presentation* tablets 100mg, ampoules 5ml con-

taining 276mg, *dose* orally 100-200mg t.d.s. reducing gradually to 100mg daily and i.v. up to 1g daily.

Conjugated Oestrogens are obtained from the urine of pregnant mares and i.v. forms are available (U.S.P.) and 'Premarin' which can be injected i.m. or i.v. the dose 25mg is contained in an ampoule. The injection is used to arrest severe uterine haemorrhage and to treat breast cancer. *Adverse effects* of oestrogens are common — nausea, anorexia, vomiting, oedema, fluid retention, heart failure, weight increase, breast fullness, headaches, uterine withdrawal bleeding and hypercalcaemia. The likelihood of venous thrombosis appears to be age and dose related and arterial thrombosis can also occur. Endometrial cancer has an increased incidence, related to dose and duration, as is gall bladder disease. Men get breast enlargement which can be prevented by radiotherapy, and experience loss of libido.

Anti-Oestrogens

Clomiphene is weak oestrogen (p. 212). **Nafoxidine** is structurally related to it and has been used for the treatment of breast cancer resistant to hormones and ablation. It also has androgenic, progestational and gonadotrophin inhibiting properties. It is taken orally at a dose 60-90mg t.d.s. daily. *Adverse effects* dry skin, hair loss from the scalp, sensitivity to sunlight and perhaps cataracts. **Tamoxifen Citrate** ('Nolvadex') is a similar compound used in postmenopausal women. *Presentation* tablets 10mg; *dose* 10-40mg b.d. It is supplanting oestrogens in the therapy of breast cancer. *Adverse effects* flushing, vaginal bleeding, gastro-intestinal intolerance, transient thrombocytopenia, occasional fluid retention, venous thrombosis. **Drostanolone Propionate** (Dromostanolone Propionate, 'Masteril') is believed to block the uptake of oestrogen by oestrogen dependent breast cancer. *Presentation* ampoules 1ml containing 100mg in a clear oily solution; *dose* 300mg weekly i.m. *Adverse effects* virilization is possible.

Progestogens

These are steroids which produce glandular or secretory changes in the oestrogen sensitized endometrium. Progesterone is made by the ovary to prepare the endometrium for reception of the fertilized ovum, enhances breast growth and helps maintain the placenta and pregnancy. Natural progesterone is ineffective orally. Substances in use are progesterone and derivatives, oral synthetic progestogens and the nor-testosterones.

Progesterone and Derivatives

Progesterone Injection Ph. Eur., B.P. ('Gestone') is an oily solution for i.m. use. *Presentation* ampoules 1ml 10, 25 and 50mg, 2ml 50mg/ml; *dose* 20-60mg. Implants 100mg and microcrystalline aqueous suspensions are available and suppositories 200 and 400mg for use in the premenstrual syndrome. By esterifying hydroxyprogesterone, compounds with prolonged i.m. action are formed. **Hydroxyprogesterone Hexanoate Injection B.P.** (Hydroxyprogesterone Caproate U.S.P. 'Proluton Depot') *presentation* ampoules 1 and 2ml 250mg/ml and pre-loaded disposable syringes 1 and 2ml; *dose* 125-500mg i.m. 1 or 2 per week. Even more prolonged **Medroxyprogesterone Acetate B.P.** ('Depot Provera') *presentation* vials 1, 3 and 5ml of an aqueous suspension 50mg/ml; *dose* 50mg weekly, or 100mg fortnightly i.m. for habitual, or threatened abortion or for short-term contraception, as a single dose 125mg i.m.

Gestronol Hexanoate (Gestonorone Caproate, 'Depostat') is a depot preparation used to treat endometrial carcinoma and benign prostatic hypertrophy. *Presentation* ampoules 2ml 100mg/ml. *Dose* 200-400mg weekly i.m.

Oral Synthetic Progestogens
The first group discussed are progesterone derivatives. These are more convenient, some such as **Megesterol Acetate B.P.** and **Chlormadinone Acetate B.P.** are, or have been used, with an oestrogen in the contraceptive pill. **Medroxyprogesterone Acetate B.P.** ('Provera') is also available for oral use and has a wider application than contraception. *Presentation* Tablets 5 and 100mg (2.5 and 10mg U.S.P.). *Dose* for threatened abortion 10-40mg daily, for infertility and uterine bleeding 2.5-10mg daily. It has also been tried for sexual precocity in girls. Inoperable uterine and renal cancers are treated with 200-400mg daily, for several months. **Dydrogesterone B.P.** is a progesterone derivative used for dysmenorrhoea and for abortion and dysfunctional bleeding.

Testosterone and Nor-Testosterone Derivatives
The first orally active progestogens **Ethisterone** and **Dimethisterone** were testosterone derivatives, but they have been superseded. Allyloestrenol is related to Testosterone. The **Nor-Testosterones** are chemically testosterones without a methyl group at position C 19 (hence, '19 nor-testosterones'). They are further modified to make them orally effective. Derivatives comprise many of the progestogens currently used in oral contraceptives Ethynodiol Diacetate B.P., Lynoestrenol B.P., Norethisterone B.P., Norethisterone Acetate B.P., Norgestrel, and Norethynodrel B.P.

TABLE 18
ORAL SYNTHETIC PROGESTOGENS

Name Approved	Proprietary	Tablet Strength (mg)	Daily Dose (mg)
Medroxyprogesterone	'Provera'	5 and 100	10-400
Dydrogesterone	'Duphaston'	10	10-30
Ethisterone	'Gestone Oral'	5, 10, 25	25-100
Allyloestrenol	'Gestanin'	5	10-20
Norethisterone (Norethindrone U.S.P.)	'Primolut N'	5	5-30
Norethisterone Acetate (Norethindrone Acetate U.S.P.)	'Norlutin A' 'SH 420'	2.5 10	2.5-15 30-60

Uses of the progesterone derivatives and oral progestogens are varied:
(1) As oral contraceptives, either alone, or with an oestrogen.
(2) For gynaecological disease such as dysfunctional bleeding, threatened or habitual abortion (if believed due to progesterone deficiency), infertility caused by deficiency (when they are prescribed from the 15th-24th day of the menstrual cycle), endometriosis, dysmenorrhoea, the pre-menstrual syndrome and the diagnosis of amenorrhoea.
(3) In inoperable renal, mammary and endometrial cancers.
(4) In blood diseases (e.g. leukaemia) daily suppressive doses have been given to prevent blood loss from menorrhagia.

FERTILITY CONTROL, 'THE PILL'

Oral contraceptives approach the ideal of a safe, acceptable, simple and cheap method of birth control. **Progestogen only** include **Ethynodiol Diacetate** ('Femulen') *dose* 500μg, **Norethisterone** ('Micronor', 'Noraday') *dose* 350μg, **Levonorgestrel** ('Microval' and 'Norgeston') 30μg and dl **Norgestrel** ('Neogest') 75μg all daily. They act on the cervical mucus making penetration by the spermatozoa more difficult. The effects lasts 24 hours so the preparation must be taken daily. Menstrual bleeding occurs and may be frequent and irregular. They may possibly have less thrombotic effects though they may be not so effective as the combined preparations. The **combined preparations** consist of a progestogen and an oestrogen. They are taken nightly from the 5th day of the menstrual cycle until the 24th inclusive. They act (1) on the pituitary inhibiting ovulation (2) on the speed of tubal transport of the ovum and (3) by affecting the quality of the cervical mucus. Within 3-4 days of stopping them withdrawal bleeding occurs like a normal period in duration, but the flow may be less. Because of the known risk of venous and arterial thrombosis with oestrogen content only low (50μg or less) forms are given (see Table 19). The added oestrogen helps to prevent break-through menstrual bleeding and allows a smaller and hence cheaper dose of progestogen to be used. Their success in dysmenorrhoea is due to the fact that they stop ovulation and anovulatory cycles are usually painless. *Adverse effects* nausea, headache, fluid retention, abdominal bloating, breast tenderness, increased weight, depression, decreased libido, genital candida, acne, chloasma, photosensitivity, diffuse alopecia, personality change, hypertension, venous and less commonly arterial thrombosis in brain or heart, and worsening or provocation of migraine. Pill amenorrhoea is common and persistent infertility may occur when the pill is stopped. If hypertension develops a low oestrogen form can be tried, or a progestogen only pill under careful observation. Here, it is probably better to try other forms of fertility control (vasectomy, laparoscopic sterilization). Benign hepatomas have been reported. Break-through bleeding occurs in 5-10%. *Precautions* concurrent therapy with barbiturates or rifampicin may make the oral contraceptive less effective. In the first cycle of use ovulation may be abnormally early so that protection should not be relied on in the first week. The risk of hypertension increases with duration on the pill and age so regular checks are indicated. *Contra-indications* patients with breast and uterine cancer, fibroids, liver disease including cirrhosis and Dubin-Johnson and Rotor syndromes, a history of venous thrombosis or emboli, or possibly a bad family history of arterial disease. Hypertension is a relative preclusion, but the pill can be given and the effects assessed. Preparations are usually stopped one month before major surgery requiring the woman to remain in bed, unless in gynaecology when withdrawal bleeding is a disadvantage. A possible foetal risk is their continuation when pregnancy has occured.

Choosing an oral contraceptive

(1) In choosing an oral contraceptive absolute and relative contra-indications should be determined. The presence of factors conducive to thrombosis should be considered such as hypertension, diabetes mellitus, cigarette smoking, age, family history, hyperlipidaemia and obesity.

(2) The lowest possible dose should be chosen providing it controls both fertility and the menstrual cycle and causes little or no adverse effects.

TABLE 19
AVAILABLE ORAL CONTRACEPTIVES

50 micrograms of Oestrogen

'Anovlar 21'	Norethisterone Acetate	4mg	Ethinyloestradiol	50µg
'Gynovlar 21'	,,	3mg	,,	,,
'Norlestrin'	,,	2.5mg	,,	,,
'Minovlar'	,,	1mg	,,	,,
'Minovlar ED'	,,	1mg(+7 inert tablets)	,,	,,
'Orlest 21'	,,	1mg(+7 inert tablets)	,,	,,
'Ovulen 50'	Ethynodiol Diacetate	1mg	,,	,,
'Demulen 50'	,,	0.5mg	,,	,,
'Minilyn'	Lynoestrenol	2.5mg	,,	,,
'Ortho-Novin 1/50'	Norethisterone	1mg	Mestranol	,,
'Norinyl - 1'	,,	1mg	,,	,,
'Norinyl 1/28'	,,	1mg(+7 inert tablets)	,,	,,
'Ovran'	Levonorgestrel	0.25mg	Ethinyloestradiol	,,
'Eugynon 50'	dl Norgestrel*	0.5mg	,,	,,

Less than 50 micrograms of Oestrogen

'Ovysmen'	Norethisterone	0.5mg	,,	35µg
'Brevinor'	,,	0.5mg	,,	,,
'Norimin'	,,	1mg	,,	,,
'Eugynon 30'	Levonorgestrel	0.25mg	,,	30µg
'Ovran 30'	,,	0.25mg	,,	,,
'Ovranette'	,,	0.15mg	,,	,,
'Microgynon 30'	,,	0.15mg	,,	,,
'Conova 30'	Ethynodiol Diacetate	2mg	,,	,,
'Loestrin 20'	Norethisterone Acetate	1mg	,,	20µg

*dl Norgestrel is a racemate of 2 optical isomers of which only the d form is active.

(3) There is no universally suitable pill and various factors are taken into consideration such as the menstrual cycle whether heavy or not, and whether the therapy is for cycle control, menorrhagia, or prevention of pregnancy. Some women are more fertile than others and need a potent preparation. If relative contra-indications are present a low oestrogen or progestogen-only pill may be required.
(4) Combined formations: Ethinyloestradiol is the usual oestrogen, but some contain mestranol. Progestogens; five varieties are in use, but comparison of their efficacy and 'potency' is not easy. All the combined pills will reduce mens-

trual loss. With higher doses of the progestogens menstrual control may be excessive and amenorrhoeic cycles can occur. Lower progestogen doses can be associated with break-through bleeding. Levonorgestrel (Norgestrel) is a powerful progestogen and can control fertility with only a small dose of oestrogen. New oral contraceptive takers are given a low-dose variety and if the cycle is not controlled higher dose forms are given.

Male Hormones (Virilizing Androgens)
Androgens are secreted mainly by the testes and induce certain male characteristics, promote protein tissue formation (anabolic) and the body and mental changes noted following puberty. *Uses* hypogonadism from testicular failure in adolescents and adults, breast cancer in post-menopausal woman, reduction of itching in obstructive jaundice, reduction of nitrogen breakdown in uraemia and by some for aplastic anaemia.

Oral and Sublingual Forms
The natural hormone testosterone is poorly absorbed from the gut. Testosterone and methyltestosterone are better absorbed sublingually. However, recent studies have shown that large amounts e.g. 400mg daily (as micronized free testosterone) give therapeutic blood levels when taken by mouth and are cheaper and have less side effects (e.g. on the liver) than testosterone derivatives. **Testosterone** ('Testoral Sublings') *presentation* tablets 10mg; *dose* 10-40mg sublingually. **Methyltestosterone Ph. Eur.** Tablets B.P. 5mg; *dose* usually 5-50mg, but up to 100mg in breast cancer. Proprietary form 'Virormone Oral' (5,10,25 and 50mg linguets). It is rarely prescribed since liver damage can occur. Androgens swallowed and absorbed are **Fluoxymesterone** ('Ultandren') *presentation* Tablets B.P. 5mg; *dose* orally 5-20mg daily. **Mesterolone** ('Pro-Viron') *presentation* tablets 25mg; *dose* initially 25mg t.d.s. or q.d.s. for several months then 25mg b.d.
Testosterone Implants B.P. are a most useful alternative since they last 4-6 months. The pellets are available in 25, 50, 100 and 200 mg strengths and they are free from the side effects of the testosterone 17 alkyl derivatives e.g. liver damage.

Injectable Forms
These are esters of testosterone and the usual one is **Testosterone Propionate Injection B.P.** ('Virormone') *presentation* ampoules 1ml 5,10,25,50 and 100mg in oil; *dose* 5-100mg i.m. once or twice weekly. Other esters are **Testosterone Phenylpropionate Injection B.P.** 25-100mg i.m. once or twice weekly, **Testosterone Enanthate Injection U.S.P.** 100-400mg i.m. every 2-4 weeks and **Testosterone Cypionate Injection U.S.P.** 100-400mg i.m. 2-4 weeks. Brand forms include 'Primoteston Depot' and 'Sustanon 100 and 250' which is a mixture of testosterone esters, '100' contains Testosterone Propionate (20mg), Phenylpropionate (40mg), Isocaproate (40mg) and '250' Propionate (30mg), Phenylpropionate (60mg), Isocaproate (60mg) and Decanoate (100mg) in 1ml.

Anabolic Non-Virilizing Androgens
Uses to build up tissue without conspicuous virilization in weak, elderly, or convalescent patients and in those with osteoporosis, but the evidence for their use is slender. They are occasionally used in renal failure to lessen catabolism,

and to slow the growth of breast cancers in young women. *Oral forms* examples are **Ethyloestrenol** ('Orabolin') Tablets B.P. 2mg; *dose* 2-4mg daily, **Methandienone** ('Dianabol') Tablets B.P. 5mg; *dose* 5-10mg, **Norethandrolone** ('Nilevar') Tablets B.P. 10mg; *dose* 20-30mg daily for adults; *dose* 0.5mg/kg B.W. Injectable forms include **Nandrolone Phenylpropionate Injection B.P.** ('Durabolin') ampoules 1ml, 25mg/ml; *dose* 25-50mg i.m. weekly and **Nandrolone Decanoate** ('Deca-Durabolin') ampoules 25 and 50mg/ml; *dose* 25-50mg every 3 weeks. *Adverse effects* of the androgens are fluid retention, virilism, polycythaemia, hypercholesterolaemia, oral methyltestosterone causes jaundice, liver cancer has been reported with oxymetholone. (see p. 195).

Anti-Androgens
Cyproterone Acetate ('Androcur') is an anti-androgen used to treat hirsutism and excessive sexuality. *Adverse effects* depression, tiredness, gynaecomastia. **Hirsutism** in women is also treated by suppressing two sites of androgen production. The ovary is suppressed by the oral contraceptive and the adrenal cortex by corticosteroid analogues such as prednisone. Other anti-androgens tried for selected patients include spironolactone (hypertension with hirsuties). Drugs can cause hirsutism (see p. 251).

IMPOTENCE
Many causes exist, only a minority will respond to drug therapy. Drugs can cause impotence (e.g. hypotensive agents, oestrogens, drugs of addiction, benzodiazepines, phenothiazines, tricyclics, diuretics, spironolactone). Endocrine and metabolic conditions can be treated (hypogonadism, thyroid dysfunction, hyperprolactinaemia, adrenal over and under activity, acromegaly, hyperoestrogenism and diabetes mellitus. A small proportion of men (with hyperprolactinaemia) will respond to **Bromocriptine** the dopamine agonist which inhibits prolactin secretion.

28   FLUIDS, ELECTROLYTES AND BLOOD

Body water: three quarters of the adult weight is water and even more in infants and children. Most is intracellular. Fluid regulation is by the kidneys. Adults need at least 700ml of fluid daily to excrete waste products. The precise amount varies with that lost from urine, stools, skin and lungs. Extra is needed in hot weather, fever and with vomiting, diarrhoea and hyperventilation. Water therapy is required in those with renal stones, particularly those with cystinuria when it has to be taken by day and at intervals during the night. Patients with overproduction of uric acid or taking probenecid, sulphonamides, certain analgesics and cyclophosphamide must take generous amounts of water. It may be of value in the prophylaxis of urinary infection.
Water deprivation is likely in the confused, weak or unconscious and in those with dysphagia. Other causes are infusion of i.v. sodium chloride, the giving of concentrated protein supplements by gastric tube and the over-indulgence of cows' milk powder, without adequate water, in feeding infants. Water loss is a feature of primary and secondary forms of diabetes insipidus. Diagnosis is aided if the fluid intake and output and the weight are charted in ill patients. Patients may lose the sensation of thirst, become confused, febrile, lose weight and have a fast pulse. Both the haematocrit and the serum sodium rise. Treatment is water by mouth or as Dextrose Injection 5% by i.v. infusion.
Water excess or intoxication arises from an excessive intake of water or substances with ADH-like activity diluting body electrolytes. Excitability, delirium, convulsions and coma occur. Causes are too much i.v. dextrose solutions, excess vasopressin injections in diabetes insipidus, excessive injections of oxytocin in pregnancy, overdrinking in mentally ill patients and the giving of enemas in patients with megacolon.
Acid-base balance: acidosis and alkalosis arise from ingesting acid or alkaline substances, their abnormal production by the body (e.g. ketones, lactic acid) or by their disproportionate loss from the bowels or kidneys. Water and electrolyte imbalance often co-exists. Treatment is by giving the appropriate acidic or basic substance by mouth, or i.v. (Table 20) and the correction of the underlying cause.

Electrolyte Disturbances

The body contains certain elements which when dissolved in water ionize and have the ability to conduct electrical charges. They are called electrolytes and have vital functions in the body. Intracellular fluid is rich in potassium and phosphate and extracellular and intravascular fluids in sodium, chloride and bicarbonate. The plasma also contains proteins which are weak electrolytes. Electrolytes in the body and in oral and parenteral fluids can be expressed as mg/dl(100ml), or, until recently, alternatively as milli-equivalents. These terms have been replaced by millimoles per litre (mmol/l). A millimole is the ionic weight expressed as milligrams. For monovalent ions the equivalent and the molecular weights are the same (Na^+, K^+, HCO_3^- and Cl^-) for divalent ions ($Fe^{2+}, Ca^{2+}, SO_4^{2-}$) for a given weight of a substance the number of millimoles is half the number of milli-equivalents.
Electrolyte deficiency arises from *intestinal loss* (steatorrhoea, infections such

as gastro-enteritis, cholera, ulcerative colitis, excessive purgation, intestinal suction after surgery), *vomiting* in pyloric stenosis and intestinal obstruction, *renal loss* from diuretic therapy, acute or chronic glomerular and tubular disorders, Addison's disease and corticosteroid therapy. Excessive sweating causes salt depletion. Potassium depletion is also likely in those with a poor appetite, anorexia nervosa, and hyperaldosteronism.

Diagnosis and Treatment

Various oral and i.v. solutions are available to treat electrolyte deficiency (Table 20). Diagnosis is made on a *history* which estimates amount and type of loss; *examination* of circulatory system, blood pressure, skin, tongue and ocular tension, plus urine constituents, specific gravity, urine output and body weight and laboratory investigations of urine and blood electrolytes, pH and E.C.G.

From the weight of the patient and the level of serum electrolytes an approximate measure of loss can be made.

TABLE 20

ELECTROLYTE SOLUTIONS (Expressed in millimoles per litre)

Injection	Na^+	K^+	Ca^{2+}	NH_4^+	Cl^-	as HCO_3^-
Sodium Chloride 0.9%	150				150	
Sodium Chloride 0.18% and Dextrose 4%	30				30	
Sodium Lactate molar/6, 1.85%	167					167
Darrow's solution	123	35			105	53
Compound Sodium Lactate (Hartmann's) solution	131	5	2		111	29
Sodium Bicarbonate 1.4% 8.4%	167 1000					167 1000
Ammonium Chloride molar/6, 0.9%				167	167	
Potassium Chloride 0.3% and Dextrose		40			40	
Potassium Chloride 0.3% and Sodium Chloride 0.9%	150	40			190	

Administration
Electrolyte solutions when possible are given orally or by gastric tube. Intravenous therapy is the only suitable alternative.

Oral Electrolyte Solutions
Electrolyte solutions are available (e.g. as 'Dioralyte') for children e.g. sodium 35 mmol/l, potassium 20mmol/l, chloride 37mmol/l, bicarbonate 18mmol/l and dextrose 200mmol/l. Under 1 year the dose is 150ml/kg/24h (Sodium Chloride and Dextrose Compound Powder B.P.C.). Ideally children require an already formulated, freshly prepared liquid solution as mothers can make mistakes. A solution (Dacca Solution) has been used in India for the oral treatment of cholera to save on i.v. infusions.

'Slow Sodium' contains 600mg or 10millimoles of ion in each tablet in a sustained release form. The dose is 4-8 tablets for prophylaxis and up to 20 daily in treatment of muscle cramps and for some patients on maintenance haemodialysis.

Magnesium Chloride and magnesium glycerophosphate have been given to correct hypomagnesaemia in malabsorption, alcoholism and endocrine disease.

Zinc Sulphate in capsules 220mg t.d.s. have been tried in skin ulcers, but their value is uncertain. Zinc is of value in acrodermatitis enteropathica. Long-continued zinc therapy as an anti-sickling agent has caused hypocupraemia. Potassium salts (p. 87), calcium (p. 217).

Injections (Infusions) of Fluids and Electrolytes
Intravenous Dextrose is a convenient way of giving water as a 5%w/v solution Dextrose Injection B.P. **Dextrose Injection Strong B.P.C.** 50% w/v in Water for Injections is used as a source of energy and to correct hypoglycaemia. Less concentrated solutions are available, which are less damaging to the veins.

Sodium Chloride Injection B.P. 0.9% w/v is used to replace salt loss. When extreme depletion occurs as in Addison's disease, salt-wasting renal disease, intestinal obstruction and diabetic coma stronger concentrations can be had. For hyperosmolar diabetic coma 0.45% and even 0.18% sodium chloride solutions have been used. **Sodium Chloride** (0.18%) **and Dextrose** (4%) **Injection B.P.** is also given to replace water without overloading the body with sodium.

Sodium Lactate Injection B.P. is 1.85% w/v a one sixth molar solution which like **Sodium Bicarbonate Injection B.P.** 1.4% w/v (a stronger 8.4% is also available) is used to combat acidosis in diabetic ketosis, cardiac arrest and after by-pass surgery. The dose depends on the hydrogen ion concentration and the duration of the cardiac arrest. The above are usually available in 500 or 1000ml packs, or in the case of sodium bicarbonate 8.4% smaller volumes to avoid excessive administration. The 'Polyfusor' range is 1.26, 1.4, 2.74, 4.2 and 8.4% of sodium bicarbonate.

Potassium Chloride Injection B.P. is presented in ampoules 1.5g in 10ml (of clear fluid which may accidentally be confused with water). It should be added to 500 or 1000ml of Sodium Chloride Injection or Dextrose Injection 5%. The potassium content is 20 millimoles. Potassium should only be given i.v. when there is adequate renal function and normally no more than up to 20mmol/h. Under conditions of extreme hypokalaemia this can be exceeded under expert guidance. **Potassium Chloride and Dextrose Injection B.P.** is a 5% w/v solution of dextrose with 0.3% w/v potassium chloride which contains 40mmol/l of

potassium and of chloride and **Potassium Chloride and Sodium Chloride Injection B.P.** 40mmol/l of potassium, sodium 150mmol/l and chloride 190mmol/l.
Magnesium Sulphate Injection U.S.P. is supplied as a 50% or a 10% solution; each gram contains 4mmol (8mEq) and is used for hypomagnesaemia as may occur following prolonged parenteral feeding or in diabetic coma.
Ammonium Chloride 0.9% w/v is a one sixth-molar solution used to correct alkalosis.

BLOOD AND BLOOD COMPONENTS

Whole blood is used to maintain blood volume after acute blood loss and in exchange blood transfusions when treating haemolytic disease of the newborn and acute liver failure (volume and red cells needed).
Red cell concentrates (packed red cells) reduce the volume infused. Plasma reduced blood should be the choice for most transfusions to improve oxygen carriage. By removing plasma less sodium is given and immunological risks are reduced. It is given when whole blood would overload the circulation in heart failure and anaemia.
Washed red cells are given to patients with circulating white cell antibodies.
Fresh blood is reserved for patients requiring massive transfusion so as to replete clotting factors and platelets.
Platelets are harvested from plasma and should be infused within a day or two of collection. They are given for thrombocytopenic purpuras.
Granulocyte concentrates are now available for neutropenic patients with infection.
Frozen thawed red cells stored in glycerol are widely available in some countries.

Risks of Blood Transfusion

These are considerable and the ready availability of blood may lead to abuse.
(1) *Incompatibility* of donor red cells and the recipient's plasma may result from errors in crossmatching or unusual antibodies (ABO, Rhesus and others). The donor's blood clumps and then haemolyses causing fever, chest pain, shock, renal failure, consumption coagulopathy and jaundice. Rhesus positive blood given to a Rhesus negative woman may prejudice future pregnancies.
(2) *Febrile reactions* may arise from antibodies to white cells, red cells, platelets and serum proteins. They occur in about 10% of transfusions and may be accompanied by headache or sickness.
(3) *Allergic reactions*, urticaria, asthma and joint pain are due to donor plasma proteins, or sensitivity to white cells.
(4) *Transmission of infections* such as viral hepatitis, malaria, brucellosis, cytomegalic inclusion disease, or syphilis, or rarely, contamination by harmful Gram-negative bacteria which cause fever, hypotension and shock. All donor blood should be tested for Australia antigen and antibody, for the exclusion of Australia antigen containing blood reduces the risk of subsequent hepatitis but does not abolish it completely. Non-A, non-B hepatitis still occurs.
(5) *Circulatory failure* may occur with cardiac disease or with chronic anaemia. It may be minimized by giving small transfusions, packed red cells and accompanying diuretics, or alternatively by an exchange transfusion. The rate of infusion (drops/min) should be told to the nursing staff and the expected time the blood container should take to empty.
(6) *Metabolic;* iron overload is possible since each pint of blood donates

250mg of iron so repeated transfusions lead to haemosiderosis. Rarer events are air-embolism and citrate and potassium intoxication. Massive transfusion of stored blood can cause hypothermia with risk of cardiac arrest unless it is warmed by coil delivery to 37°C. Acid Citrate Dextrose B.P. solutions have a low pH (7), raised potassium, sodium, lactate and citrate levels and lowered levels of calcium, platelets and Factors V and VIII. They have been replaced in some centres by **Citrate Phosphate Dextrose B.P. (CPD)** with a pH of 7.2 and which causes less potassium leak and maintains better levels of diphospho-glycerate (2,3-DPG). Adenine added to the storage medium increases ATP content and lengthens red-cell life (citrate phosphate dextrose adenine).

Plasma is obtained from pooled donor blood which has become time-expired in the blood bank. *Uses* for plasma depletion in burns and to replace protein in malabsorption states, hunger oedema and after fractures, crush injuries, shock and haemoconcentration. Plasma can be stored when dried for long periods and is reconstituted by dissolving in Water for Injections B.P. Plasma supplies albumin so maintaining plasma oncotic pressure (see below).

Fresh Plasma or **Fresh Frozen Plasma** can be transfused to patients with reduced clotting defects. Its use in haemophilia has virtually been superseded. Plasma can transmit viral hepatitis although storage in individual plastic units (i.e. unpooled) reduces the risk.

Albumin Fractions

These can be heat treated and so prevent the transmission of viral hepatitis.

Human Albumin Fraction (Saline) B.P. or Human Plasma Protein Fraction is supplanting plasma. It is a 4.5g/dl protein solution with the same colloid osmotic pressure as freeze-dried plasma reconstituted with sterile water. Albumin comprises 90% of the protein, the rest is alpha and beta globulins. It is conveniently ready for i.v. infusion (or it may be stored freeze-dried). 'Buminate' is a 5% w/v solution in saline.

Low Salt Albumin (Low in sodium, potassium and citrate ions per gram of protein). It is available as a concentrated solution or freeze-dried.

Human Albumin B.P. is a solution containing 15-25% protein used for hypoalbuminaemia in liver disease, nephrotic syndrome and for blood volume expansion. Human Albumin Injection B.N.F. is a 20% solution in Water for Injections in vials 100ml and available as 'Buminate' 20%.

Dried Human Albumin B.P. made by freeze-drying human albumin of protein concentration up to 10% is supplied as a powder (e.g. in 25g amounts) which is made up to give a concentration of 5-25g/dl in Water for Injections.

Clotting Factors

Dried Human Antihaemophilic Fraction B.P. or **Dried Factor VIII** concentrate (anti-haemophilic globulin) and **Dried Human Factor IX Fraction B.P.**, which is rich in clotting factors II, IX, X and may contain factor VII are specially derived from fresh plasma. **Cryoprecipitate** is a concentrate of human anti-haemophilic globulin (AHG) made in transfusion centres by a precipitation process using fresh frozen plasma so that the vital, but labile AHG is contained in a small volume of 10ml, or so. The content of AHG is variable. Single doses of the cryoprecipitate are given i.v. for therapeutic, rather than prophylactic reasons, since the product is in short supply. There is still a slight risk of hepatitis. It is stored at −20°C. **Lyophilized Human AHG** is a freeze-dried preparation originally obtained from a few centres, but it is now commercially available ('Profilate', 'Koate', 'Hemofil', 'Kryobulin'). It has the advantage that it is easier to store (at 4°C). The Factor VIII content is known and predictable so dose schemes are simpler. It is easier to reconstitute so it has been used in self-administration schemes at home. The risk of hepatitis is greater than with cryoprecipitate. Fresh blood or plasma contains a low concentration of AHG.

Human Fibrinogen as Dried Human Fibrinogen B.P. is also available.

Plasmapheresis

This is a method whereby plasma can be skimmed off and red cells returned to the donor. The immunoglobulins such as anti-D globulin (p. 60) and also the anti-HBsAg immunoglobulin (to protect against viral hepatitis) can be obtained from those with high titres. The procedures may also be helpful to remove high molecular weight viscous globulins in macroglobulinaemia.

Artificial or Synthetic Plasma-Like Solutions

These have been introduced to avoid either the hazards of viral hepatitis seen with plasma, or the expense of human albumin. These solutions contain no clotting factors and are plasma or blood expanders only.

Dextran is a complex carbohydrate formed by the coalescence of simple glucose sugars to make a large molecule or polymer. These polymers exert an osmotic or water attracting effect. It is antigenic and some (e.g. Dextran 110) interfere with blood crossmatching which must be done before administration. Since they potentiate the action of heparin the dose of this must be reduced otherwise bleeding can occur.

Uses **Dextran Injections** are used i.v. as blood volume expanders when blood or plasma is not available or unsuitable and also as a prophylaxis against arterial and venous clotting post-operatively and in sickle cell crises. The types are Dextran 40 Injection B.P. ('Gentran 40', 'Lomodex 40', 'Rheomacrodex') with a low molecular weight of 40 000, Dextran 70 Injection B.P. ('Gentran 70', 'Lomodex 70', 'Macrodex'), Dextran 110 Injection B.P. ('Dextraven 110') and Dextran 150 ('Dextraven 150') with an average molecular weight of 150 000. The low molecular weight forms do not interfere with crossmatching of blood (whereas this is a particular problem with Dextran 150). They inhibit red cell aggregation and decrease blood viscosity, but these low molecular forms can impair renal function during excretion. Dextran 40 is a 10% w/v solution in Dextrose Injection 5% or Sodium Chloride Injection. The higher molecular weight dextrans have similar uses and 500-2000ml daily are infused for those with haemorrhage or burns. Their concentrations are 6% w/v in Dextrose 5%, or Sodium Chloride 0.9%. *Adverse effects* allergy, sodium and fluid overload, impairment of renal function with low molecular weight dextran.

Modified Gelatin Solutions

'Gelofusine' is gelatin 4%, calcium chloride 0.05% and sodium chloride 0.85% and has an average molecular weight of 30 000 and is used to restore blood volume in shock, haemorrhage and burns. It has the claimed advantage that large quantities can be given (e.g. up to 4000ml) without affecting haemostasis and it is less antigenic. 'Haemaccel' is a similar 3.5% gelatin infusion in an electrolyte solution.

Intravenous Foods

These are prescribed when medical or surgical patients cannot eat normally, before, during or after major surgery in selected cases. Their use anticipates the marked catabolism of burns, injury, infection and surgery. The prescription covers water, electrolytes, the need for proteins, calories and vitamins and the amounts which can be metabolized daily. Care is needed over asepsis during prolonged i.v. therapy and that sodium overload is avoided. Aminoacids are given as 'Synthamin', or 'Vamin'. Energy is provided by ethanol, dextrose (glucose), laevulose (fructose) 10, 20 and 40% strengths, sorbitol 30%, or as fats as 'Intralipid' 10 and 20%—the latter provides 2000 kcalories/litre. The best sources of energy are dextrose and lipids. 'Aminoplex 5' in 3 litres of fluid contains 15g of utilizable nitrogen and 3000 kcalories.

Oral synthetic foods include 'Vivonex' (6 packets daily) which provides total nutrition, contains no milk or milk products and has no exogenous residue. It is suitable for malabsorption states or Crohn's disease, but is expensive. These highly concentrated foods should be sipped and not drunk as they are hyperosmolar. Patience and persistence are required and the patients should be warned that the bowels may only open once weekly. 'Vivonex HN' is a high nitrogen form. 'Flexical' is another low-residue diet. 'Isocal' is an iso-osmolar lactose and gluten free liquid diet, (supplied in tins). The protein is in the form of sodium caseinate and soy protein isolate. Fat is supplied as soy oil and medium chain triglycerides. Corn syrup provides the carbohydrates and minerals and vitamins are added. The formulation is designed for tube feeding. 'Trisorbon' is another liquid diet taken orally or by tube and supplied as powder in sachets.

Electrolytes and Food

A list of potassium, sodium and calcium content in food is of value. Potassium in significant amounts is present in milk, potatoes, meat, beans, tomato and orange juice, melons, bananas, apricots, strawberries, celery and spinach.

TABLE 21
SOME PARENTERAL FEEDING SOLUTIONS

Product	Pack presentation (ml)	Kcalories per litre	Water per litre	Glucose	Sorbitol	Fructose	Amino Acids	Fat	Glycerol	Ethanol	Na$^+$	K$^+$	Cl$^-$	pH	Uses
Dextrose 50%	500	2000 (8.4MJ)	680	500										3.5-6.5	Energy source in liver and renal failure
Sorbitol 30%	500	1200 (5MJ)	800		300										
Intralipid 10% Intralipid 20%	500 100	1100 2000	850 750					100 200	25 25					7-7.5	Energy Energy
Aminoplex 5	1000	1000 (4.2MJ)	769		125		31			50	35	15	62	7.4	Protein source Energy
Vamin-Fructose	500	650 (2.6MJ)	920			100	70				50	20	55	5.2	Protein source Energy
Vamin-Glucose	100 500	650 (2.6MJ)	920	100			70				50	20	55	5.2	Protein source Energy
Vamin-N	500	250 (1MJ)	980				70				50	20	55	5.2	Nitrogen source also contains calcium 2.5mmol 1/^{l} magnesium 1.5mmol 1/^{l}

29 DRUGS USED IN RHEUMATOLOGY

Rheumatic disorders are a major cause of disability and loss of working ability. Anti-inflammatory drugs are principally used for active rheumatoid arthritis and similar arthritides (e.g. Reiter's syndrome), ankylosing spondylitis and the simple analgesics mainly for the degenerative osteo-arthritis and burnt-out rheumatoid arthritis. It is not usually possible to eradicate the prime cause so that drugs are used which by their chemical and cellular action modify tissue injury and inflammation and reduce body temperature. Chemically they are usually organic acids. The aim of treatment in the absence of cure is to relieve symptoms, suppress active disease, halt progression and preserve joint function.

ANTI-INFLAMMATORY AGENTS
Salicylic acid compounds
Salicylates are still widely used in the control of the inflammatory arthritides such as rheumatoid disease. Aspirin is the drug of choice, but other than its cheapness leaves much to be desired. Effective blood levels are necessary.
Soluble Aspirin (see p. 96) is of value in the rapid relief of pain, but in view of the side effects, especially indigestion, overt blood loss, or deafness its use is limited. A usual dose is 1g 4-6 hourly controlled by blood levels. Over 5g daily is advised to get anti-inflammatory effects. **Enteric Coated Tablets** will reduce stomach discomfort, but occult bleeding can still occur from the small bowel. The dose (e.g. 300 or 600mg of 'Nu-Seals') is adjusted to give a salicylate level of 20-30mg/dl ideally in 6 hourly divided amounts so as to give continuous therapeutic levels, or 2-4 at night with 10-12 soluble aspirins by day.
Aloxiprin ('Palaprin Forte') is aspirin condensed with aluminium oxide and releases aspirin in the small bowel. It is generally acceptable to patients, especially children, as the tablets can be suspended in water to give a pleasant-tasting mixture.
Benorylate (see p. 97) releases salicylate in the bowel and probably after absorption. It is expensive, but may be of use in patients who have indigestion with other forms of aspirin. The usual dose is 10ml b.d. Nausea and vomiting limit its usefulness and paracetamol interferes with the monitoring of blood levels. All the above drugs are contra-indicated in aspirin sensitivity and may cause gastro-intestinal symptoms and blood loss or interfere with blood clotting. All anti-inflammatory analgesics should be taken with food. When aspirin is ineffective, or unacceptable, other agents are tried. Patients should be warned about black motions indicating blood loss.

Anthranilic Acid Compounds
These have trivial anti-inflammatory actions.
Mefenamic Acid ('Ponstan') has a mild, but rapid and prolonged action. *Presentation* Capsules B.P. 250mg, tablets 500mg, suspension 50mg/5ml; *dose* 500mg initially then 500mg 8 hourly. Children over 6 months can be given 6.5mg/kg B.W. 6-8 hourly for up to a week.
Flufenamic Acid ('Meralen') *presentation* Capsules B.P. 100mg; *dose* 300-600mg daily for adults. *Adverse reactions* the fenamates can cause nausea,

vomiting, diarrhoea, rashes and haemolytic anaemia. They are *contra-indicated* in patients with intestinal disease, in pregnancy, or if lactating. They may potentiate anticoagulants.

Propionic Acid Derivatives
Ibuprofen ('Brufen') is long established but a minor anti-inflammatory agent. *Presentation* tablets B.P. 200 and 400mg, suspension 20mg/ml 200ml bottles; *dose* 400mg t.d.s. up to 1600mg daily. It is more expensive than aspirin or phenylbutazone, but less gastro-intestinal side effects are claimed. Other derivatives are stronger and preferred by many to aspirin. **Fenoprofen Calcium** ('Fenopron') *presentation* tablets 300 and 600mg; *dose* 300-600mg 3 or 4 times daily for adults only. **Ketoprofen** ('Alrheumat', or 'Orudis') *presentation* capsules 50mg; *dose* 50mg 2 or 4 times daily with food. **Naproxen** ('Naprosyn') is a naphthalene propionic acid derivative. *Presentation* Tablets B.P. 250 and 500mg, suspension 25mg/ml, suppository 500mg; *dose* orally 250-750mg daily in 2 or 3 divided amounts; 500mg is said to be equivalent to 4g of aspirin. **Flurbiprofen** ('Froben') *presentation* tablets 50 and 100mg; *dose* 50-100mg t.d.s. has proved a useful alternative to phenylbutazone in ankylosing spondylitis. *Adverse effects* of the group. Dyspepsia and epigastric pain occur and they are not advised in those with peptic ulcer symptoms or diagnosis. They interact with aspirin and they may potentiate anticoagulants, hydantoins, sulphonamides and other protein-bound drugs. Rashes have occurred with naproxen and occasionally severe gastro-intestinal haemorrhage. Bronchospasm has been reported particularly with ibuprofen and asthma may be worsened. Thrombocytopenia can also occur.

Acetic Acid Derivatives
Indomethacin ('Imbrilon', 'Indocid') an indole derivative is an effective anti-inflammatory analgesic, expensive, but often a second choice after salicylates. It is also useful for the night pain of osteoarthritis of the hip. *Presentation* Capsules B.P. 25 and 50mg, suspension 25mg/ml and Suppositories B.P. 100mg. *Dose* 75-150mg daily in 3 divided amounts with food. The suppository is useful taken at night to relieve morning stiffness. *Adverse effects* are common with doses above 150mg daily. They are severe headaches, giddiness, unsteadiness, drowsiness, vertigo, blurred vision, impaired concentration, nausea, diarrhoea, vomiting, gastric antral ulcers, gastro-intestinal bleeding, depression, hallucinations, epilepsy, coma, confusion and a variety of rashes including urticaria. It is the treatment of choice for gout. *Contra-indications* migraine, epilepsy, peptic ulcer. 'Indocid R' is a slow release form. **Tolmetin Sodium** ('Tolectin') is related to indomethacin. *Presentation* tablets 200mg; *dose* 200mg t.d.s. up to a maximum of 9 tablets daily. **Fenclofenac** ('Flenac') *presentation* capsules 300mg; *dose* up to 1400mg daily taken morning and night. **Diclofenac Sodium** ('Voltarol') *presentation* tablets 25 and 50mg; *dose* 25-50mg t.d.s. has similar actions and uses. The adverse reactions, precautions and warnings are as for propionic acid derivatives and salicylates.

Indene Derivatives
Sulindac ('Clinoril') is a fluorinated sulphoxide compound metabolized into the active sulphide with a long action. *Presentation* tablets 100 and 200mg; *dose* 100-200mg twice daily. Precautions are as for salicylates and propionic acid derivatives.

Pyrazolone Derivatives

These protonated compounds are acidic and have a strong anti-inflammatory, immunosuppressive and antipyretic action. The originals, amidopyrine and aminopyrine, proved too dangerous and have been replaced.

Phenylbutazone Ph. Eur. ('Butacote' designed to dissolve in the alkaline media of the small intestine and 'Butazolidin', 'Butazone', 'Flexazone'). *Presentation* Tablets B.P. 100 and 200mg, Suppositories B.P. 250mg, ampoules phenylbutazone sodium 600mg in 3ml. *Dose* orally 400mg daily reduced to 200-300mg daily for long-term use. Phenylbutazone was originally used in 1949 as a solvent for amidopyrine and was found to be an effective inexpensive antirheumatic substance. From the family doctor point of view it is widely prescribed and few complications are seen in short term use. However, precautions are needed—the patient should be weighed regularly to detect sodium and water retention, sodium intake is restricted, the blood pressure is regularly measured, the lowest dose possible is given for the shortest time, an accurate record is made of the total prescribed and blood checks should be made. From the hospital aspect complications are common and, at times, fatal. *Adverse effects* fatalities from agranulocytosis, aplastic anaemia, haematemesis, perforation of peptic ulcer, renal failure, exfoliative dermatitis, masking of infection, precipitation of heart failure, toxic hepatitis. Other symptoms are nausea, oedema, melaena and rash. Suppositories reduce the risk of bleeding from direct contact with gastric mucosa. They may cause bleeding from proctitis. *Contra-indications* are cardiac, liver, kidney or stomach disease and severe hypertension. 'Butacote' tablets are enteric coated and not B.P. tablets.

Oxyphenbutazone ('Tanderil', 'Tandacote') tablets 100mg dose and uses as for phenylbutazone. **Feprazone** ('Methrazone') *presentation* capsules 200mg; *dose* 200-600mg daily and **Azapropazone** ('Rheumox') *presentation* capsules 300mg; *dose* up to 300mg 4 times daily are new additions. They all potentiate coumarin anticoagulants, sulphonylurea hypoglycaemics and sulphonamides.

Long-term Anti-inflammatory Agents

Antimalarials take 4-6 weeks to work; they are useful in systemic lupus erythematosus and post-pregnancy exacerbations of rheumatoid arthritis. Chloroquine Phosphate ('Aralen', 'Avloclor', 'Resochin') *presentation* Tablets B.P. 250mg; *dose* 250-500mg daily, or Chloroquine Sulphate ('Nivaquine') Tablets B.P. 200mg; *dose* 200-400mg daily, and Hydroxychloroquine Sulphate ('Plaquenil') Tablets B.P. 200mg; *dose* 800mg-2g daily reduced later to 200-400mg daily. *Adverse effects* long-term use has ocular side effects, so patients should be seen for evidence of corneal and of retinal damage (which is irreversible). Other complications are psychosis, giddiness, aplastic anaemia, thrombocytopenia, nausea, vomiting, diarrhoea, itching, rashes, bleaching of hair and neuro-muscular weakness. Chloroquine overdosage is like that for quinine and quinidine with cardiac and respiratory arrest, arrhythmias and renal and liver damage. It is a protoplasmic poison; 1g or so can kill a child. Ocular damage precludes long-term use.

Corticosteroids and ACTH

These very potent drugs are only used when anti-inflammatory drugs of the type used above, fail. They interfere with hypothalamic, pituitary and adrenal function and have many other side effects (see p. 81). The corticosteroids tend to be used for those with marked systemic features (such as arteritis). Prednisone 20-40mg, or an equivalent of another type, is given initially and this is reduced to the smallest amount that keeps the patient comfortable, usually 5-15mg daily, or 5-7.5mg at night. Some authorities prefer ACTH. Both corticosteroid and ACTH dosage can be monitored by measuring blood cortisol levels. ACTH need not be given daily. The eye complications of sero-negative arthritides are better controlled by corticosteroids than ACTH. The benefit in the short-term has to be balanced against the long-term adverse effects and erosions still continue.

Gold and Penicillamine are not analgesics, nor anti-inflammatory, but modify by unknown means the course of rheumatoid arthritis. They are used if there is continuous progression of the disease such as erosions, inability to work, or disabling or chronic disease.

Sodium Aurothiomalate ('Myocrisin') will induce remissions and is usually tried before corticosteroids. No benefit is expected for several months. *Presentation* Injection B.P. a solution in ampoules 0.5ml containing 1,5,10,20 or 50mg; *dose* various schemes are given—initially a test dose 2.5-10mg i.m. then increasing by 10mg each week to 50mg if no ill-effects; others jump straight to 50mg weekly after the test dose. A weekly 50mg i.m. can be given until clinical remission and fall in ESR and then the intervals are increased to every 2, then 3 weeks and finally, monthly. Alternatively, some give 50mg weekly until a total dose of 1g has been given. Whereas in the past it was customary to have a rest period of 6 months between courses now monthly or 2-monthly injections are given for a number of years. *Adverse effects* are common (often after months of trouble-free therapy) namely diarrhoea, dermatitis, renal, hepatic, marrow, brain and nerve damage. *Contra-indications* severe anaemia, renal or liver disease, or marrow depression and dermatitis from previous therapy. During treatment the urine is tested for protein and the blood for ESR, white cell and platelet count, at first weekly, and the mouth and skin are checked. Gold poisoning is treated by dimercaprol (p. 241).

D. Penicillamine (see p. 241) is given initially 250mg daily as the base at least for 2 weeks with an increase of 250mg as base at similar intervals. The eventual dose if side effects do not occur can be up to 2g, but most rheumatologists prefer to keep below 1g. Reactions usually reverse if the drug is stopped or reduced in amount. Like gold it is slow to act. It mobilizes gold by chelation; whether an interval of a few months should occur before following gold by penicillamine is unclear. Precautions are as for gold. Thrombocytopenia is common, but purpura and bleeding are rare. Nephropathy is of the immune complex type and is said usually to reverse on stopping penicillamine but it may be slow. Rheumatological patients have many other drugs (e.g. analgesics); this and their immunological responses may account for why adverse reactions are seen by experienced observers more frequently than in the treatment of cystinuria or Wilson's disease with penicillamine.

Cytotoxics
The antiproliferative drugs **Cyclophosphamide** and **Azathioprine** have been used, and shown to retard erosions, to spare the dose of corticosteroids and to be as effective as gold in early rheumatoid arthritis. Cyclophosphamide 100mg daily seems better, but produces azoospermia in males. The effects of marrow depression and on the ovary, foetus and bladder also limit their use and the

long-term hazards of malignancy and mutagenesis are not ruled out. Cyclophosphamide can also be injected into joints.

Supportive Measures
Bed rest, skilled nursing and physiotherapy are needed in the acute stage in some patients. As the disease progresses antidepressives, iron, folic acid and vitamins, wax baths, splints and physiotherapy are often required, as well as surgery to joints and tendons. An optimistic and involved doctor helps in the chronic phase. Corticosteroids may occasionally be injected with relief into joints, capsules or tendons and radioactive yttrium in those past reproductive life.

GOUT
Acute symptoms respond to **Indomethacin** 50-100mg initially then 25-50mg 6 hourly (first choice), **Phenylbutazone** 400-600mg daily for 1 or 2 days orally, or 250mg i.m., **Naproxen** 750mg initially then 250mg 8 hourly, or the long-established **Colchicine**. *Presentation* Tablets B.P. 250 and 500µg; *dose* orally 1000µg (1mg) initially then 500µg (0.5mg) every 2-3 hours until the pain is relieved, or diarrhoea, or vomiting occurs. Most attacks subside after 4-5mg. Salicylates can be given concurrently. Pseudogout (chondrocalcinosis) as synovitis, or arthritis, from calcium pyrophosphate crystals may also be relieved by colchicine. Colchicine 0.5mg twice or three times daily has improved familial Mediterranean fever. *Adverse effects* nausea, vomiting, abdominal pain and diarrhoea; rarely, blood disorders, neuritis or alopecia.

Interval Treatment
Between attacks substances promoting renal excretion of uric acid, i.e. uricosuric drugs, are used. Their indications are recurrent gout, gouty tophi and a persistently high (e.g. more than 10mg/dl) serum uric acid. They reduce the body total of uric acid as well as the visible deposits, the frequency of gout and the chances of renal damage. While taking them the patient is given plenty of fluids, sodium bicarbonate to keep the urine alkaline, and, since in the first 6 weeks the mobilization of uric acid can actually provoke acute gout, daily colchicine. It is traditional to avoid foods rich in nucleoproteins like sweetbreads and to curtail alcohol which blocks renal uric acid excretion, but it is no longer obligatory.

Uricosuric Drugs
Probenecid ('Benemid') a sulphonamide derivative, inhibits renal excretion of organic acids and has been used to prevent penicillin and rifampicin excretion as well as preventing reabsorption of tubular uric acid. *Presentation* Tablets B.P. 500mg; *dose* 250mg twice daily for a week then 1-2g daily indefinitely. *Adverse effects* anorexia, nausea, vomiting (reduced by taking tablets with food), occasionally renal colic, haematuria, nephrotic syndrome and hypersensitivity reactions. Probenecid increases the excretion of calcium, magnesium, and citrate and leads to calcium loss, but reduces the excretion of conjugated sulphonamides. If an analgesic is needed paracetamol and not aspirin is prescribed, since it does not block the action of probenecid. Probenecid is combined with colchicine in 'Colbenemid'.
Sulphinpyrazone ('Anturan') is related to phenylbutazone, but is safer. *Presentation* Tablets B.P. 100 and 200mg; *dose* 200-800mg in divided doses after

meals. *Adverse effects* as for pyrazolones including potentiation of warfarin. It also inhibits platelet aggregation (p. 138).

Reduction of uric acid synthesis
Allopurinol ('Zyloric') reduces uric acid formation by interfering with xanthine oxidase. It is probably now the drug of choice. *Presentation* Tablets B.P. 100 and 300mg; *dose* 200-900mg daily in single or divided amounts. *Adverse effects* rashes sometimes exfoliative, fever, nausea, gastro-intestinal symptoms, allergic vasculitis. It is useful for gout with renal failure (the dose is reduced to 100-200mg daily), or stones, as well as in patients excreting large amounts of uric acid following cytotoxic and radiation therapy. Allopurinol potentiates the action of mercaptopurine so the dose of the cytotoxic drug is reduced if the two are given together.

Many drugs e.g. thiazide diuretics (see p. 253) provoke gout. Uric acid is bound to plasma proteins and contrast media injected i.v. may displace uric acid and provoke gout.

Osteoarthritis and ankylosing spondylitis. Simple analgesics are tried first (e.g. aspirin, paracetamol) and later indomethacin or phenylbutazone (especially for ankylosing spondylitis). The pain relief produced by indomethacin in osteoarthritis of the hip may be followed by increased activity and repeated microtrauma to the hip joint with further damage.

CONNECTIVE TISSUE DISORDERS
Rheumatic fever: this is still a major health problem in many parts of the world (Asia, Oceana) in the acute stage, bed rest and nursing are important. **Salicylates,** usually aspirin, are given in large doses unless there is cardiac enlargement with failure since they may induce pulmonary oedema. They usually relieve pain quickly, but they do not prevent cardiac damage. *Dose* is 1g of aspirin or 2g of sodium salicylate 4 hourly, until the pain and fever have settled. **Corticosteroids** are tried first in severe illness with myocardial, valvular or pericardial involvement. Antibiotics like **Penicillin** are advisable initially to treat streptococcal infection and for a lengthy period (until adult life or longer) afterwards to prevent subsequent streptococcal infection, but may prove inadequate in eradication in overcrowded and poor countries.

Systemic lupus erythematosus: in the acute stage corticosteroids may be helpful and in selected patients with renal or brain involvement. In others, cytotoxics are useful.

Dermatomyositis is also treated with corticosteroids, or if resistant, with azathioprine, cyclophosphamide or methotrexate. **Polymyalgia rheumatica** and **temporal arteritis** respond excellently to long-term corticosteroids.

Muscular rheumatism: fibrositis, sprains and lumbago are often treated by counter-irritants which promote warmth and relieve pain and spasm. Preparations include non-staining iodine ointment (ung. iodi denigrescens), methyl salicylate ointment, turpentine liniment and white liniment. Numerous proprietary remedies exist, e.g. 'Algipan'. Local steroid injections are helpful in soft tissue lesions such as tennis elbow and capsulitis of the shoulder.

Polyarthropathy may co-exist with hypogammaglobulinaemia and immune deficiency, and immunoglobulin injections (p. 60) at a dose of 25mg/kg i.m. may be helpful.

Levamisole has been used as an immunological modulating drug to control rheumatoid arthritis in a dose of 150mg daily. Its use is associated with a high incidence of adverse drug reactions including agranulocytosis, rash and fever.

30 DRUGS USED IN METABOLIC DISORDERS

Chelating agents combine with (literally 'claw out') metallic substances in the body. The resulting combinations are water soluble and excreted by the kidneys. *Uses* poisoning by heavy metals and for diseases caused by accumulation of metals.

Desferrioxamine Mesylate ('Desferal') combines with iron. *Uses* acute iron poisoning, iron storage diseases of secondary origin e.g. transfusion haemosiderosis. Primary haemochromatosis is treated by de-ironing with repeated venesections. *Presentation* Injection B.P. vials containing 500mg dissolved in Water for Injections (2ml); *dose* 2g i.m. initially, then 2g i.m. b.d. It may also be given i.v. at a dose up to 15mg/kg B.W. hourly to a total of 80mg/kg B.W. as well as 5g dissolved in 100ml of water being left in the stomach after washout with dilute bicarbonate solution. It has been used prophylactically in the prevention of iron overload or haemosiderosis in sickle cell anaemia and thalassaemia; 1-3g is added to a pint of blood and then 500mg is given i.m. daily by the patient, relative or nurse. It has recently been shown that iron excretion is greater with prolonged i.v. or s.c. infusions. The cost is several thousand pounds yearly.

De-ironing by venesection, or desferrioxamine, has been used in forms of porphyria.

D-Penicillamine B.P. ('Cuprimine', 'Distamine') is a sulphur containing aminoacid originally obtained as a metabolite from penicillin and used to reduce the body stores of copper in Wilson's disease by increasing the excretion of urinary copper; it also splits the large (macro) globulins present in macroglobulinaemia and has been used for this purpose and it does the same for the rheumatoid factor (see uses for rheumatoid arthritis). It may also help other heavy metal poisoning and possibly cystinosis and cystinuria. It is very expensive. *Presentation* as penicillamine base Capsules B.P. 250mg ('Cuprimine'), Tablets B.P. 50, 125 and 250mg ('Distamine'). *Dose* 300-2000mg in terms of base starting at a low dose e.g. 2 tablets and increasing slowly at intervals of 2-4 weeks or so. *Adverse effects* are common; gastro-intestinal—anorexia, nausea, vomiting, loss or distortion of sense of taste; renal damage—proteinuria (if mild can continue therapy), nephrotic syndrome haematuria, rashes—maculopapular (early in treatment and may only need a reduction in dosage), exfoliative dermatitis, allergies such as urticaria, thrombocytopenia, neutropenia, aplastic anaemia, fever, joint pain and muscle weakness and myasthenic symptoms.

Dimercaprol (BAL) is used for antimony, arsenic, bismuth, gold and mercury poisoning. *Presentation* Injection B.P. contained in ampoules 2ml of a solution 50mg/ml in benzylbenzoate and arachis oil. *Dose* 8-16ml in divided doses during the first day then according to the patient's needs, or 3mg/kg B.W. 4 hourly for 48 hours, 6 hourly the third day, thereafter, twice daily. *Adverse effects* nausea, vomiting, headache, facial flushing, tears and salivation.

Edetates: Sodium Calciumedetate ('Calcium Disodium Versenate Injection', 'Ledclair', Calcium Disodium EDTA) is used for lead poisoning. *Presentation* Injection B.P., U.S.P. a 20% solution (200mg/ml) in 5ml ampoules and a 10%

cream. *Dose* up to 40mg/kg B.W. twice daily i.v. given over 1 hour in a 5 day course. The 20% solution is diluted with Dextrose Injection B.P. 5% to a concentration of 2-3%.

Disodium Edetate B.P., U.S.P. is used in hypercalcaemia and as eye drops for lime burns. *Presentation* Injection B.P.C. a solution 200mg/ml in ampoules 5ml or the equivalent **Trisodium Edetate Injection B.P.** ('Limclair'). *Dose* adult 5g daily by slow i.v. infusion in Sodium Chloride or Dextrose Injections; children 60mg/kg B.W. *Adverse effects* renal damage, haemorrhage, hypocalcaemia, nausea, cramps and rashes.

Idiopathic Hypercalciuria
The **Thiazides** e.g. bendrofluazide 5mg daily reduce calcium excretion and may be supplemented by a low calcium diet.

Sodium Cellulose Phosphate adsorbs calcium ions within the intestine and so prevents over-absorption. Since sodium is exchanged for calcium and this is absorbed care is needed in cardiac and renal failure.

Hyperlipidaemia
The hyperlipidaemias are grouped by blood analysis into 5 main groups whether hyperchylomicronaemia, hypercholesterolaemia or hypertriglyceridaemia alone, or mixed is present, so typing is essential for proper therapy.Treatment in the short term eases pain (e.g. abdominal pain), skin eruptions and hyperlipidaemia, and, in the long run may help prevent vascular disease. For **Type I** hyperchylonmicronaemia reduction of fat intake is needed and median chain triglycerides. The other types are seen in adults and in all the ideal weight should be achieved. In **Type II** the serum cholesterol is raised (alone in IIa and with elevated triglycerides in IIb). Saturated animal and vegetable fats are restricted and fat should only comprise 30-35% of the energy intake and the ratio of polyunsaturated to saturated fats is 2:1. Safflower or corn oil can be added to food and special margarine bought. Skimmed milk, cottage cheese, soft margarine (to replace butter), fish, chicken and turkey trimmed of fat (rather than steaks) are permitted but no shell fish, egg yolks or full cream cheese. In hypertriglyceridaemia e.g. **Type IV** a low carbohydrate diet is given, simple sugars are excluded, alcohol is forbidden and starches decreased. If both cholesterol and triglyceride are raised both diets must be combined.

Secondary factors (diabetes mellitus, hypothyroidism, alcohol, gout, porphyria) are corrected as well as other risk factors (obesity, hypertension, cigarettes, oral contraceptives).

Medication
Hypercholesterolaemia (Hyperbetalipoproteinaemia)
Cholestyramine ('Questran') is the chloride salt of a basic anion-exchange resin which exchanges chloride for bile salts. The bound bile acids are insoluble and excreted so reducing the body pool. At the same time cholesterol formation is increased and because of lack of available bile acids fat absorption is decreased and steatorrhoea can result. Fat soluble substances are poorly absorbed and so may be various drugs (digitalis, anticoagulants, nitrofurantoin). *Presentation* a powder in sachets; *dose* 16-32g daily. It is also used to relieve itching partial biliary obstruction and biliary cirrhosis. Bile salts are normally absorbed in the terminal ileum. If unabsorbed they irritate the colon

and cause diarrhoea e.g. in Crohn's disease and here cholestyramine may help. *Adverse effects* nausea, heartburn, constipation and nasty taste (made acceptable by mixture with fruit juices). **Polidexide** a dextran derivative had a similar function, but was withdrawn in 1976.

Colestipol Hydrochloride ('Colestid') is an alternative available in 5g sachets. The dose is 15-30g daily in 2 or 4 divided doses in liquid. **Probucol** ('Lorelco') is available in the U.S.A. Under trial are gemfibrozil and halofenate.

Nicotinic Acid 3-6g daily has been used starting with a small dose first. *Adverse effects* are common e.g. flushing, nausea, vomiting, hyperglycaemia and abnormal liver function so it is of secondary importance.

Neomycin impairs absorption of fat micelles and cholesterol. *Dose* 1-2g daily. *Adverse effects* malabsorption, and if absorbed, renal impairment.

D-Thyroxine ('Choloxin') increases cholesterol metabolism. Cardiac side effects are still possible, especially in those with extrasystoles. The medication, if prescribed at all should be given to those under 35 years of age. *Dose* up to 8mg daily with 10-20mg of propranolol 8 hourly to counter cardiac stimulation.

Hypertriglyceridaemia (with or without hypercholesterolaemia)

Clofibrate ('Atromid S', 'Liprinal') is used for Type III and IV hyperlipidaemia after weight reduction and diet. It may act synergistically with polidexide in Type IIb. It also increases platelet survival. *Presentation* Capsules B.P. 500mg; *dose* 4 capsules daily in divided doses after meals. *Contra-indications* pregnancy, renal and liver disease e.g. with hypoalbuminaemia. It potentiates oral anticoagulants. *Adverse effects* nausea, water retention, indigestion, loose motions, weight gain, alopecia, thigh muscle pain and liability to gallstones caused by the increased biliary excretion of cholesterol.

Drugs for Alcoholism

Disulfiram ('Antabuse 200') causes an unpleasant reaction when alcohol is drunk. *Presentation* Tablets B.P. 200mg; *dose* 800mg first day, 600mg second day, 400mg third day. On the fourth and fifth days 200mg daily, thereafter 100-200mg daily. It is excreted mainly by the kidneys. *Adverse effects* thrombocytopenia and after alcohol flushing, arrhythmia and occasionally death. The mode of action is that alcohol breaks down to toxic levels of acetaldehyde which cannot be metabolized to acetate. Alcohol should only be given under strict medical and nursing supervision. If a bad reaction occurs the foot of the bed is blocked and treatment is for shock. Ephedrine, and injections of an antihistamine and ascorbic acid should be available. *Contra-indications* diabetes mellitus, cardiac disease, pregnancy, epilepsy, cirrhosis of the liver and nephritis.

Citrated Calcium Carbimide ('Abstem') *presentation* tablets 50mg; *dose* 50mg b.d. or t.d.s. has similar uses. *Adverse effects* drowsiness, fatigue, tinnitus, rash and possibly hypothyroidism with prolonged use.

Chlormethiazole Edisylate ('Heminevrin') related to vitamin B_1 (the thiazole part) is a sedative, hypnotic and anticonvulsant. *Presentation* tablets 500mg, syrup 50mg/ml for hypnotic use in bottles 300 and 500ml, capsules 192mg of the base and therapeutically equal to the tablet which is chlormethiazole edisylate; solution 8mg/ml for injection, or infusion of chlormethiazole edisylate bottles 100 and 500ml. *Uses* to ease the withdrawal symptoms of alcohol, including delirium tremens, agitation, restlessness in acute mania, status epilepticus and pre-eclampsia and eclampsia with convulsions. Its widest use is as a night-time hypnotic. *Dose* orally initially 1-2g 2 hourly up to a total of 8g daily. In the treatment of alcohol withdrawal it should only be used for 7 days otherwise addiction to it can occur. *Dose* i.v. initially 30-50ml at 60 drops/min until the patient is sedated then 10-15 drops/min. *Adverse effects* of oral therapy—nasal irritation, gastro-intestinal upset; i.v. hypotension and respiratory depression.

Eclampsia was treated by some with **bromethol** rectally 0.1ml/kg B.W. in solution, which is first tested with Congo Red to check safety. Other agents used are anticonvulsants, anaesthetic agents, hypotensives and tranquillizers e.g. diazepam.

ERYTHROPOIETIC PROTOPORPHYRIA
Beta carotene a carotenoid pigment allied to vitamin A has been shown to protect against the phototoxicity seen in this disorder. *Dose* 30-300mg daily.

31 ADVERSE DRUG REACTIONS

An adverse reaction is defined here as any unwanted effect of a drug including allergy, side effects, toxicity, idiosyncrasy and interactions. They are major problems and certain rules may help reduce their incidence.

(1) Before prescribing any drug its necessity should be queried. Many illnesses are self-limiting and not all symptoms warrant therapy. Many die from prophylactic penicillin. Some patients are intolerant of most drugs, even placeboes.

(2) Five drugs or more concurrently, increase the risks. Most hospital in-patients have a startling number of drugs. Some may be antagonistic e.g. antidepressives which may cancel the effect of many hypotensive agents.

(3) Know what is in the drug prescribed. This will help to avoid drug potentiation, antagonism, or interaction and will aid recognition of side effects.

(4) To reduce sensitivity-reactions applications to the skin should not be of substances also given systemically. (Important exceptions are corticosteroids, tetracycline and chloramphenicol.)

(5) Choose the oral route when possible.

(6) Ask the patient about previous drug intolerance or allergy and who diagnosed it. Unless there is no alternative life-saving drug as in endocarditis, it is best to avoid the same preparation and try not to desensitize.

(7) Ask about previous alcohol intake and medication. Phenobarbitone administration may influence subsequent therapy with other drugs by stimulating liver enzymes.

(8) Consider the physiological state of the patient.

Age: neonates often have immature liver enzymes which cannot adequately detoxicate drugs by conjugation. In general, the incidence of adverse drug reactions increases with age since in the elderly metabolic and excretory processes are impaired.

Weight: some adults may be very small e.g. Indian women and orthodox doses may be too much.

Sex: in women cyclical hormonal changes, reproduction and lactation may contra-indicate, or restrict drug or hormone therapy. Drugs may put the foetus at risk during all stages of pregnancy.

Race: Negroes and Mediterranean peoples may have red cell enzyme defects which make their cells easily damaged or oxidized by many drugs. Glucose 6 phosphate dehydrogenase deficiency occurs in 3% of the world population. Other races may only detoxicate hydrazines (e.g. isoniazid) slowly and this may cause toxic blood levels.

Families: certain kindreds cannot adequately metabolize drugs including warfarin, phenylbutazone, monoamine oxidase inhibitors and suxamethonium.

Diurnal changes: variations in plasma volume can make hypotensives more potent in the morning.

(9) **Pathological conditions:** these may indicate a higher risk of adverse reactions. Previous or past allergy, eczema or asthma or a family history of such may raise the possibility of hypersensitivity antigen:antibody reactions. *Impaired absorption* in coeliac disease affects absorption of glucose, xylose, fusidic acid and digoxin. In obstructive jaundice bile salts are necessary for fat

soluble drug and vitamin absorption. *Impaired metabolism* is seen with hepatic disease which may make oral anticoagulants and cyclophosphamide therapy hazardous, and also increases sensitivity to sedatives, narcotic analgesics and some diuretics. *Impaired excretion* by the kidney can cause toxic levels in the blood, but also ineffective therapy in renal infection. The presence of infectious mononucleosis and lymphatic leukaemia makes an ampicillin rash very likely. A low blood pressure may make syncope probable with many fluid depleting agents, or those that interfere with vessel tone. Addison's disease and hypothyroidism potentiate narcotic analgesics. In patients with cerebral arteriosclerosis dementia, confusion or hallucinations are likely events with therapy. Previous temperament may explain why depression or euphoria has occurred with the use of corticosteroids. A greasy skin or acne may determine the choice of a suitable oral contraceptive.

(10) Treatment should be stopped when no longer needed, or pruned in long term use where possible. Many elderly patients are better when their therapy is stopped under medical guidance. Surveys show that digoxin, diuretics, tranquillizers and antidepressants are continued too long.

(11) Certain therapy such as immunosuppression and anticoagulation require close surveillance and laboratory control in hospital and in out-patients. The family doctor must be informed of drug regimes and up-to-date laboratory tests.

RECOGNIZING ADVERSE DRUG REACTIONS

The first thing is to always consider their possibility in any unexplained illness. Then to determine which drugs are responsible. The mechanisms are varied.

(1) **Allergic;** here antibodies are formed and an immunological process, which may be immediate or delayed, is responsible for the hypersensitivity (altered degree of susceptibility). Usually there is an initiating dose, a latent period, then a sensitivity eliciting or provoking dose.

(2) **Toxic;** this results from a pharmacological dose or an overdose (i.e. is dose dependent) and depends on the blood and tissue levels, the duration of effect and the patient's ability to excrete or break down the drug.

(3) **A side effect** is an unwanted action of a drug accompanying its desired pharmacological effect.

(4) **Idiosyncrasy;** here there is an abnormal reaction to a usually harmless amount of the drug (extreme sensitivity to small dose). The basis is usually a biochemical genetic defect involving hydrolysis, dehydrogenation, oxidation, acetylation or conjugation, or other synthetic defect or enzyme lack. It is not allergic or antibody mediated. The variation in drug response determined by heredity is studied in **pharmacogenetics.** Common pharmacogenetic traits are glucose-6-phosphate dehydrogenase defects of red cells (e.g. primaquine), acetyl conjugation of hydrazines (e.g. isoniazid), dapsone and sulphadimidine, and the intra-ocular pressure response to corticosteroids. Patients with hepatic porphyria, hyperbilirubinaemia from defects in liver cell uptake or conjugation, bleeding disorders (e.g. von Willebrand's disease and aspirin), osteogenesis imperfecta (suxamethonium hyperthermia), periodic paralysis, and some forms of gout with enzyme defect may react abnormally to drug therapy.

(5) Interactions between drugs are highly important. They may occur pharmaceutically in the drug formulation and in solutions given i.v. In the body potential sites are in the gut preventing absorption, after absorption by inter-

fering with protein carriage and distribution within the body compartments, metabolization by liver and other organs and during excretion.
(6) Carcinogenesis, teratogenesis and mutagenesis.
(7) Drug alteration of flora with superinfection and drug resistance.
(8) Suppression or prolongation of diseases (e.g. masked by antibiotics or corticosteroids).
(9) Tolerance, abuse, dependence and withdrawal syndromes.

History taking is important; questions are asked about self-prescription for bowels, tonics, sleep, nerves, periods, rheumatism and headaches, plus medical or dental prescribing. Investigational substances, anaesthetics and pre- and post-operative medications may be incriminated in adverse reactions.
Examination may reveal fever, rash, itching, jaundice, lymphadenopathy, or derangement of any organ. Clues to a drug aetiology are marrow depression, neutropenia, thrombocytopenia, or haemolysis with Heinz bodies. Liver function may be abnormal and a chest x-ray may show infiltration due to pulmonary eosinophilia.
   The final diagnosis depends on knowing what has been prescribed and if it is known to cause the relevant reaction. The following tabulates some important adverse drug reactions.

ALIMENTARY
Constipation; analgesics (codeine, morphine, opiates), antacids, (calcium and aluminium salts), anticholinergic and antiparkinsonian drugs, ganglion blocking hypotensives (mecamylamine, pempidine), iron salts, tricyclic antidepressants, vincristine.
Diarrhoea; antibiotics (cephalosporins, colistin, lincomycin, clindamycin, tetracyclines), antirheumatics (colchicine, flufenamic and mefenamic acid), chemotherapy (para-aminosalicylic acid, nitrofurantoin), digitalis glycosides, hypotensives (guanethidine, guanoxan, mecamylamine, methyldopa, reserpine), parasympathomimetics (e.g. neostigmine), deliberate purgation.
Dry mouth and dental caries; hypotensives (e.g. clonidine, prazosin, methyldopa), narcotics, anticholinergics, antihistamines, antidepressants, phenothiazines, benzodiazepines.
Gastric irritation, discomfort, nausea or vomiting; antibiotics (cephalosporins, colistin, oral penicillins, rifampicin, tetracyclines) cytotoxics (nitrogen mustards, antifolates, antipurines, vinca alkaloids, antibiotics), anthelmintics (bephenium hydroxynaphthoate, dichlorophen, filix mas, niclosamide, niridazole, tetrachloroethylene, tetramisole, thiabendazole), antimalarials (primaquine, proguanil), analgesics (heroin, morphine, pethidine), cardiac glycosides, phenylbutazone, chemotherapy (metronidazole, para-aminosalicylic acid, sulphonamides, emetine, ethacrynic acid, anticonvulsants (sulthiame), ergotamine, anti-inflammatory (aspirin, indomethacin, naproxen, fenoprofen, ibuprofen, ketoprofen, alclofenac).
Gastric ulcer; aspirin, corticosteroids, indomethacin.
Gastro-intestinal haemorrhage; anticoagulants, aspirin, ethacrynic acid, marrow suppressants (cytotoxic agents causing thrombocytopenia), pyrazoiones (phenylbutazone, oxyphenbutazone), indomethacin, alcohol particularly with analgesics.
Gastro-intestinal pain; methysergide, parasympathomimetics (e.g. carbachol, neostigmine), vasopressin, purgative abuse.

Ileus; tricyclic antidepressants, drugs causing hypokalaemia.

Intestinal stenosis and stricture; potassium salts in solid form.

Malabsorption; neomycin, colchicine (large continuous doses), cholestyramine, colestipol, biguanides (metformin, phenformin), antacids (e.g. phosphorus depletion) para-aminosalicylic acid, chronic laxative abuse.

Pancreatitis; colaspase, corticosteroids, hypervitaminosis D, oral contraceptives, thiazide diuretics, frusemide.

Stomatitis and proctitis; broad spectrum antibiotics, corticosteroids, cytotoxic therapy.

Tongue ulceration; sublingual isoprenaline. Mouth ulcers; emepronium bromide.

BLOOD

Marrow Function—Underproduction

Total (aplastic anaemia), or partial (agranulocytosis and thrombocytopenia) marrow suppression is caused invariably and unavoidably by cytotoxic drugs (e.g. alkylating agents) and at times with the following:

antibiotics; chloramphenicol (1:20 000 approx), rifampicin, streptomycin, methicillin, ampicillin, sulphonamides.

anticoagulants; indandiones (phenindione).

anticonvulsants; carbamazepine, ethosuximide, phenytoin, ethotoin, methoin, paramethadione, phenacemide, pheneturide, troxidone.

antidiabetic agents; chlorpropamide, tolbutamide (sulphonylureas).

antihistamines

antimalarials; pyrimethamine, dapsone, chloroquine, mepacrine.

antiarrhythmics; quinidine, procainamide, ajmaline.

antirheumatics; amidopyrine (aminopyrine), gold, indomethacin, oxyphenbutazone, phenylbutazone, penicillamine, rarely aspirin.

antithyroid; carbimazole, thiouracils, potassium perchlorate.

diuretics; ethacrynic acid, thiazides, frusemide, chlorthalidone, acetazolamide.

hypnotics; barbiturates (rare), benzodiazepines (rare), carbromal.

chemotherapy; para-aminosalicylic acid, sulphonamides, thiacetazone, cotrimoxazole, levamisole.

tranquillizers; phenothiazines (e.g. chlorpromazine), meprobamate, dichloralphenazone. Alcohol-induced thrombocytopenia is common.

Drugs causing megaloblastic anaemia by an antifolate action are alcohol, barbiturates, primidone, pyrazolones (phenylbutazone, oxyphenbutazone), cotrimoxazole, triamterene, pentamidine, proguanil, pyrimethamine, methotrexate, possibly nitrofurantoin and the oral contraceptives. Cytotoxic drugs (e.g. cytarabine, hydroxyurea) interfere with DNA synthesis, so causing megaloblastosis.

Thrombocytosis—increased numbers of platelets may be seen after stopping alcohol and cytotoxic therapy and sometimes during vincristine therapy.

Drugs Affecting Erythrocyte Survival

Haemolysis occurs in several ways:

(1) Toxic by oxidizing drugs such as the sulphones and phenacetin in normal pharmacological doses.

(2) Enzyme deficient red cells (glucose 6 phosphate dehydrogenase). There may be a deficiency of glutathione reductase, synthetase, or peroxidase. Such

cells are susceptible to oxidation by small doses of drugs. The drugs change haemoglobin to methaemoglobin. Negroes and Mediterranean people are liable to this.

analgesics; acetylsalicylic acid, phenacetin (acetophenetidin) phenazopyridium ('Pyridium').

antimalarials; primaquine, pamaquine, mepacrine, quinine.

antimicrobials; chloramphenicol, nitrofurans (furazolidine, nitrofurantoin, nitrofurazone), para-aminosalicylic acid, sulphonamides.

others; dimercaprol, probenecid, quinidine, the water soluble analogues of vitamin K, sulphones, nalidixic acid.

Abnormal haemoglobins e.g. haemoglobin Zurich; haemolysis occurs with sulphonamides.

(3) **Abnormal immunological mechanisms.** Drugs can induce antibody formation and so lead to destruction of red cells. Type I immune haemolysis results from hypersensitivity to the drug usually attached to the red cell and antibodies (IgG) are formed against them e.g. penicillin. In Type II the drug combines first with an antibody and the immune complex including complement is adsorbed on to cells which are involved as 'innocent bystanders'. The classic example is stibophen, but this mechanism also applies to isoniazid, para-aminosalicylic acid, phenacetin, quinidine, quinine, sulphonamides and sulphonylureas. In the third type typified by methyldopa (and also mefenamic acid, chlordiazepoxide and levodopa) antibodies are directed against the red cell antigen and it is an auto-immune haemolytic anaemia closely resembling the idiopathic form except for the history of drug exposure. The positive Coombs' reaction and haemolytic anaemia produced by methyldopa are the commonest adverse drug reaction. Both the cephalosporins (e.g. cephalothin) and rifampicin cause immune haemolytic anaemia and positive Coombs' reaction, but the mechanisms are not as clear.

Drugs Affecting Erythrocyte Function

Methaemoglobinaemia; phenacetin, phenazone, sulphonamides, nitrates.

Lymphadenopathy; para-aminosalicylic acid, methoin, phenytoin, pyrazolones, dapsone, serum sickness.

Anticoagulant potentiation of oral indandiones and coumarins with enhanced action and bleeding occur with:

(1) antibiotics suppressing vitamin K formation in the gut e.g. broad spectrum tetracyclines, neomycin, oral streptomycin, ampicillin, sulphonamides.

(2) displacement of bound anticoagulants from plasma proteins by anabolic steroids (ethyloestrenol, methandienone, methandriol, methenolone, nandrolone, norethandrolone, oxymetholone, stanolone, stanozolol), clofibrate, indomethacin, pyrazolones (phenylbutazone, oxyphenbutazone, nifenazone), chloral, ethacrynic acid, phenytoin, nalidixic acid, mefenamic acid, salicylates, triclofos.

(3) inhibition of liver enzyme function by alcohol, allopurinol, chloramphenicol, disulfiram, phenylbutazone.

(4) uncertain action; quinidine, paracetamol, thiouracil, cimetidine.

(5) increase in clotting factor metabolism—thyroid hormones.

If any drug has to be given concurrently the dose of anticoagulant may be reduced and the monitoring of tests should be more frequent. The physician must therefore know all the other drugs the patient is taking and what he has taken recently.

The action of oral anticoagulants **is reduced by** drugs promoting liver enzyme activity which metabolize them (inducers) e.g. barbiturates, corticosteroids, phenytoin, glutethimide, ethchlorvynol, griseofulvin, meprobamate and the phenothiazines. The danger is when they are stopped there can be a disastrous rebound increase in anticoagulant action. Vitamin K and oral contraceptives also counteract anticoagulants, as will drugs which interfere with their absorption such as cholestyramine.

Sideroblastic anaemia; chloramphenicol, cycloserine, alcohol, isoniazid, pyrazinamide, phenacetin.

CARDIOVASCULAR

Anaphylactic shock; i.v. antitoxins, aminophylline, contrast media, iron; parenteral penicillin (rarely oral or even topical), injected allergens in desensitization therapy.

Angina; adrenaline, isoprenaline and other sympathomimetics, emetine, hypotensive therapy (occasionally), insulin and oral hypoglycaemics, methysergide, pentamidine, antimony sodium tartrate, ergotamine tartrate, thyroxine, vasopressin, vasodilators (which increase the pulse and cardiac output reflexly), sudden withdrawal of beta-blocking drugs 'rebound angina'.

Arrhythmias; bradycardia—digitalis, beta-blockers, methyldopa, reserpine. Tachycardia—alcohol, caffeine, nicotine, digitalis, atropine, tricyclic antidepressants, phenothiazines, sympathomimetics (adrenaline, isoprenaline, orciprenaline, salbutamol, terbutaline), thyroxine. Other arrhythmias —quinidine, digitalis, anaesthetic agents, suxamethonium, drugs causing hypokalaemia, tricyclic antidepressants.

Fluid and sodium retention; carbenoxolone, adrenal corticosteroids and analogues, androgens, oestrogens, anabolic steroids, fludrocortisone, cyanocobalamin, hydroxocobalamin, indomethacin, insulin, chlorpropamide, carbamazepine, clofibrate, hypotensives (via secondary aldosteronism-methyldopa, reserpine and most others), vasodilators, minoxidil, beta-blockers, diazoxide, monoamine oxidase inhibitors, analgesics (aspirin, pyrazolones e.g. phenylbutazone, indomethacin), lithium salts, i.v. and oral sodium chloride, lactate or bicarbonate solutions, certain parenteral feeding solutions containing salt, sodium salts of penicillin and cephalosporins e.g. cephalothin, carbenicillin. Pulmonary oedema i.v. sodium, salicylates, paradoxical reaction to heroin. 'Fybogel' and 'Complan' contain sodium.

Hypertension; amphetamines, monoamine oxidase inhibitors (iproniazid, isocarboxazid, mebanazine, nialamide, pargyline, phenelzine, tranylcypromine) if given with amphetamines, foods containing dopamine or tyramine (cheese, 'Marmite') or sympathomimetics such as ephedrine; oral contraceptives, corticosteroids, ergotamine.

Hypotension and syncope; antidepressants, fluid-depleting diuretics, hypotensives, monoamine oxidase inhibitors, particularly with hypotensives and diuretics; barbiturates, tranquillizers, phenothiazines, benzodiazepines (e.g. diazepam, chlordiazepoxide), chlormethiazole, levodopa, quinidine, procainamide, injections of suramin, emetine, pentamidine, antimony sodium tartrate, nalorphine, morphine; trinitrin, bromocriptine.

Myocarditis; antimony compounds, emetine, phenothiazines, alcohol, tricyclic antidepressants, doxorubicin, daunorubicin, vincristine, anaesthetics (cyclopropane, halothane), sensitivity to sulphonamides, sera and vaccines.

Vasculitis; polyarteritis—iodides, penicillin, sulphonamides, alclofenac.

Lupus erythematosus—griseofulvin, hydrallazine, penicillin, procainamide, practolol, sulphonamides.
Gangrene; ergotamine tartrate. **Raynaud's disease;** beta-blockers, bromocriptine.
Thrombophlebitis; i.v. dextrose, antibiotics, alkylating agents, colchicine, vincristine, vinblastine.
Venous thrombosis; oral contraceptives, oestrogens.
ENDOCRINE
Adrenal suppression; corticosteroids.
Amenorrhoea; oral contraceptives.
Breast secretion; methyldopa, phenothiazines, reserpine, clomiphene, digoxin, oral contraceptives.
Flushing; alcohol, sulphonylureas, furazolidine, disulfiram, metronidazole.
Gynaecomastia; digitalis glycosides, oestrogens, spironolactone, phenothiazines, guancydine, cyproterone acetate, cimetidine.
Hirsutism and hypertrichosis; androgens, diazoxide, phenytoin, hydrallazine, minoxidil, corticosteroids.
Hyperglycaemia; corticosteroids, pyrazinamide, diuretics (ethacrynic acid, frusemide, thiazides), phenytoin, diazoxide, pentamidine, colaspase.
Hypoglycaemia; alcohol, insulin and oral hypoglycaemics, salicylates, pyrazolones (phenylbutazone); sulphonamides and monoamine oxidase inhibitors potentiate sulphonylureas.
Hypothyroidism; antithyroid drugs, chronic intake of iodine powders or elixirs, oral hypoglycaemics, para-aminosalicylic acid, radio-iodine, lithium salts, calcium carbimide.
Hyponatraemia; inappropriate ADH secretion with phenytoin, chlorpropamide, thiazide diuretics, carbamazepine, vincristine, cyclophosphamide.
Hyperthyroidism; iodine, thyroxine.
Sterility; antimitotics (alkylating agents, antimetabolites).
EYES
Cataract; busulphan, corticosteroids, ecthiopate iodide and demecarium bromide eye drops, phenothiazines, piperazine.
Corneal damage; chlorpromazine, chloroquine, hydroxychloroquine, indomethacin, mepacrine, practolol.
Focusing; paralysis of parasympathetic fibres by atropine, ganglion blockers, anticholinergics and antidepressants.
Glaucoma (shallow anterior chamber and narrow angles); atropine eye drops, anticholinergics, antidepressants, corticosteroids—topically or systemically.
Optic neuritis; alcohol, chloramphenicol, clioquinol, ethambutol, digitalis, isoniazid, para-aminosalicylic acid, tryparsamide, sulphonamides, penicillamine, quinine, disulfiram.
Retinal damage; chloroquine, organic arsenicals, phenothiazines (chlorpromazine, thioridazine), quinine.
Visual disturbances; coloured vision (yellow, green) and scotomata with digitalis, nalidixic acid, tryparsamide; visual defects, light glare with clomiphene, ethosuximide, paramethadione, troxidone, night blindness; troxidine; blurred vision, salicylates; perceptual visual hallucinations and illusions; propranolol.
LIVER
Drug administration has increased dangers in prematurity, neonates, pregnancy, in alcoholics and in the malnourished.

Hepatic coma may be induced by thiazide diuretics; coma from hypoglycaemia is seen in cirrhotic diabetics given hypoglycaemics.
Impaired liver function tests; lincomycin, oral contraceptives, phenothiazines, pyrazinamide, rifampicin, isoniazid, paracetamol, perhexiline.
Jaundice. The mechanisms by which drugs cause jaundice vary and overlap.
(1) Defective uptake of bilirubin by liver cells (filix mas).
(2) Defective intracellular conjugation (novobiocin).
(3) Interference with canalicular biliary excretion (rifampicin, rifamycin).
(4) Direct hepatoxicity, dose-related and predictable; chlorinated hydrocarbons (carbon tetrachloride, chloroform), i.v. tetracycline, especially in pregnancy or post-operatively, mercaptopurine, methotrexate, ferrous sulphate and paracetamol poisoning.
(5) Hepatitis-like hypersensitivity reactions in general unrelated to dose or duration; antituberculous therapy (cycloserine, ethionamide, isoniazid, para-aminosalicylic acid, pyrazinamide, rifampicin, thiacetazone), benzodiazepines (diazepam), amitriptyline, iprindole, halothane inhalation, phenothiazines, phenacemide, indandiones, sulphonamides, penicillins, methyldopa, monoamine oxidase inhibitors (hydrazine type—iproniazid, isocarboxazid, phenelzine, pheniprazine, phenoxypropazine), troxidone, dapsone, oxyphenisatin, perhexiline, phenytoin.
(6) **Cholestatic or intrahepatic obstruction** of the steroid type, dose and duration related occurs with C_{17} substituted testosterones or nortestosterones e.g. methyl testosterone, norethandrolone, methandienone, oral contraceptives. Erythromycin estolate given for 10 days or more produces cholestasis, usually reversible. Idiosyncratic, and not dose or duration related, are para-aminosalicylic acid, phenothiazines including the antihistamines promethazine and trimeprazine, phenylbutazone, nitrofurantoin, thiouracil, chlorpropamide, sulphonamides, chlordiazepoxide, methimazole, phenindione.
Liver cancer; anabolic steroids (oxymetholone) androgens, **cirrhosis** (methotrexate).
Liver adenoma; oral contraceptives.

LOCOMOTOR
Joint pain and swelling; serum sickness (antitoxins, penicillin), arthralgia (barbiturates, carbimazole), haemorrhage into joints with anticoagulants; secondary gout.
Myopathy; corticosteroids, hypokalaemic drugs (diuretics, carbenoxolone).
Muscle pain; clofibrate, oral contraceptives, alcohol. **Cramps;** diuretics, salbutamol.

MALIGNANCIES
Reticuloses-immunosuppressives (e.g. bowel, brain), cancer—anabolic steroids (liver), oestrogens given to pregnant women (cervical and vaginal cancer in daughters).

METABOLIC
Acidosis; alcohol, acetazolamide, i.v. fructose.
Bromidism; bromides, carbromal.
Hypercalcaemia; thiazides, vitamin D, calcium carbonate, oestrogen therapy in cancer.
Hyperkalaemia; potassium salts, spironolactone, amiloride, triamterene.
Hypokalaemia; carbenoxolone, corticosteroids, diuretics including

acetazolamide, cyanocobalamin therapy initially, insulin and dextrose i.v., amphotericin B, purgatives, intravenous salbutamol.

Hyperuricaemia and gout; ethanol (alcohol) diuretics (thiazides, frusemide, ethacrynic acid), pyrazinamide, cytotoxic therapy, cyanocobalamin, drugs causing haemolysis, uricosuric agents mobilizing uric acid, starvation therapy.

Hyperthermia; tricyclic antidepressants, monoamine oxidase inhibitors, drug fever (e.g. quinidine, methyldopa, phenindione), suxamethonium, phenothiazines in hot weather by altering temperature regulation.

Hypothermia; alcohol (ethanol), phenothiazines by reducing shivering, chloramphenicol in neonates (grey baby syndrome), diazepam in neonates when given to mother at birth.

Osteomalacia; phosphate depletion with aluminium hydroxide, prolonged anti-epileptic therapy (barbiturates and phenytoins).

Porphyria; barbiturates, chloroquine, griseofulvin, oral contraceptives, sulphonamides, alcohol, sulphonylureas, methyldopa.

NEUROPSYCHIATRIC

Abnormal movements; bromocriptine, levodopa, phenothiazines, oral contraceptives (chorea), phenytoin.

Ataxia; alcohol, aminoglycosides (e.g. gentamicin, streptomycin), barbiturates, carbamazepine, benzodiazepines (e.g. chordiazepoxide, diazepam), ethopropiazine, lithium salts, pethidine, phenothiazine, pheneturide, phenytoin, primidone, tricyclic antidepressants, dichlorphenamide, polymyxins e.g. colistin, chloroquine, minocycline.

Confusion and delirium; alcohol, amphetamines, antiParkinsonian drugs (e.g. benzhexol), atropine, barbiturates, indomethacin, levodopa, lignocaine, lithium, nalidixic acid, opiates, phenothiazines, tricyclic antidepressants, quinacrine, cycloserine, digitalis glycosides, phenytoin, bromocriptine.

Convulsions; amantadine, baclofen, chloroquine, cycloserine (accentuated by alcohol), isoniazid, glutethimide, nalidixic acid, niridazole, monoamine oxidase inhibitors with tricyclic antidepressants, phenothiazines, i.v. penicillin and cephalosporins in large amounts, withdrawal of alcohol and barbiturate type drugs; dilution overhydration and hyponatraemia with ADH, i.v. glucose, drugs depressing serum calcium, drugs depressing blood sugar, insulin, oral hypoglycaemics, excitation of cortex (lignocaine, isoniazid, amphetamines, theophyllines), vaccines, melarsoprol, morphine, ethionamide, levodopa.

Dependence; amphetamines, barbiturates, opiates.

Depression; barbiturates, beta-blockers, antihypertensives (e.g. guanethidine, methyldopa, reserpine), corticosteroids, fenfluramine, oral contraceptives, oral hypoglycaemics, cardiac glycosides, levodopa, sulphonamides, phenytoin, phenothiazines.

Drowsiness; alcohol, antihistamines, barbiturates, fenfluramine, hypnotics, sedatives, methyldopa, phenytoins, procarbazine, clonidine.

Headache; adrenaline, codeine, griseofulvin, indomethacin, monoamine oxidase inhibitors, orciprenaline, vasopressin, trinitrin.

Interference with penile erection and ejaculation; most hypotensives (not the beta-blockers or diuretics, although libido may be reduced as it may equally well be by placeboes).

Priapism; phenothiazines.

Neuromuscular blockade; polymyxins (potentiate non-depolarizing agents e.g. ether, curare), colistin sulphate and methosulphate, polymyxin B sulphate, aminoglycosides act pre-synaptically and displace calcium needed for the enzymatic release of acetylcholine, kanamycin, neomycin, streptomycin; others—suxamethonium, quinine. Tetracyclines should be avoided in myasthenia gravis.

Nightmares; methyldopa, beta-blockers e.g. propranolol, levodopa, withdrawal of barbiturates, alcohol, benzodiazepines.

Paraesthesiae; hydrallazine, polymyxins, thalidomide, ethionamide, oral hypoglycaemic agents, insulin.

Parkinsonism; haloperidol, hypotensives (e.g. methyldopa, reserpine), phenothiazines, tetrabenazine, metoclopramide, tricyclic antidepressives.

Polyneuritis; allopurinol, colistin, ethionamide, isoniazid, gold, nitrofurantion, vincristine, vinblastine, perhexiline.

Raised intracranial pressure (papilloedema); corticosteroids, tetracyclines, vitamin A overdosage in children, nalidixic acid, oral contraceptives, perhexiline.

Spinal cord damage; clioquinol, ethambutol, intrathecal methotrexate.

Stimulation of cortex causing insomnia, excitement or hallucinations; aminophylline, amphetamines, atropine, barbiturates in the elderly, benzhexol, bromocriptine, caffeine, corticosteroids, cycloserine, ephedrine, isoniazid, methysergide, orphenadrine, thyroxine, pentazocine, hypoglycaemic agents, monoamine oxidase inhibitors, amantadine.

Tremor; sympathomimetics, amphetamine, thyroxine, alcohol, lithium salts.

OTOLOGICAL

Deafness and tinnitus; aspirin, i.v. frusemide (transient), ethacrynic acid, kanamycin, quinidine, quinine, neomycin, streptomycin, vancomycin, viomycin, gentamicin. Ototoxicity tends to be permanent when damage is to the sensory cells of the inner ear for if destroyed they have little ability to regenerate themselves.

PREGNANCY

It is best to avoid drug therapy unless vital. Nausea and vomiting are treated with antacids and some obstetricians to prevent hyperemesis allow antiemetics. Anaemia, epilepsy, infection and hypertension should be treated in pregnancy. Drugs are dangerous when, as with fat soluble drugs, they cross the placenta. Probable or possible danger may arise from the following.

Antibiotics; streptomycin may damage foetal ears, tetracyclines are deposited in growing teeth and bones. They can cause deformity, enamel hypoplasia and discolouration of teeth.

Anticoagulants; oral forms are more likely to cause placental haemorrhage. At birth heparin is safer.

Anticonvulsants; phenytoin may cause folate depletion, foetal malformation (rare) and neonatal and intra-uterine haemorrhage.

Antimalarials; quinine has caused abortion and deafness, pyrimethamine congenital abnormalities, chloroquine neurological damage and deafness. In malarial areas these minute risks are accepted.

Antithyroid drugs; hypothyroidism, goitre. The drugs are usually stopped in the last month of pregnancy.

Antimitotics; death and malformation, but some foetuses are unscathed.

Barbiturates and anaesthetics; sedation.

Corticosteroids; hare-lip reported.

Diuretics (thiazides); thrombocytopenia, haemolytic anaemia.
Narcotics; respiratory distress and narcotic withdrawal syndrome. Foetal heart rate is depressed by opiates, pethidine, diazepam, barbiturates, promazine, local anaesthetics (buvicaine, mepivacaine).
Hypoglycaemia may be caused by propranolol.
Progestogens and androgens; virilization of female foetus.
Smallpox vaccination; abortion and vaccinial infection.
Sulphonamides; interference with bilirubin binding leading to hyperbilirubinaemia and kernicterus.
Vitamin D; hypercalcaemia, aortic valve deformity, hypercholesterolaemia.
Vitamin K; haemolysis.

NEWBORN
Certain drugs are excreted in the breast milk, usually the amounts do not matter clinically. Others have to be noted namely antithyroid agents (e.g. thiouracils, carbimazole), bromides, iodides, nalidixic acid, oral anticoagulants, penicillin, phenobarbitone, pyrimethamine and propranolol.

THE NEONATE
Many enzymes metabolizing drugs in the neonate are deficient. Liver glucuronyl tranferase cannot deal with chloramphenicol or morphine properly. Other enzymes fail to detoxicate sulphonamides, isoniazid, barbiturates, pethidine and succinylcholine. High-concentration oxygen may cause retrolental fibroplasia (leads to blindness) and death from lung bleeding. Too little oxygen may kill by inducing hyaline membrane disease.

RENAL
Haematuria; cyclophosphamide, hexamine, penicillin (methicillin) in large doses in uraemia, anticoagulants, sulphonamides.
Nephrotic syndrome; bismuth, gold and other heavy metals, organic and inorganic mercurials, paramethadione, penicillamine, phenindione, potassium perchlorate, probenecid, smallpox vaccine, serum sickness, troxidone, tolbutamide, pyrazolones e.g. phenylbutazone.
Pyelonephritis (papillary necrosis 'analgesic kidney', interstitial nephritis); phenacetin, possibly aspirin.
Retention of urine; sudden increase in flow and amount following diuretics in patients with prostate enlargement. Lack of awareness of a full bladder due to analgesics and narcotics. Interference with autonomic nerves by atropine, and anticholinergics (used as antacids, and in the treatment of Parkinsonism), tricyclic antidepressants and ephedrine.
Renal damage; dysfuntion results (see p. 252) from hypercalcaemia, hypokalaemia, hyperuricaemia or hypovolaemia. Tubular damage—vitamin D overdose, amphotericin B, vancomycin, aminoglycosides (gentamicin, kanamycin, neomycin, streptomycin, paromomycin, viomycin), polymyxin B, cephaloridine, methicillin, ampicillin, colistin, tetracycline. Renal failure from plasma volume depletion—potent diuretics, tubular blockage by sulphonamides (sulphathiazole, sulphamerazine), uricosuric drugs. Renal failure is of relevance since it interferes with drug absorption, metabolism, pharmacological action and excretion. In urinary infection it may prevent adequate antibiotic therapy. Potassium salts and diuretics may be dangerous, though frusemide can be effective. Digoxin dosage should be curtailed. Phenobarbitone and the phenothiazines need reduction of dose, but the short and

medium acting barbiturates, nitrazepam, chloral, dichloralphenazone and diazepam, can be given in normal amounts. Antibiotics are the main concern.
(1) **Those potentially dangerous** and largely excreted by the kidneys. If they must be given either the dose, or the frequency of administration is markedly reduced and blood levels are monitored. Examples are amphotericin B, colistin, cycloserine, gentamicin, kanamycin, para-aminosalicylic acid, polymyxins, streptomycin, vancomycin.
(2) **Renally excreted but less toxic.** Here the dose is reduced to a lesser extent, though blood level measurements are not obligatory, e.g. carbenicillin, cephaloridine, cephalexin or cephalothin (*never with frusemide*), lincomycin, clindamycin, isoniazid, co-trimoxazole, benzylpenicillin, ampicillin.
(3) **Excretion extrarenal** can be given in normal amounts; sodium fusidate.
(4) **Normal dosage** in renal failure; sulphadimidine, sulphamethoxazole, nalidixic acid, novobiocin, erythromycin.
(5) **Never used;** chloramphenicol, tetracyclines (possibly doxycycline is an exception), nitrofurantoin.

RESPIRATORY
Airways. Asthma; inhalants (pituitary snuff, acetylcysteine), allergic reactions to antibiotics (cephaloridine, erythromycin, ethionamide, griseofulvin, neomycin, penicillin, streptomycin, tetracycline), monoamine oxidase inhibitors, local anaesthetics, mercurials, iron dextran, heparin, antisera, vaccines, pollen extracts. Asthma as part of the serum sickness reaction—betalactam antibiotics, streptomycin, sulphonamides, griseofulvin, thiouracils. Aspirin, pyrazolones, mefenamic acid, pentazocine, and indomethacin by unknown mechanisms; bronchoconstriction by beta-blockers e.g. propranolol, histamine, nitrofurantoin, prostaglandins. Tartrazine colouring agents in capsules.
Parenchymal lesions. Eosinophilic infiltration; imipramine, mephenesin, nitrofurantoin, penicillin, para-aminosalicylic acid, sulphonamides, sulphonylureas.
Fibrosis; busulphan, hexamethonium, hydrallazine, methysergide, procainamide, methotrexate, cyclophosphamide, bleomycin, inhalation of pituitary snuff, sulphasalazine, nitrofurantoin.
Oedema; nitrofurantoin, i.v. diuretics (rare), i.v. sodium solutions, mineralocorticoid overdose, prolonged high oxygen therapy, heroin overdose.
Opportunistic infections e.g. fungi, antibiotic and immunosuppressive therapy. Quiescent disease, such as tuberculosis, may be provoked by corticosteroids.
Lipoid pneumonia; inhalation liquid paraffin and other oily medicines.
Pulmonary vessels. Polyarteritis nodosa suspicion rests on organic arsenicals, iodides, mercurials, hydantoins, penicillin, gold salts, thiouracils, phenothiazines, and sulphonamides.
Pulmonary hypertension has followed certain anti-anorexic drugs.
Respiratory depression of central origin; diphenoxylate, hypnotics, narcotics, polymyxin, narcotic antagonists (not naloxone), oxygen in above air concentrations given to certain patients with obstructive airway disease. Respiratory muscle paralysis; suxamethonium.
Rhinitis or nasal stuffiness; abuse of nasal sprays and drops, hypotensive therapy (e.g. reserpine, phenoxybenzamine) and the contraceptive pill.
Hypoxia; sympathomimetics by a paradoxical effect e.g. when inhaled and which increase perfusion of underventilated lung.

SKIN

The most common complication of systemic drug therapy (other than a toxic or irritant effect on the gastro-intestinal tract) is to cause a rash. The mechanisms are allergy, toxicity, idiosyncrasy, and phototoxicity. One drug can evoke various types of rashes and conversely different drugs can cause the same rash. The skin responses are those which may be caused by natural disease. The rashes are erythema; erythema and oedema; erythema, oedema and bullae; erythema, oedema, bullae and necrosis; urticaria, eczema; lichenification; nodules; purpura and combinations of the above. Drug rashes (dermatitis medicamentosa) have been recognized for centuries even in the age when galenicals and alkaloids were the only therapy. A drug rash is suggested by its appearance during therapy (from doctor, nurse e.g. enema, pharmacist, self-prescribed or from food additives). A note should be made of all medications taken before and at the time the rash appeared. The rash is often a vivid bright colour, extensive over the body and fades eventually after stopping therapy. Some drugs have a bad reputation or are used so widely that rashes are not infrequent e.g. co-trimoxazole, ampicillin and methyldopa. Rashes may arise unsuspectedly in drugs used for years as with practolol. Types of disorders are:

Acne; ACTH, adrenocorticosteroids, androgens, anti-tuberculous therapy, bromides, chloral, ethionamide, iodides, isoniazid, oral contraceptives, progestogens, prothionamide, quinine, troxidone.

Alopecia; anticoagulants (heparin, phenindione), antithyroid agents, clofibrate chloroquine, cytotoxics (e.g. cyclophosphamide, melphalan; alkaloids—colchicine, vincristine, vinblastine; antimetabolites; antibiotics (daunorubicin), dextrans, diethylcarbamazepine, levodopa, mephenesin, oral contraceptives, para-aminosalicylic acid, troxidone, vitamin A.

Angioneurotic oedema and urticaria; antitoxins (e.g. horse sera), aspirin, barbiturates, bromides, carbamazepine, codeine, heparin, insulin, morphine (a histamine liberator), penicillin, procaine, quinine, salicylates, streptomycin, sulphonamides, sulphones. Serum sickness and penicillin allergy cause urticarial rash plus fever, joint pain and synovial effusion.

Bullous eruptions; (these include bullous erythema multiforme, bullous urticaria, dermatitis herpetiformis), acetazolamide, barbiturates (including barbiturate blisters in coma), bromides, chloral, glutethimide, imipramine, iodides, meprobamate, methadone, nalidixic acid, nitrazepam, pentazocine, phenolphthalein, phenylbutazone (and oxyphenbutazone), phenytoin, salicylates, sulphonamides, sulphones, thiazide diuretics. Special forms are Lyell's syndrome ('scalded skin') and Stevens-Johnson syndrome (bullae in mouth. body, involvement of conjunctivae and urethra).

Cancer; squamous from long-continued arsenic.

Contact dermatitis; antibiotics (gentamicin, neomycin, penicillin, streptomycin, sulphonamides), antihistamines, local anaesthetics.

Eczema; allopurinol, ethionamide, gold, methyldopa, penicillin, quinine, salicylates, sulphonamides, thiazides.

Erythema nodosum; allopurinol, oral contraceptives, phenylbutazone, sulphonamides, sulphonylureas, thiouracil.

Erythematous (scarlatiniform or morbilliform); allopurinol, antibiotics (especially ampicillin if given in infectious mononucleosis, lymphatic leukaemia or cytomegalovirus infection), streptomycin, antihistamines, barbiturates, belladonna, benzodiazepines, carbamazepine, chloral, chloroquine, co-trimoxazole, digitalis, diuretics, gold salts, griseofulvin, iodides, isoniazid,

mercurials, para-aminosalicylic acid, phenazone, phenindione, phenothiazines, phenylbutazone, phenytoin, quinine, salicylates, sulphonamides, sulphones, tetracycline.
Exfoliative dermatitis can be fatal. Many drugs can cause it especially if they are not stopped in time—allopurinol, anticonvulsants, arsenic, barbiturates, codeine, chloroquine, chlorpropamide, co-trimoxazole, gold salts, melarsoprol, para-aminosalicylic acid, penicillamine, penicillins, phenothiazine, phenylbutazone, phenytoin, practolol, propranolol, salicylates, sodium antimony tartrate, streptomycin, sulphonamides, suramin, thiacetazone.
Fixed eruptions; antibiotics (penicillin, tetracycline), antihistamines (cyclizine, dimenhydrinate), anticonvulsants, barbiturates, chlordiazepoxide, phenacetin, phenazone, phenolphthalein, phenylbutazone and oxyphenbutazone, quinine, rauwolfia alkaloids, sulphonamides, tetracyclines.
Lichenoid; amphenazole, arsenic, bismuth, chloroquine, chlorothiazide, chlorpropamide, gold, mepacrine, methyldopa, mercury, para-aminosalicylic acid, phenothiazines, quinine.
Lupus erythematosus; drug forms occur equally in the sexes, renal disease is unlikely and positive anti-nuclear factor and LE cells are present, but no DNA antibodies. The condition is usually (?always) reversible. Causes are antibiotics (griseofulvin, penicillin, streptomycin, tetracycline), chemotherapy (isoniazid, para-aminosalicylic acid, sulphonamides), anticonvulsants (carbamazepine, ethosuximide, methsuximide, phenytoin, primidone, troxidone), thiouracils, hypotensives (hydrallazine, guanoxan, methyldopa), antiarrhythmics (practolol, procainamide), antirheumatics (gold, phenylbutazone).
Photosensitivity (allergy and toxicity); antihistamines, chlordiazepoxide, chloroquine, chlorpromazine, chlorpropamide, griseofulvin, nalidixic acid, oral contraceptives, penicillin, protriptyline, tetracyclines (e.g. demeclocycline, doxycycline), sulphonamides, thiazide diuretics. Visitors to sunny climates are at risk.
Pigmentation; ineffective steroid therapy in Addison's disease with ACTH and MSH oversecretion, arsenic, bleomycin, busulphan, bromides, clofazimine, chloroquine, griseofulvin, mepacrine, metals (bismuth, gold, mercury), oral contraceptives causing chloasma, phenazone, phenothiazines, sulphones, treosulfan.
Psoriasiform; arsenic, antimalarials, gold, practolol, salicylates.
Purpura (allergic thrombocytopenic and normopaenic and toxic thrombocytopenia); acetazolamide, amphetamines, antihistamines, barbiturates, carbromal (Apronal or 'Sedormid' is no longer available), chlorpropamide, desipramine, digitoxin, ethacrynic acid, gold, indomethacin, meprobamate, penicillamine, phenacetin, phenylbutazone, quinine, quinidine, sulphonamides including co-trimoxazole, tolbutamide, thiazide diuretics. Marrow depression from cytotoxic agents. Occasionally tetracycline, ampicillin and the benzodiazepines. Bruising from anticoagulants and corticosteroids.
Striae; systemic corticosteroids and topical steroids, especially fluorinated causing atrophy and telangiectasia.

32 THE LAW AND DRUGS

Medical staff should be familiar with the following.

(1) Classes of persons authorized to order, possess, prescribe and supply substances controlled by law.

(2) Regulations concerning; the ordering, storage and administration of these substances.

The control of medicines which fall into the above categories is vested in the Secretary of State for Home Affairs, who is responsible for the details of enforcement of (a) The Misuse of Drugs Act (1971). (b) The Pharmacy and Poisons Act and Rules. Other medicinal substances, not necessarily classed as poisons, are controlled by the provisions of the Therapeutic Substances Act, for which the responsible authority is the Minister of Health.

Controlled Drugs are dangerous drugs now under the control of the Misuse of Drugs Act (1971) and its Regulations which came into force on 1st July 1973. These Controlled Drugs include narcotic and non-narcotic drugs which may be abused. The narcotic drugs opium, morphine and its derivatives, diamorphine (heroin), codeine, dihydrocodeine ('DF 118'), levorphanol, pethidine and methadone come into this category plus the stimulating and euphoric substances cocaine, cannabis indica and marihuana. Also included are methaqualone (in 'Mandrax'), methylphenidate ('Ritalin'), phenmetrazine ('Preludin'), the amphetamines (e.g. 'Dexedrine', 'Drinamyl', 'Methedrine'), benzphetamine, mephentermine and chlorphentermine. Other habit-forming drugs such as the barbiturate and non-barbiturate hypnotics (except methaqualone), are controlled by the Pharmacy and Poison Act. Certain preparations such as cocaine eye drops, analgesic oral preparations containing codeine and remedies for coughs and diarrhoea containing small amounts of morphine are listed in *Schedule* I of the Regulations. These formulations of Controlled Drugs are allowed the least stringent control providing the quantity of drug supplied does not constitute a risk to health. (*Schedule* II mainly contains the narcotics and amphetamine, *Schedule* III the amphetamine-like drugs and *Schedule* IV cannabis and cannabis resins, mescaline, lysergic acid and raw opium among others). Certain injurious substances, including alcohol and aspirin can be purchased without medical control. **Dependence** is a condition in which persons resort to drugs continuously to such an extent that they find life intolerable without them. The addict is physically and emotionally dependent on them and tends to take increasing amounts to satisfy his craving. Deprivation leads to illness and severe withdrawal symptoms. The urgent need for regular supplies often brings the addict into antisocial activities. They may also steal prescriptions and attempt to forge them. **Habituation** is defined as a psychological dependence which produces a desire (but not a compulsion) to continue drug taking for the sense of well-being it produces. Drug abuse as defined by W.H.O. is the sporadic excessive taking of drugs not in accordance with medical practice. **People at risk** to misuse of drugs include medical and nursing staff and pharmacists because of their availability. The taking of heroin, cannabis, intravenous amphetamine and methaqualone may be an illegal social, or cultural fashion. Others liable to addiction are those with personality disorders and those with severe pain and crippling disease.

Treatment of Drug Dependence

In Britain addicts are notifiable and treatment with morphine, heroin and cocaine is only permitted in hospital and special prescribing clinics. Drugs may be withdrawn and replaced by less harmful ones. In the U.S.A. methadone given orally and daily is prescribed from clinics and substituted for heroin which is illegal. The number of addicts is increasing in Britain.

Prevention of Drug Dependence and Misuse of Drugs

(1) Precisely worded and specific prescriptions. In order to comply with the Regulations all prescriptions of Controlled Drugs have to be:

(a) Written in the practitioner's own handwriting in ink or other indelible marking.

(b) The dose to be taken must be specified and in the case of a prescription containing a Controlled Drug which is a preparation (e.g. tablet or injection) the form and where appropriate, the strength of the preparation and either the total quantity (in both words and figures) of the preparation or the number (in words and figures) of dosage units, as appropriate to be supplied. In any other case (e.g. for a mixture) the total quantity (in both words and figures) of the Controlled Drug to be supplied.

(c) All prescriptions (except for in-patients which are written on a standard Prescription Form) must include the name and address of the patient in the practitioner's own handwriting.

(d) Dentists must write 'for dental treatment only' on the form. Unless the prescription is complete as above it cannot be issued or dispensed.

(2) Persons authorized to possess Controlled Drugs include registered medical, dental and veterinary practitioners, registered pharmacists, ward sisters and acting ward sisters.

(3) All Controlled Drugs must be stored locked in hospital in the 'Dangerous Drugs Cupboard' and the key kept on the person of the sister or acting sister in charge of the ward, theatre or department.

Supplies of Controlled Drugs may only be obtained as stock from the hospital pharmacy on production of a requisition signed and dated by sister or acting sister. Controlled Drugs may not be supplied from stock other than to administer to a patient in the ward, theatre or department in accordance with the directions of a doctor or dentist. No Controlled Drugs may be destroyed, or disposed of, without prior arrangement with the authorized personnel. All transactions involving Controlled Drugs are to be recorded in the ward Dangerous Drugs Record Book and the entry signed by two people one of whom shall be a State Registered Nurse. Each General Practitioner is required to have a Register in which he enters receipts, issues and administrations of all Controlled Drugs.

Poisons Act

There are now no schedules in the United Kingdom. All schedules are now covered in the New Medicines Act 1968. It lists drugs as

1. G.S.L. (General Sales List)

2. P. (Pharmacy only)

3. P.O.M. (Prescription Only Medicines)

Hospital and Scheduled Drugs

The hospital pharmacist is authorized to purchase, store and supply poisons. Nursing staff obtain ward supplies by production of the patient's treatment card on which a prescription has been written, name, strength and quantity of drug, dose and signature of prescriber are given. The ward sister may also order stock preparations by the use of a signed order. *Storage* of poisons is obligatory in the locked cupboard provided for this purpose. The key must be kept in a safe place determined by the ward sister. *Administration* of poisons is only in accordance with the written and signed prescription of a registered practitioner.

Therapeutic Substances Act

This controls antibiotics, insulin, sera, vaccines, heparin, ACTH and blood products. The manufacture is limited to licensed premises and the Minister of Health has the power to define details of the tests for purity, strength and toxicity. The general public may obtain these substances only by prescription, and in hospital the same conditions apply as to scheduled poisons except for storage. Most of these products are stored in a refrigerator and at present it is impracticable to keep them under lock and key.

The Medicines Act 1968 consolidates the legislation dealing with medicines irrespective of their toxicity.

GLOSSARY OF TERMS

Agonist: a substance with activity on a receptor site, causing a reaction to occur.

Alkaloid: plant substance containing nitrogen, their names usually end with letter 'ine', e.g. morphine.

Allergy: a state of abnormal sensitivity to a substance which enters the body by ingestion, inhalation, injection or by contact with skin.

Ampoule: a heat sealed glass container, for single dose injection.

Analeptic: a drug which stimulates the medullary nerve centres thereby improving the circulation or respiratory rate or decreasing the depth of unconsciousness.

Analgesic: a pain reliever.

Analogue: a drug similar in structure or function.

Anaphylaxis: an increased sensitivity to drugs the basis of which is an antibody antigen reaction in which histamine is produced. The blood vessels dilate and there is shock, hypotension, syncope and at times death.

Antagonist: a substance with opposing action.

Antibiotics: chemical substances which act against living organisms. They are usually produced by bacteria or fungi, but some are synthesized.

Antigen: a substance usually of protein origin which causes the body to produce a neutralizing chemical called an antibody.

Bacterial resistance: the ability of bacteria to withstand antibiotics.

Bactericidal: the ability to kill bacteria.

Bacteriostatic: the ability to prevent bacteria from multiplying.

Bioavailability: percentage of a drug absorbed into the systemic circulation.

Booster dose: a reinforcing dose to promote extra immunity.

Broad-spectrum antibiotic: one with a wide range of activity, affecting different types of bacteria often unselectively.

Cross-resistance: when bacteria are uninfluenced or resistant to several related antibiotics.

Cytotoxic: a drug which kills actively growing (usually cancer) cells.

Dangerous Drugs: as covered by the Dangerous Drugs Act are narcotics, i.e. like morphine and are substances which cause or have been shown to be capable of causing true addiction or dependence.

Decongestant: that which reduces mucosal swelling or congestion.

Desiccated: dried, free of water.

Diuresis: increased production, or flow of urine.

Diuretic: a drug which increases urinary output.

Drug: a substance used for the specific (curative), symptomatic, or preventative treatment of disease.

Electrolyte: a chemical which in solution carries an electrical charge and has the ability to conduct electricity.

Endogenous: coming or produced from within the body.

Ethical drug: is one advertized to the medical or pharmaceutical profession only.

Euphoriant: a substance producing a cheerful contented mood.

Exogenous: derived or coming from outside the body, an external factor.

262

Food: is that which is taken into the body for the purpose of the normal processes of life. Vitamins can be considered food or drugs.

Hormone: a substance secreted by a gland into the blood stream which acts as a chemical messenger and has some special action on another part of the body known as the target organ.

Idiosyncrasy: an abnormal or unusual response given to a drug in normal dosage.

Intolerance: is an undue susceptibility to small or normal amounts of drugs.

Intrathecal injection: is one made by lumbar puncture into the cerebrospinal fluid.

Materia medica: those remedies used in medicine. It refers to their origin, physical, chemical and economic properties.

Milli equivalent (mEq): is the equivalent weight of an ion in milligrams. Equivalent weight can be defined as that weight of a substance that will combine with 1g of hydrogen or 8g of oxygen.

Miotics: constrictors of the pupil.

Molar solution: is one containing the molecular weight, in grams per litre. Various proportions can be made, e.g. one-sixth molar solution. A millimole is a thousandth part.

Mutation: is a transformation of an organism usually by genetic means whereby it changes its characteristics and abilities, sometimes becoming more harmful.

Mydriatrics: dilators of the pupil.

Overdosage: an amount of a drug too great for therapeutic purposes.

Oxytocic drug: one which causes contraction of the uterus.

Parenteral: the giving of a drug by injecting it into the body.

Passive immunity: a process whereby foreign proteins (antibodies) are injected into patients conferring on them temporary protection against disease.

Pharmacology: is the study of the action of drugs, i.e. their absorption and distribution within the body, and the manner of their action.

Pharmacopoeia: a reference book of standards and dosage for drugs and pharmaceuticals.

Pharmacy: is the art and science of preparing drugs for medicinal use.

Placebo: a harmless medicine which makes the patient feel better by suggestion.

Plasma half-life of a drug; the time it takes for concentrations to fall by 50%.

Poison: any substance, usually in small quantities, which when taken into the body causes serious illness or death. Any substance on the Poisons List.

Presentation: the form in which a drug is prescribed, e.g. tablet or capsule and the strength of the active ingredient.

Pressor-agent: substances raising the blood pressure.

Prophylaxis: the prevention of disease.

Sensitivity: when applied to bacteria is when they are inhibited in growth or destroyed by drugs.

Sensitivity: in patients is when they react abnormally or in an 'allergic manner' with rashes, or liver, gut or cardiovascular disturbances.

Serum sickness: an illness characterized by fever, rash or joint pain coming on about a week after the injection of a foreign protein.

Side effects: actions not medically of value and an unwanted by-product of the drug's activity; also referred to as adverse effects.

Super-infection: the production of an illness or carrier state which is the result of eradicating the normal bacterial inhabitants of a part of the body, e.g. gut.

Synthetic: a substance prepared chemically or artificially from basic ingredients.

Systemically: acting through the body by way of the blood stream.

Therapeutics: is concerned with the action of remedial agents such as drugs in the treatment and prevention of disease.

Tolerance: a condition which arises when repeated administration of a drug produces a decreasing result or when increasing doses are needed to achieve the original effect.

Topical: the application of a medicament to act directly on a surface such as the skin, or inserted into an orifice such as the mouth, ear, vagina, or rectum.

Toxoids: detoxified or harmless toxins.

Vaccines: are preparations of dead organisms, or living organisms, made harmless.

Vial: a rubber capped glass container usually multidose.

THE PERCENTAGE METHOD FOR ESTIMATING PAEDIATRIC DOSES†

This is a more realistic way of calculating a dose than the mg/kg body weight basis.

Approx. age	Weight kg	lb	Surface area m²	Percentage of Adult Dose
Premature	1.1	2½	—	2.5—5*
Premature	1.8	4	—	4—8*
Premature	2.5	5	0.17	5—10*
Full-term	3.2	7	0.21	12.5
2 months	4.5	10	0.26	15
4 months	6.5	14	0.34	20
12 months	10	22	0.42	25**
18 months	11	25	0.50	30
3 years	15	33	0.56	33⅓
5 years	18	40	0.68	40
7 years	23	50	0.85	50
10 years	30	66	1.00	60
11 years	36	80	1.20	70
12 years	40	88	1.28	75
14 years	45	100	1.36	80
16 years	54	120	1.53	90
20 years	65	145	1.70	100

*The smaller percentage applies during the first two to three weeks of life; the larger percentage applies after this period provided that baby is not jaundiced.

**At 10 kg Butler and Richie give the percentage of the adult dose as 28%. I have altered this to 25% for the convenience of remembering that an infant of 1 year requires 25%, or one quarter, of the adult dose. The difference of 3% is neglible.

†Reproduced with permission from *Paediatric Prescriber* 3rd ed. (1966), P. Catzel: Blackwell.

ABBREVIATIONS USED IN TEXT

A.C.T.H.	adrenocorticotrophic hormone
B.A.L.	British antiLewisite
B.C.G.	bacillus Calmette Guérin
b.d.	twice daily
b.i.d.	twice daily
B.N.F.	British National Formulary
B.P.	British Pharmacopoeia
B.P.C.	British Pharmaceutical Codex
Ci	Curie
C.N.S.	central nervous system
C.S.F.	cerebrospinal fluid
dl	100ml
E.C.G.	electrocardiogram
Ph. Eur.	European Pharmacopoeia
Eq	equivalent
e.g.	for example
g	gramme or gram
h	hour
i.e.	that is to say
i.m.	intramuscular(ly)
i.v.	intravenous(ly)
K	potassium
kg/B.W.	kilogram per body weight
l	litre
μg	microgram
mEq	milliequivalent
min	minute
mg	milligram
ml	millilitre
mmol	millimole
pH	hydrogen ion concentration
q.d.s.	four times daily
s.c.	subcutaneous(ly)
t.d.s.	thrice daily
u	unit
U.S.N.F.	United States National Formulary
U.S.P.	United States Pharmacopoeia
vac	vaccine

A capital letter is used for an official preparation (B.P., B.P.C., U.S.P., Ph. Eur.), e.g. Tablet or Injection.

BACTERIA

Esch. coli	Escherichia coli
H. influenzae	Haemophilus influenzae
Ps. aeruginosa	Pseudomonas aeruginosa
Staph. pyogenes	Staphylococcus pyogenes
Str. pyogenes	Streptococcus pyogenes

WEIGHTS AND MEASURES

Metric System

M	mega 10^6	d	deci 10^{-1}
k	kilo 10^3	m	milli 10^{-3}
c	centi 10^2	μ	micro 10^{-6}

MASS (weight)

1000 micrograms (μg) = 1 milligram (mg)
1000 milligram (mg) = 1 gram (g)
1000 gram (g) = 1 kilogram (kg)

CAPACITY

1000 millilitres (ml) = 1 litre (l)

ENERGY

1 calorie = 4.2 joules   1 kilocalorie (Calorie) = 4200 joules

All medicines are prescribed in the metric system. Liquid medicines are prescribed as one, two or more 5ml spoonfuls. The dosage of linctuses, elixirs and paediatric mixtures is 5ml and the dosage of adult mixtures is 10ml.

N.B. Mass (weight) per m² refers to the body surface area of the patient e.g. the dose is proportional to the body surface area.

FURTHER READING

Chapter 1

Laurence, D. R. *Clinical Pharmacology*, Fourth edition. Churchill Livingstone, Edinburgh and London (1974).

Meyers, F. H., Jawetz, E. and Goldfien, A. *Review of Medical Pharmacology*, Fifth edition. Lange, California (1978).

Smith, S. E. and Rawlins, M. D. *Variability in Human Drug Response*. Butterworth, London (1973).

Costrini, N. V. and Thompson, W. M.(Eds.). *Manual of Medical Therapeutics*, Twenty second edition, Little, Brown and Company, Boston (1977).

Melmon, K. L. and Morrelli, H. F. (Ed.) *Clinical Pharmacology*, Second edition. Macmillan, New York and Baillière Tindall, London (1978).

Alstead, S. *Textbook of Medical Treatment*, Fourteenth edition. Churchill Livingstone, Edinburgh and London (1978).

Prescribers' Journal, published biomonthly.

Drug and Therapeutics Bulletin, published fortnightly by Consumers' Association.

Havard, C. W. H. (Ed.). *Current Medical Treatment*, Fourth edition. John Wright, Bristol (1976).

Turner, P. and Richens, A. *Clinical Pharmacology*, Third edition. Churchill Livingstone, Edinburgh and London (1978).

Chapter 2

Kucers, A. and McBennett, N. *The Use of Antibiotics*, Third edition. William Heinemann Medical Books Ltd., London (1979).

Garrod, L. P., Lambert, H. P. and O'Grady, F. *Antibiotics and Chemotherapy*, Fourth edition. Churchill Livingstone, Edinburgh and London (1973).

Chapter 5

Catterall, R. D. *Short Textbook of Venereology*, Second edition. Hodder and Stoughton Ltd., London (1975).

Catterall, R. D. *Venereology and Genito-Urinary Medicine*, Second edition. Hodder and Stoughton Ltd., London (1979).

Chapter 7

Woodruff, A. W. (Ed.). *Medicine in the Tropics*. Churchill Livingstone, Edinburgh and London (1974).

Chapter 8

Perkins, F. T. (Ed.). *Symposia Series in Immunological Standardization*, Volume Twenty-Two. S. Karger, London and New York.

Chapter 13

Wood-Smith, F. G., Vickers, M. D. and Stewart, H. C. *Drugs in Anaesthetic Practice*, Fifth edition. Butterworth, London (1978).

Chapter 14

Day, M. D. *Autonomic Pharmacology*. Churchill Livingstone, Edinburgh and London and New York (1979).

Calne, D. B. *Therapeutics in Neurology*, Second edition. Blackwell Scientific Publications. Oxford, London, Edinburgh, Melbourne (1979).

Chapter 15

Silverstone, J. T. and Turner, P. *Drug Treatment in Psychiatry*, Second edition. Routledge and Kegan Paul, London and Boston (1978).

Chapter 16
Eadie, M. J. and Tyrer, J. H. *Anticonvulsant Therapy*, Second edition. Churchill Livingstone, Edinburgh and London (1978).
Chapter 17
Mathew, H. and Lawson, A. A. H. *Treatment of Common Acute Poisonings*, Fourth edition. Churchill Livingstone, Edinburgh and London (1979).
Chapter 25
Oakely, W. G., Pyke, D. A. and Taylor, K. W. *Diabetes and its Management*, Third edition. Blackwell, Oxford (1978).
Chapter 28
Dickerson, J. W. T. and Lee, H. A. *Nutrition in the Clinical Management of Disease*. Edward Arnold, London (1978).
Walker, W. F. and Johnston, I. D. A. *The Metabolic Basis of Surgical Care*. William Heinemann Medical Books Ltd., London (1971).
Wilkinson, A. W. *Parenteral Nutrition*. Churchill Livingstone, Edinburgh and London (1972).
Notes on Transfusion. Issued by the Department of Health and Social Security with the Scottish Home and Health Department and Welsh Office.
Gorst, D. W. *The Rational Use of Blood Products*. Hospital Update Vol. 4, 711 (1978).
Chapter 30
The Dietary Management of Hyperlipoproteinaemia. National Heart and Lung Institute, Bethesda, Maryland (1971).
Drugs and Hematologic Reactions. Nikolay V. Dimitrov and John H. Nodine, Editors. The Twenty-Ninth Hahnemann Symposium. Grune and Stratton, New York and London (1974).
Chapter 31
Beeley, L. *Safer Prescribing*. Blackwell Scientific Publications, Oxford, London, Edinburgh, Melbourne (1976).
Davies, D. M. (Ed.). *Textbook of Adverse Drug Reactions*. Oxford University Press, New York, Toronto (1977).
Wade, O. L. and Beely, L. *Adverse Reactions to Drugs*, Second edition. William Heinemann Medical Books Ltd., London (1976).

APPENDIX OF U.S. APPROVED NAMES

The following list of official drugs (U.S.P. and U.S.N.F.) is the equivalent or near-equivalent of medicinal agents mentioned in the text. The presentation and dose range may not always be identical in the United States and the British Pharmacopoeias. Included for informational purposes are a selected number of registered or proprietary drugs available in North America (U.S.A. and Canada).

Acenocoumarol U.S.N.F. Sintrom
Acetaminophen U.S.P. Datril, Tempra,.Tylenol, Voladol
Acetazolamide U.S.P. Diamox
Acetohexamide U.S.P. Dymelor
Acetylcysteine U.S.N.F. Mucomyst
Agar U.S.P.
Normal Human Serum Albumin U.S.P. Albuminar, Albuspan, Albutein
Alcohol (Ethanol) U.S.P.
Allopurinol U.S.P. Zylorim
Aloe U.S.P.
Aluminium Hydroxide Gel U.S.P. Amphojel
Dried Aluminium Hydroxide Gel U.S.P.
Amantadine Hydrochloride U.S.N.F. Symmetrel
Ambenonium Chloride U.S.N.F. Mysuran, Mytelase
Aminocaproic Acid U.S.N.F. Amicar
Aminophylline U.S.P. Lixaminol
Aminophylline Enema U.S.P.
Amitriptyline Hydrochloride U.S.P. Elavil, Endep.
Ammonium Chloride U.S.N.F.
Amobarbital U.S.N.F. Amospan, Amytal
Amobarbital Sodium U.S.P.
Amodiaquine Hydrochloride U.S.P. Camoquin
Amphotericin B. U.S.P. Fungizone
Ampicillin U.S.P. Alpen, Amcill, Ampen, Ampicin, Omnipen, Penbritin, Polycillin
Ampicillin Sodium U.S.P.
Human Antihemophilic Factor U.S.P.
Antimony Potassium Tartrate U.S.P.
Apomorphine Hydrochloride U.S.N.F.
Anti-Rabies Serum U.S.P.
Antitoxin Botulism U.S.P.
Antitoxin Tetanus U.S.P.

Ascorbic Acid U.S.P.
Aspirin U.S.P. Aspro
Atropine U.S.N.F.
Atropine Sulfate U.S.P. Atropisol
Aurothioglucose U.S.P.
Azathioprine U.S.P. Imuran

Bacitracin U.S.P. Baciquent
Bacitracin Zinc U.S.P.
Belladonna Leaf U.S.P.
Belladonna Tincture U.S.P.
Bendroflumethiazide U.S.N.F. Benuron, Naturetin
Gamma Benzene Hexachloride U.S.P. Gexane, Kwell, Lindane
Benzoic and Salicylic Acid U.S.P.
Benzthiazide U.S.N.F. Aquatag, Exna, Hydrex
Benztropine Mesylate U.S.P. Cogentin
Benzylbenzoate U.S.P.
Bephenium Hydroxynaphthoate U.S.P. Alcopara
Betamethasone U.S.N.F. Colestone
Betamethasone Acetate U.S.N.F.
Betamethasone Sodium Phosphate U.S.N.F. Colestone Soluspan
Betamethasone Valerate U.S.N.F. Valisone
Betazole Hydrochloride U.S.P. Histalog
Bethanechol Chloride U.S.N.F. Urecholine, Myotonachol
Biperidin U.S.N.F. Akineton
Biperidin Hydrochloride U.S.N.F.
Biperidin Lactate Injection U.S.N.F.
Bisacodyl U.S.P. Dulcolax
Whole Human Blood (Citrated) U.S.P.
Packed Human Red Blood Cells U.S.P.
Botulism Antitoxin U.S.P.
Brompheniramine Maleate U.S.N.F. Dimetane, Disomer

Busulfan U.S.P. Myleran
Caffeine U.S.P.
Calamine U.S.P.
Precipitated Calcium Carbonate U.S.P.
Calcium Chloride Injection U.S.P.
Calcium Gluconate U.S.P.
Calcium Lactate U.S.P.
Candicidin U.S.N.F. Candeptin, Vanobid
Sterile Capreomycin Sulfate U.S.P. Capastat Sulfate
Carbachol U.S.P.
Carbamazepine U.S.P. Tegretol
Carbasone U.S.N.F.
Carbenicillin Disodium U.S.P. Geopen, Pyopen
Carboxymethylcellulose Sodium U.S.P.
Cascara Sagrada U.S.P.
Castor Oil U.S.P.
Oxidised Cellulose U.S.P.
Cephalexin U.S.P. Keflex, Keforal
Cephaloglycin U.S.N.F. Kafocin
Cephaloridine U.S.N.F. Loridine
Cephalothin Sodium U.S.P. Keflin
Activated Charcoal U.S.P.
Chloral Hydrate U.S.P. Aquachloral, Amylophe, Felsules, En-Chlor, Hydral, Kessodrate, Lycorol, Noctec, Rectules, Somnos
Chlorambucil U.S.P. Leukeran
Chloramphenicol U.S.P. Amphicol, Chloromycetin, Mychel
Chloramphenicol Palmitate U.S.P.
Sterile Chloramphenicol Sodium Succinate U.S.P.
Chlordiazepoxide Hydrochloride U.S.P. Librium
Chlorophenothane U.S.N.F. Topocide
Chloroquine U.S.P.
Chloroquine Hydrochloride U.S.P.
Chloroquine Phosphate U.S.P. Aralen, Resochin

270

Ergotamine and Caffeine Suppositories U.S.N.F.

Ergotamine Tartrate and Caffeine Tablets U.S.N.F.

Erythromycin U.S.P. E-Mycin, Erypar, Eryprogran, Eryroguent, Ethril, Erythrocin, Ilotycin

Erythromycin Estolate U.S.N.F. Ilosone

Erythromycin Ethylsuccinate U.S.P. Erythrocin Ethylsuccinate, Pediamycin

Erythromycin Gluceptate U.S.P. Ilotycin Gluceptate

Erythromycin Lactobionate U.S.P. Erythrocin Lactobionate

Erythromycin Stearate U.S.P. Bristamycin, Ethril, Erythrocin Stearate

Esterified Estrogens U.S.P. Amnestrogen, Evex, Glyestrin, Menest, SK-Estrogens

Estradiol U.S.N.F. Aquadiol, Femogen, Microdial, Progynon

Estradiol Benzoate U.S.N.F. Progynon-Benzoate

Estradiol Cypionate U.S.P.

Estradiol Dipropionate U.S.N.F. Dep-Estrogen

Estriol U.S.P.

Conjugated Estrogens U.S.P. Conestron, Menotabs, Premarin

Estrone U.S.N.F. Menformon, Theelin, Urestrin

Ethacrynate Sodium Injection U.S.P. Edecrin Sodium

Ethacrynic Acid U.S.P. Edecrin

Ethambutol U.S.P. Myambutol

Ethchlorvynol U.S.N.F. Placidyl

Ethinamate U.S.N.F. Valmid

Ethinyl Estradiol U.S.P. Feminone, Estinyl, Lynoral

Ethionamide U.S.P. Trecator-SC

Ethopropazine Hydrochloride U.S.P. Parsidol

Ethosuximide U.S.P. Zarontin

Ethynodiol Diacetate U.S.P.

Fentanyl Citrate U.S.P. Sublimaze

Ferrous Fumarate U.S.P. C-Ron, Fumasorb, Ircon, Prematinic, Toleron

Ferrous Gluconate U.S.N.F. Fergon

Ferrous Sulfate U.S.P. Feosol, Ferralyn

Human Fibrinogen U.S.P. Parenogen

Flucytosine U.S.P. Ancobon

Fludrocortisone Acetate U.S.P. Florinef Acetate

Fluocinolone Acetonide U.S.P. Fluonid, Synalar

Fluorouracil U.S.P. Adrucil

Fluoxymesterone U.S.P. Halotestin, Oral Testryl, Ultandren

Fluphenazine Enanthate U.S.P. Prolixin Enanthate

Fluphenazine Hydrochloride U.S.P. Permitil, Prolixin, Trancin

Flurazepam Hydrochloride U.S.N.F. Dalmane

Folic Acid U.S.P. Folacine, Folvite

Fructose U.S.N.F. Levugen

Furosemide U.S.P. Lasix

Gallamine Triethiodide U.S.P. Flaxedil

Gentamicin Sulfate U.S.P. Garamycin

Immune Human Serum Globulin U.S.P.

Rho(D) Immune Human Globulin U.S.P.

Vaccinia Immune Human Globulin U.S.P. Gamastan, Gamulin

Glucagon U.S.P.

Glutethimide U.S.N.F. Doriden

Glyceryl Trinitrate U.S.P.

Glycobiarsol U.S.N.F. Amoebicon, Broxolin, Milibis

Gold Sodium Thiomalate U.S.P. Myochrysine

Gramicidin U.S.N.F.

Griseofulvin U.S.P. Fulvicin U/F, Grifulvin, Grisactin, Grisovin

Guanethidine Sulfate U.S.P. Ismelin

Haloperidol U.S.P. Haldol

Heparin Sodium U.S.P. Hepathrom, Lipo-Hepin, Liquaemin, Panheprin

Hexobarbital U.S.N.F.

Hexylresorcinol U.S.N.F. Caprokol, Crystoids

Histamine Phosphate U.S.P. Histapon

Homatropine Hydrobromide U.S.P. Homatrocel

Hydralazine Hydrochloride U.S.P. Apresoline

Hydrochlorothiazide U.S.P. Esidrex, HydroDiuril, Oretic, Thiuretic

Hydrocodone Bitartrate U.S.N.F. Dicodid, Mercodinone

Hydrocortisone U.S.P.

Hydrocortisone Acetate U.S.P. Cortef Acetate, Hydrocortone Acetate

Hydrocortisone Sodium Phosphate U.S.P. Hydrocortone Phosphate

Hydrocortisone Sodium Succinate U.S.P. Solu-Cortef

Hydroflumethiazide U.S.N.F. Diucardin, Saluron

Hydromorphone Hydrochloride U.S.N.F. Dilaudid, Hymorphan

Hydroxocobalamin U.S.N.F. alpha-Redisol, Sytobex-H

Hydroxychloroquine Sulphate U.S.P. Plaquenil Sulfate

Hydroxyprogesterone Caproate U.S.P. Corlutin, Delalutin, Hylutin, Lutate

Hydroxystilbamidine Isethionate U.S.P.

Hydroxyurea U.S.P. Hydrea

Hydroxyzine Hydrochloride U.S.N.F. Atarax

Hydroxyzine Pamoate U.S.N.F. Vistaril

Hyoscyamine U.S.N.F.

Hyoscyamine Hydrobromide U.S.N.F.

Ichthammol U.S.N.F.

Idoxuridine U.S.P. Dendrix, Herplex, Stoxil

Imipramine Hydrochloride U.S.P. Presamine, 'sk-Pramine', Tofranil

Indomethacin U.S.N.F. Indocin

Influenza Virus Vaccine U.S.P.

Insulin Injection U.S.P.

Globin Zinc Insulin U.S.P.

Isophane Suspension U.S.P.

Insulin Zinc Suspension U.S.P.

Extended I.Z.S. U.S.P.

Prompt I.Z.S. U.S.P.

Protamine Zinc Insulin Injection U.S.P.

Iodine U.S.P.

Ipecac U.S.P.

Iodochlorhydroxyquin U.S.N.F. Vioform

Iron Dextran Injection U.S.P. Imferon

Iron Sorbitex Injection U.S.N.F. Jectofer

Isocarboxazid U.S.N.F. Marplan

Isoniazid U.S.P. Hydrazid, Hyzyd, Isonico, Laniazid, Niconyl, Nydrazid, Rimifon

Isproterenol Hydrochloride U.S.P. Aerotrol, Iprenol, Isuprel, Norisodrine, Proterenol, Vapo-N-Iso

OFFICIAL NAMES DIFFERING IN THE U.S.A. AND U.K.

U.S.A.	U.K.
Acenocoumarol	Nicoumalone
Acetaminophen	Paracetamol
Acetophenetidin	Phenacetin
Amobarbital	Amylobarbitone
Amoxicillin	Amoxycillin
Barbiturates end in -al	Barbiturates end in -one
Betazole Hydrochloride	Ametazole Hydrochloride
Butethal	Butobarbitone
Chlorophenothane	Dicophane
Colistimethate Sodium	Colistin Sulphomethate
Cosyntropin	Tetracosactrin
Cromolyn Sodium	Disodium Cromoglycate
Deferoxamine	Desferrioxamine
Desoxycorticosterone	Deoxycortone
Dextroamphetamine	Dexamphetamine
Diiodohydroxyquin	Diiodohydroxyquinoline
Diethylstilbestrol	Stilbestrol
Diethylstilbestrol Diphosphate	Fosfestrol Sodium
Epinephrine	Adrenaline
Ergonovine Maleate	Ergometrine Mˆleate
Furosemide	Frusemide
Gold Sodium Thiomalate	Sodium Aurothiomalate
Iron Sorbitex	Iron Sorbitol
Isoproterenol	Isoprenaline
Leucovorin Calcium	Calcium Folinate
Levarterenol Bitartrate	Noradrenaline Bitartrate
Lidocaine Hydrochloride	Lignocaine Hydrochloride
Menadione Sodium Bisulfite	Menaphthone Sodium Bisulphate

Meperidine — Pethidine
Mephenytoin — Methoin
Mephobarbital — Methylphenobarbitone
Metaproterenol — Orciprenaline
Methandrostenolone — Methandienone
Methyprylon — Methyprylone
Mineral Oil — Liquid Paraffin
Niacin — Nicotinic Acid
Norethindrone — Norethisterone
Nylidrin — Buphenine
Oxytriphylline — Choline Theophyllinate
Phytomadione — Phytomenadione
Propoxyphene — Dextropropoxyphene
Quinacrine Hydrochloride — Mepacrine Hydrochloride
Rifampin — Rifampicin
Salicylazosulfapyridine — Sulphasalazine
Secobarbital — Quinalbarbitone
Succinylcholine Chloride — Suxamethonium Chloride
Sulfamethazine — Sulphadimidine
Sulfisoxazole — Sulphafurazole
Scopolamine — Hyoscine
Triflupromazine — Fluopromazine
Trihexyphenyl Hydrochloride — Benzhexol Hydrochloride
Trimethadione — Tridione
Trimethaphan — Trimetaphan
Trimethoprim-Sulfamethoxazole — Co-Trimoxazole
Uracil Mustard — Uramustard

SOME NON-OFFICIAL DRUGS AND THEIR PROPRIETARY NAMES

Alseroxylon; Rauwiloid
Amiloride; Colectril
Amoxicillin; Amoxil, Larotid, Polymox
Aminoglutethimide; Cytadren
Beclomethasone Dipropionate; 'Vanceril, Viarex'
Bethanidine; 'Tenathan'
Bleomycin Sulfate; Blenoxane
Carbenicillin Indanyl Sodium; Geocillin
Cefazolin Sodium; Ancef, Kefzol
Cephapirin Sodium; Cefadyl
Cephradine; Anspor, Velosef
Clonazepam; Clonopin
Clopamide; Aquex
Clotrimazole; Lotrimin
Colestipol; Colestid
Doxepin; Adapin, Sinequan
Fenfluramine; Pondimin
Fenoprofen; Nalfon
Hetacillin; Veraspan
Ibuprofen; Brufen, Motrin
Mefenamic Acid; Ponstel
Methenamine Hippurate; Hiprex, Urex
Miconazole Nitrate; Mica Tin, Monistat
Mitomycin; Mutamycin
Nicotinyl Alcohol Tartrate; Roniacol
Concentrated Opium Alkaloids; Pantopon
Pheniramine Maleate; Inhiston, Trimeton
Phentermine; Ionamine, Wilpo
Prazosin Hydrochloride; Minipress
Protirelin; Thypinone
Terbutaline Sulfate; Brethine, Bricanyl
Timolol; Timoptic
Triclofos Sodium; Triclos
Trimethoprim-Sulfamethoxazole; Bactrim, Septra
Valproic Acid; Depakene

DRUG INDEX

'Yutopar', 213

Zagreb Antiserum, 61
'Zarontin', 126
'Zinacef', 16
'Zinamide', 30
Zinc Oxide, 181
Zinc Sulphate, 229
'Zyloric', 240

GENERAL INDEX*

*This index comprises all entries which are not specific drug names. The reader should also refer to the Glossary of Terms (pp. 262-264) where appropriate.